"Dr. Bland is a remarkable visionary who sees the greatest potential in human life through the intricate interaction between genetics and the environment. His words will inspire people to empowerment and transformation in a time of broken health-care models and undeniable despair. He is ushering us into the medicine we've all been waiting for—moving us from the frantic chaos of revolution into a network of evolution in how we think about our health."
—DEANNA MINICH, PhD, FACN, CNS
Nutritionist and Author

"No one has done more to advance nutritional medicine throughout the world than Dr. Jeff Bland. He has served not only as a teacher but also as an inspiration to so many doctors who realized the old disease diagnosis and treatment model failed most of their patients. Readers will find wisdom and hope in this excellent book."
—JOSEPH PIZZORNO, ND
Founder, Bastyr University
Co-author of *Encyclopedia of Natural Medicine*
Editor in Chief of *Integrative Medicine: A Clinician's Journal*

"Dr. Jeff Bland, the most significant medical educator of our generation, has authored one of the most important books on health and disease in this decade. I am recommending it to all my patients, family, and colleagues. Dr. Bland presents innovative proposals, all supported by scientific research, to win the battle against chronic disease."
—SCOTT RIGDEN, MD, PRIVATE PRACTICE
Diplomate, American Board of Family Practice
Diplomate, American Board of Obesity Medicine
Fellow, American Academy of Family Physicians
Fellow, American Society of Bariatric Physicians

"Dr. Jeff Bland has been teaching a better way of delivering health care to doctors for the last thirty years. He now shares his brilliance and wisdom with the general public. Essential reading for all those interested in their health."
—FRANK LIPMAN, MD
Founder and Director of Eleven-Eleven Wellness Center

"A tour de force that could have been written only by this visionary scientist, *The Disease Delusion* will radically transform not just how you think about 'disease' and human health, but how society thinks about them, and indeed how our health-care system approaches them."
—MICHAEL STROKA, JD, MS, CNS, LDN
Executive Director
Certification Board for Nutrition Specialists

"As a doctor trained in 'old medicine' and intrigued by 'new medicine,' I recommend *The Disease Delusion* to everyone in the health-care world who is struggling with why our patients are suffering and dying from preventable and recoverable illnesses that seem perplexingly impervious to modern medicine."
—STACIE J. MACARI, DC, CNS
Chairman of Functional Medicine, Cancer Treatment Centers of America

"A new paradigm shift is taking root, sprouting more healthy people through the functional medicine paradigm. Self-management is now 'king' more than ever before, as elucidated in this outstanding book of science, statistics, and evidence."
—GRAHAM REEDY, MD
Founder, Sports Activity Medicine
Personal Physician

"*The Disease Delusion* provides a brilliant blueprint for changing the way we deal with our modern chronic disease epidemic, coming from the ultimately authoritative source—the founder of functional medicine, Dr. Jeffrey Bland."
—WOODSON MERRELL, MD, ScD(HC)
Director, the Integrative Medicine Consortium Center for Health and Healing

"*The Disease Delusion* establishes a practical, evidence-based foundation for functional medicine through the pioneering work of Dr. Jeff Bland. This is a requisite book for both professionals and the general public seeking optimal health and well-being."
—KENNETH R. PELLETIER, PhD, MD(HC)
Clinical Professor of Medicine and Professor of Public Health, University of Arizona

"*The Disease Delusion* provides critical insight into our understanding of the genesis of diseases and promises to provide us with completely new approaches for preventing and treating human pathological conditions in the twenty-first century."
—RANDY JIRTLE, PhD
Professor of Epigenetics at the Department of Sport and Exercise Sciences, University of Bedfordshire, Bedford, UK, and a Senior Scientist at McArdle Laboratory for Cancer Research, University of Wisconsin

"Dr. Bland illustrates the fallacy of the pharmaceutical reductionist approach to treat the symptoms of chronic disease, while offering can-do nutritional and lifestyle strategies to treat the causes."
—ROGER S. NEWTON, PhD
Esperion Therapeutics, Inc. (co-discoverer of Lipitor)

"We live in the best of times, we live in the worst of times—we are living longer, but we are not living healthier. Dr. Bland presents us with a unique and much-needed new lens for viewing the rising tide of chronic disease that is flummoxing our current health-care system. But more than this, his book presents us with an elegant system for stemming this flood of disease and enabling us to live lives that are vital and healthy."
—BRIAN BERMAN, MD
President of the Institute for Integrative Health

"A global visionary and champion for personalized lifestyle medicine—the expert of all experts and one of the world's leading authorities on health and chronic disease—has just written the ultimate book, sharing his biological breakthrough secrets, drawing on his knowledge and synthesis of the latest scientific evidence, which is changing the management of chronic illness forever. This book is an absolute must-have for anyone interested in understanding how to, once and for all, win the battle, conquer chronic disease, and achieve true health."
—SHEILA DEAN, DSc,RD,LD,CCN,CDE
Integrative Medicine Nutritionist and Author

"Dr. Bland has spent his career searching for solutions based on the functional nature of medicine. In *The Disease Delusion*, he brilliantly lays the groundwork for new solutions, ones that appreciate the complexity of the human state, the intricacies of our genetic network, and the importance of our individual experiences."
—ROBERT BONAKDAR, MD, FAAFP
Director of Pain Management, Scripps Center for Integrative Medicine

"Jeff Bland is legendary for his big-picture thinking. He has an uncanny knack for making sense of complex disease processes and developing innovative approaches that are light-years ahead. For more than thirty years he has warned of the coming pandemic of chronic disease and the need for an integrated, systems biology approach. In this book he shows how functional medicine offers us the opportunity to thrive and flourish—not just managing existing disease but restoring health and preventing future disease. Finally we have an effective, scientifically sound approach to achieving vibrant health in this era of chronic disease."
—RUTH DEBUSK, PhD, RD
The Family Medicine Residency Program
Tallahassee Memorial Healthcare

"Jeff Bland has explained how medicine has advanced from a focus on antibiotics treating bacteria and drugs treating symptoms to a focus on health and living a healthy life free of chronic disease. What I especially appreciate is that Jeff has done it using language that someone from the world of business, not science, can clearly understand."
—BROOKE WADE
President, Venture Capital and Private Equity
Wade Capital Corporation

"Dr. Bland offers us amazing insight into the health-care challenges facing the world today. Recognizing the limits of reductionist thinking, he calls for a revolution in how we approach health and chronic disease. By breaking out of the silo of disease naming and focusing on health from a systems medicine approach, Dr. Bland offers solutions for individual and global health challenges that will sustain not only the individual but the planet."
—MIMI GUARNERI MD, FACC
President the American Board of Integrative and Holistic Medicine

"Genomics begot systems biology and then systems medicine. But the true value of genomics will be in 'systems wellness,' and Jeff Bland is its most prominent creator. Read this book to see how medicine will finally enter the twenty-first century."
—WAYNE B. JONAS, MD
Samueli Institute, President and CEO

The Disease Delusion

The
Disease
Delusion

CONQUERING THE
CAUSES OF CHRONIC ILLNESS FOR A
HEALTHIER, LONGER, AND HAPPIER LIFE

Dr. Jeffrey S. Bland

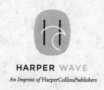

HARPER WAVE

An Imprint of HarperCollinsPublishers

This book is written as a source of information only. The information contained in this book should by no means be considered a substitute for the advice of a qualified medical professional, who should always be consulted before beginning any new diet, exercise, or other health program.

All efforts have been made to ensure the accuracy of the information contained in this book as of the date published. The author and the publisher expressly disclaim responsibility for any adverse effects arising from the use or application of the information contained herein.

HarperCollins books may be purchased for educational, business, or sales promotional use. For information, please e-mail the Special Markets Department at SPsales@harpercollins.com.

A hardcover edition of this book was published in 2014 by HarperWave, an imprint of HarperCollins Publishers.

FIRST HARPERWAVE PAPERBACK EDITION PUBLISHED 2015

Designed by Renato Stanisic

Library of Congress Cataloging-in-Publication Data has been applied for.

ISBN: 978-0-06-229074-8 (pbk.)

23 24 25 26 27 LBC 25 24 23 22 21

To Susan Bland, who has lovingly held
me to the highest standards of dedication to
excellence, and to my family, which has supported
me in what it takes to make this happen

Get More Out of *The Disease Delusion*!

This Book Features Multimedia Content Beyond the Printed Page

Some of the pages in *The Disease Delusion* feature special icons you can use to activate and discover additional content on your smartphone, mobile, or tablet device.

How Does It Work?

1. Visit www.harpercollinsunbound.com to download the free app for your iOS or Android device.

2. When you see this icon on pages throughout the book, open the app on your device and scan the page.

3. The app will do the rest, bringing multimedia and interactive content that relates to the page you're reading right onto your device.

Download the free app at www.harpercollinsunbound.com.

Contents

Imagine a time when people died or suffered from incurable acute infections. Imagine a time before antibiotics when women died of simple childbirth fever, when a bad chest infection could lead to death, when a strep throat caused heart failure, when limbs were amputated because of an infected wound. Those commonplace occurrences seem unimaginable now.

Yet that is the exactly the state of medicine today as we face the tsunami of chronic diseases that will cost our global economy $47 trillion over the next twenty years and kill twice as many people around the world as infectious disease.

As we spend more and more for health care, we get less and less. The United States has worse health-care outcomes and lower life expectancy than almost every other developed nation. Heart disease, diabetes, cancer, autoimmune diseases, digestive disorders, dementia, allergies, asthma, arthritis, depression, attention deficit disorder, autism, Parkinson's disease, hormonal problems like early puberty and infertility—these and more cause endless suffering and drain our financial resources. Chronic diseases now affect one in two Americans and account for 80 percent of our health-care costs. Yet despite a host of new drugs and procedures, the incidence of chronic disease continues to rise, not only in the United States but around the globe as developing countries adopt the worst of our food and culture.

The answer to this paradox should be obvious to all of us: what we are doing is not working. Our current medical model was constructed to treat acute disease, which we have mostly vanquished. We identified a single agent for illness—a microbe—and a single agent to treat it: antibiotics. Since then, medicine has pursued a quest: to find a pill for every ill. This quest has failed. We need a different paradigm, a different model for diagnosing and treating this new epidemic of chronic disease.

The Disease Delusion dissects the failure of medicine to solve our health crisis and lays out a new map for understanding and treating illness based on functional medicine, a fundamental paradigm shift from medicine by symptom to medicine by cause, from medicine by disease to medicine by system, from medicine by organ to medicine by organism. It is an ecological view of the body where all the networks of our biology intersect and interact in a dynamic process that creates disease when out of balance and creates health when in balance. It takes all the component parts of science, all the puzzle pieces, all the data about how we get sick and what makes us well, and reorganizes them into a narrative that makes sense, one that has the capacity to fix our health-care crisis nearly overnight if it was applied widely.

Medicine is the youngest science. There is no theory of medicine. There are no organizing principles that help us navigate the territory of chronic disease. Functional medicine is that breakthrough theory, the biggest breakthrough idea in medicine since the discovery of the microbe and antibiotics.

It is a cataclysmic shift in our view of biology. There are moments of awakening in science that are not incremental but transformational—Columbus proving the earth was round, not flat, Galileo showing us the earth was not the center of the universe, Darwin explaining that species evolved and didn't arise fixed in their current form, and Einstein shattering our notions of time and space. Functional medicine is a paradigm shift of equal magnitude and significance.

Disease appears real and fixed, just as the earth seems flat and time and space seem linear and solid. In *The Disease Delusion*, the father of functional medicine, Dr. Jeffrey Bland, the man who has synthesized more medical science from more fields of study than any other human in the past thirty years, shatters our notion of disease. Disease as we think about it is a false idol. It does not exist in the way we think about it. The names we give diseases are useful for finding the right medication but not for truly getting to the cause or creating a healing response.

When we tell a patient who has symptoms of sadness and hopelessness, who can't sleep, who lacks interest in daily activities, food, or sex that he has depression, this is not helpful. Depression is not the *cause* of his misery; it is merely the name we give to this constellation of symptoms. We then treat these symptoms with an antidepressant, which works only a little better than chance.

The actual cause of the depression may vary greatly from patient to patient. It may be a leaky gut caused by gluten that activates the immune system to produce antibodies against the thyroid, leading to low thyroid function and depression. It may be a vitamin B12 deficiency resulting from long-term use of an acid-blocking drug for reflux, or a folate deficiency caused by a gene called MTFHR, or a vitamin D deficiency resulting from inadequate sunlight. It may be a mercury toxicity from a diet too high in tuna, or an omega-3 deficiency from a diet too low in fatty fish, or prediabetes brought on by a diet high in sugar. The symptoms may arise from changes in brain chemistry brought on by life trauma or stress, or even by alterations in the gut flora resulting from antibiotic use. Each of these factors— dietary, environmental, lifestyle—creates a different imbalance, yet all cause depression. Knowing the name of a disease tells us nothing about its true cause; nor does it lead us to the right treatment. This is the disease delusion.

As a student of functional medicine for twenty years, and as a practitioner who daily faces the failures of our current medical model and witnesses the miracles of treating illness using this new medical paradigm, I feel strongly that we are on the verge of a true transformation in medicine.

Functional medicine is not simply about improving diet or getting more exercise or managing stress or reducing exposure to environmental toxins, all of which are critical foundations for creating a healthy human. Above all, functional medicine is the science of creating health. Disease goes away as a side effect.

Functional medicine is a personalized method for getting to the root of symptoms and restoring balance. It is the story of a little girl, Elise, who had suffered from intractable psoriasis, with red, weeping, raw skin from head to toe, since she was six months old. Her parents had taken her to the top medical schools, and she had been given the most advanced drugs, including powerful immune suppressants and chemotherapy to shut off inflammation. When I first saw Elise she was four years old. She had just emerged from a month in the intensive care unit after fighting a life-threatening staphylococcus infection triggered by her medication, Enbrel, which suppressed her immune system. Rather than inquiring about the root cause of her inflamed skin, doctors used medication to suppress symptoms. Still she was no better. No one asked about her diet or thought about how her history of antibiotics as a baby affected her delicate gut flora, thus setting up the conditions for inflammation.

Functional medicine led me to a different set of questions. Rather than asking what drug I should use to treat the symptoms, I asked what caused the inflammation in the first place—a simple idea that is foreign to our medical training. The causes of inflammation are few—microbes, allergens, toxins, poor diet, stress. And I asked what her immune system needed to regain balance. Then I applied these principles to her by removing a common cause of inflammation in our diet—gluten, known to be linked to psoriasis—and cleared out bad microbes (yeast) in her gut that resulted from years of antibiotics and steroids. I also added a few ingredients needed to support proper immune function—omega-3 fats, zinc, vitamin D, and probiotics to help balance her gut flora.

Within two weeks her skin, red and raw for over three years, was clear. Not a miracle, but a repeatable result that is a natural outcome of breaking our disease delusion and employing a new framework for solving our chronic disease epidemic.

Paradigm shifts are hard, detractors abound, yet the evidence is in and the failure of our current approach is evident to any student of health care. The time is ripe for a radical transformation in health care with the power to end needless suffering for millions of people. *The Disease Delusion* is the manifesto for the new medicine. Every medical student, every stakeholder in health care, and every government leader involved in health policy should read it. For the rest of us, it is our road map to true health and healing.

Mark Hyman, MD
Chairman, Institute for Functional Medicine
November 19, 2013
West Stockbridge, Massachusetts

The Disease Delusion

Chronic Concerns

Travel back in time with me to the late nineteenth century—to the years, in the United States, just after the Civil War, when peace, albeit imperfect, had settled in. What did people in that era worry about?

If you were a parent, you worried that your children would succumb to one of the numerous infectious diseases that routinely swept away infants and toddlers in those days—diphtheria, whooping cough, pneumonia. If you were a woman about to become a mother for the first or third or fifth or last time, you worried that you yourself might die of postpartum sepsis, the blood infection that killed so many women just after childbirth, and thus not be there to nurse your children in their illnesses. Like your parents and grandparents before you and their parents and grandparents before them, you worried that an epidemic would break out—an influenza, a plague—and decimate or destroy your family, your community, the world as you know it.

Such worries were very real four generations ago, and they were wholly justified. Down the centuries, hundreds of millions of people had been wiped off the face of the earth by infectious diseases, caused, it was believed, by miasmas—noxious vapors from decayed matter—that were carried on the air or spread via physical contact. The medical response to the diseases caused by miasmas was to suggest the patient go somewhere else where the miasma would not be present. It was a typically ineffectual remedy.

Yet before the nineteenth century was over, scientists like Joseph

Lister, Robert Koch, Louis Pasteur, and others would revolutionize the way illness was perceived and, in turn, transform the way medicine was practiced. The germ theory that these scientists elucidated advanced the idea that submicroscopic organisms, not vapors, caused these infectious diseases. Once the particular submicroscopic organism causing a specific disease was identified, the body could be immunized against the organisms.

The theory gave rise to what we would today call a paradigm shift in the health-care universe—the bacteriological revolution. Everything changed—medical training, surgical techniques, standards of sanitation and public health—and a whole new industry was spawned, the pharmaceutical industry, with its steady stream of vaccines for immunization and, throughout the twentieth century, of antibiotics, drugs that could treat infections for which there were no immunizations.

It has been a spectacular success story. In the United States alone, life expectancy rose from forty-seven years in 1910 to seventy-four years as I write this, thanks to germ theory and the paradigm shift it brought about. It means that unlike your nineteenth-century forebears and all the generations of your family before them, you do not need to worry unduly about the deadly infectious diseases that constituted such a scourge down the ages. If the diseases haven't been totally wiped out—like smallpox—there are remedies available for those that still infect us.

But unfortunately, that doesn't mean you don't have to worry at all. While immunization and antibiotic treatment have made infectious diseases less prevalent and less frightening, another family of illnesses has been growing in importance and impact: chronic diseases.

By chronic diseases, I mean all those conditions, ailments, and illnesses that make you sick and then never really go away. That's not their nature. Their nature is to stay or to come back again and again. We can manage their effects and find occasional relief from them, but we tend not to be able to zap them the way we can zap infectious disease, so one way or another, they enfeeble and disable us, and they drain the life out of us.

What are these diseases? They are familiar, and they run the gamut of misery and danger. They include:

- Heart and blood-vessel diseases like type 2 diabetes, gout, high blood pressure, and dementia
- Autoimmune inflammatory diseases like arthritis
- Neurological disorders such as depression, attention deficit disorders, and autism
- Digestive diseases: gastric reflux, duodenal ulcer, and inflammatory bowel
- Bone loss diseases like osteoporosis
- Obstructive pulmonary disease and asthma
- Muscle pain and weakness from chronic fatigue syndrome and fibromyalgia
- Kidney and liver ailments
- Vision problems like macular degeneration and retinopathy
- Cancer

What do such illnesses have in common that qualify them all under the "chronic disease" rubric? Four characteristic features distinguish them:

First, chronic illnesses do not heal by themselves; the term of art is that they are not "self-limiting." The common cold is self-limiting; it runs its course and then it's gone. Not so with chronic illnesses.

Second, chronic illnesses grow worse over time. Since we can only palliate but not obliterate these illnesses—at least, so far—there is no return to health, just an ongoing management of recurring episodes.

Third, a chronic disease doesn't have a single cause one can point to; rather, several factors or agents give rise to it.

Fourth, chronic illnesses tend to have complex symptom profiles; that is, the sick person has numerous different complaints and there are varying indications of illness.

Complex and common, with numerous hard-to-specify causes but no single origin, chronic illnesses are increasingly conditions we have to live with. More and more of us are doing so, and it is an expensive proposition. In fact, unless we can implement drastic change, the numbers tell us we are all on a headlong course toward a frail, sick old age in which we will spend much of our time going to doctors and popping pills.

It doesn't have to happen. As you'll learn in the pages that follow, dramatic scientific discoveries have put in our hands the power to avoid the collision with debilitation and illness, setting the stage for a veritable revolution in health care. We can now identify the causes of chronic illness in an individual, and using the approach described in this book, we can then put an end to the illness; even better, we can identify the causes of a chronic illness before it becomes a disease and avert it through early intervention. This is transformational. It is equivalent to the paradigm shift in medicine brought about by the discovery of immunization and antibiotics for the management of infectious disease. I call it the "functional medicine revolution." And for the past forty years, as a researcher in biological and clinical sciences and a medical educator, I have been in the forefront of the effort to bring it about.

What do I mean by "functional medicine"? As you know, your body is a network of systems. We speak of the circulatory system, the digestive system, the nervous system, the endocrine system, the immune system, the reproductive system, the respiratory system—the list goes on. Each system is composed of organs that work together to perform a biological function: the heart and blood vessels of your circulatory system pump blood to your body; the brain, spinal cord, and nerves of your nervous system receive and process information that tells your body to do various things; the lungs, bronchi, and larynx of your respiratory system send oxygen throughout your system to keep your body operating. It takes a lot for each of these systems to continue to work smoothly and at peak performance. In addition, the systems interact with one another via complex networks; this adds yet more intricacy to the dynamics of all the biological functioning going on. So when we think about how our bodies work—something we usually do when they're not working very well—we ought to be thinking about how the component parts of these systems relate to one another and to all the other systems.

Yet our current medical model—the way health-care professionals are trained and the strategy of therapy they apply—is not based in such systems thinking. Precisely because it derives from the germ theory, it is based in reductionist thinking: find the bug and nuke it with a drug developed for just that purpose. Period. As brilliantly as the model works in providing acute care, it clearly does nothing to restore or maintain balance among functional systems or the networks that connect them.

But functional medicine does exactly that. It looks at the patterns of dysfunction underlying the chronic diseases that are shadowing all our lives, and it offers a model of care that can prevent or reverse these illnesses. How does that model of care work? You'll learn more about it in subsequent chapters of this book, but suffice it to say that it is based on the way our genes are stimulated by and respond to what is going on around us and the kinds of behaviors we practice. Basically, if we can change the latter—our environment and our behavior—we can change the former. That is, we can change the way our genes get stimulated and the way they respond, and since genes regulate or direct our biological functions, that can also change our pattern of health.

This is new science. It comes out of the genomic revolution that is rewriting our understanding of how our genes form our individuality, of how we get from genotype to phenotype, from the latent genetic possibilities we're born with to the unique individuals we become, sporting the particular observable characteristics that make us who we are. The new science tells us that this does not happen according to a fixed blueprint incised at conception into our genes; rather, it happens because of the way our genotype interacts with our environment, stimulating responses in our core physiological processes throughout our lifetime.

So profound a change in understanding surely requires a new model of medical care, one focused on that interaction and on how and how well those core processes are functioning.

That is what functional medicine does. Where the standard medical model addresses the symptoms of illness and focuses on coming up with a diagnosis, and where integrative or alternative models offer a cafeteria list of historical healing approaches to health problems, functional medicine accesses the newest scientific biomedical discoveries to focus on the underlying causes of an individual's health problems.

Compellingly, functional medicine matches those discoveries and technologies against *the* health issue of our time—chronic illness—as it searches for underlying causes in the interaction between the individual's genetic uniqueness and his or her lifestyle, environment, and diet. Functional medicine then engages patient and practitioner in designing a personally tailored health-management program that couples pharmaceutical science, where necessary, with changes in the patient's environment, diet, and lifestyle—not just to bring relief to the individual but to realize his or her full genetic potential for vitality and longevity.

It works. I've seen it work time after time after time over the past forty years. To the people for whom it has worked, it has been a miracle. I know what they mean. My son Justin is such a miracle.

Born prematurely in 1982, Justin was half the birth weight of his two older brothers and needed special care in the neonatal intensive care unit before being allowed to come home. But even when he did, something just didn't seem right with him, and at three months it became obvious that he had developed hydrocephalus—water on the brain—with its associated swelling of the brain. Even after a surgical procedure to implant a shunt in his brain in order to reduce the pressure, it was not clear how Justin would develop, and although over the ensuing years, he received the best of traditional medical care from very skilled and compassionate professionals, there were continued signs of perceptual and learning challenges. There just seemed to be something Justin needed that excellent medical care was not able to deliver.

Then by chance I met Glenn Doman, founder of the Institutes for the Achievement of Human Potential in Philadelphia, which helps brain-injured children achieve high function through a personalized program that the IAHP developed, a program the kids' parents have the basic responsibility to apply.

What followed was a life-changing experience for our family and for Justin. He graduated from a prominent high school and then from a well-regarded university where he majored in political science. One of the most remarkable experiences of my life was hearing Justin deliver a lecture to the staff at the IAHP describing how he felt during the stages of his own development, starting as a child who wondered if he would be able to succeed, given his mental challenges, addressing those challenges, and becoming a high-performing adult who recognizes his uniqueness but now has numerous skills he can call upon as he moves independently through life. Call it what you will; as a father, I call it a miracle.

Nor is Justin the only member of my family to benefit from the program. A nephew diagnosed with an autism-spectrum disorder was able to move from what appeared to be a future in special education to graduation from a mainstream high school and then on to a successful experience in college.

No wonder I became a member of the institutes' scientific advisory board. Every spring, when the cherry blossoms are blooming in Philadelphia, I attend the IAHP Graduation to Life ceremony and watch as "brain-injured" children perform at amazing levels—synchronized gymnastics, ensemble concerts of complex pieces of violin music played from memory, and a Shakespeare play, performed from memory and of course in full costume. The Graduation to Life never fails to move me to tears as I see confirmation each year that what seems impossible can become possible with the right personalized program, aided by the dedication and love of parents, family, and friends.

How does it happen? Through an intensive regimen of personalized health management incorporating specific physical training and conditioning, mental training and pattern development, and structured nutrition and diet. The program has the rigor of routine and repetition along with the flexibility to be individualized to the specific needs of the child based upon his or her health status, environment, and genetics. In essence, this is a pediatric functional medicine program; it focuses on improving cognitive, emotional, and physical function. The kids are basically creating new ways for their genes to interact with their environment, and over time, that changes the course of both their physical and their mental functioning. They eat diets that are rich in whole foods and low in sugars and processed fats; they take specific nutritional supplements that help protect the brain from injury and support its repair; and they engage in physical and mental training exercises that build strength, endurance, and flexibility. As their bodies change from the often crippled, spastic form of brain-injured infants to that of strong and athletic teenagers, their cognitive function enjoys a parallel improvement until what seemed an irreversible illness is altered to a state of health. It is a testament to the power of a functional medicine approach to chronic illness.

And it has taught me about the plasticity of health and disease. There are many stories locked into our genes. Some of these are health tragedies while others are health miracles. A functional medicine program focuses like a laser on finding the personalized key that unlocks those stories in an individual's genes that will result in improved function. This improved function in one individual becomes in turn a lesson that can lead to improvement for others. That has always been the way medical science works. You perceive the illness in a fresh way, and you adjust the way you confront that illness. That's how revolutions in health care happen. Once they do, we wonder how we ever could have perceived the illness or administered the cure any other way.

Earlier, I mentioned the postpartum sepsis that was so deadly for so many women in the time of our great-great-grandparents. It was a young woman suffering from this disease—and on the brink of death—who would become the first critically ill human to be injected with penicillin at what was virtually the point of death. Identifying who that first recipient would be was a weighty decision for the medical research team that had developed penicillin, the first of the antibiotics to be ready for human testing. The team members knew that if Recipient One had a bad outcome, it could doom the future development of the drug; at the same time, a good outcome had to be dramatic enough to be seen to work. For this new mother afflicted with the condition that had killed millions of new mothers throughout history, there was really no choice. Either the penicillin would save her life or she would die by morning. It was decided: she received the first dose of penicillin ever administered to a dying human. The next day she was free of infection.

That was less than eighty years ago, yet what was considered a miracle back then has become the expected standard of care, and today it is extremely rare for any woman—at least in the developed world—to die of postpartum sepsis. That was a revolution; it changed the way we thought about illness, and it changed the way we administered health care.

Another case in point: not long ago people who had suffered a heart attack were told to rest completely; it was assumed that any form of exercise would trigger another heart attack. A few pioneering doctors, however, asked whether a program of personalized exercise might not be helpful in rebuilding heart function, and in doing so, they revolutionized cardiology. Today it is standard procedure to get patients up and moving and on a cardiac rehabilitation program as soon as possible precisely to *prevent* a second heart attack. Custom-tailored to the lifestyle of the individual patient, cardiac rehab doesn't change the genes in the heart; what changes is the patient's behavior and lifestyle. Those changes redefine the environment sending messages to the genes of the heart, which in turn changes how they express their responses to the messages—that is, how they direct the cardiac patient's biological functioning. The result improves the operation of the heart and circulatory system; this not only helps to prevent a second heart attack but actually improves all aspects of health. Thus do the miracles of one age become the expected standards of another.

I believe functional medicine is no miracle; rather, it is proven science, as you will learn in this book. It's the kind of health care that addresses the illnesses we confront today—the chronic diseases that are burdening our lives and killing us before our time.

In 2012, I founded the Personalized Lifestyle Medicine Institute to advance the functional medicine model as an operating system for transforming our entire approach to chronic illness. Headquartered here in Seattle, the institute is a not-for-profit educational organization. Its aim is to serve as a meeting place—both virtual and actual—for health professionals, researchers, health educators, and health-conscious consumers to share ideas and engage in conversation about how functional medicine can be delivered to every individual. The institute's website, at www.plminstitute.org, teems with posts from researchers and physicians and patients, questions to our staff and answers from them, updates on the latest developments in personalized lifestyle health care, and a steady stream of information from individuals about the application of their own personalized health programs. It's a vehicle for participation in today's health-care revolution, and I invite readers to climb aboard and join in.

Getting functional medicine to where it is the daily standard of medical care may constitute a revolution, but you can get a head start on the revolution now, as you learn how to personalize your own health-management program, then manage it to reverse or avert chronic illness and live your personal life span to the fullest.

Take the first step to your personal health-management plan by answering the questions in this health self-assessment.

MY HEALTH SELF-ASSESSMENT

1. Do you feel that your health has gotten worse over the past two years?
2. Have you lost or gained more than 10 percent of your body weight over the past five years—even though you weren't intentionally dieting?
3. Do you have trouble going to sleep or staying asleep?
4. Does pain in your joints or muscles limit your physical activity or mobility?

5. Do you commonly feel fatigued for no apparent reason?
6. Are you frequently depressed or anxious?
7. Do you have problems with memory?
8. Is there a consistent ringing in your ears?
9. Do you feel that you are losing your strength?
10. Do you take any prescription medications? Do you take more than two?
11. How about over-the-counter medications? Do you commonly take any of these?

   a Anti-inflammatories
   b Antacids
   c Analgesics
   d Sleeping remedies

12. Do you suffer from allergies?
13. Do you occasionally have episodes of poor concentration or confusion?
14. Do you commonly suffer from shortness of breath or feel winded?
15. Have you lost any of your sense of taste or smell over the past few years?
16. Do you feel that you have lost a significant amount of muscle mass over the past few years?
17. Have you heard from your doctor that you have any of the following?

   a Elevated blood pressure
   b Elevated blood cholesterol
   c Elevated blood glucose

18. Has your dentist told you that you have gum or periodontal disease?
19. Do you frequently alternate constipation and diarrhea or feel pain or discomfort in your digestive area?

20. Have you been told that you have chronic bad breath?
21. Are you shorter than you used to be? Had any evidence of calcium deposits?
22. Do you catch every cold and flu that's going around?

This is the first of eight self-assessments this book asks you to do, and it is the one that will give you a general idea of your overall health. Later, in Part 2, you'll home in on how each of your core physiological processes is functioning, and in Part 3, you'll put all the self-assessments to work in creating your personalized health-care program.

But let's begin by considering the wider context of health and illness.

PART ONE

THE CONTEXT

Disease is a delusion, one that has been shattered by the still-emerging science of genomics. Breakthrough discoveries over the last decade of the twentieth century and the first decade-plus of the twenty-first have demonstrated that your heart disease is not the same as mine, that everyone with type 2 diabetes is not just like everyone else with type 2 diabetes, that the people with rheumatoid arthritis or Alzheimer's disease are not all similar to others with the same diagnosis. Rather, these so-called diseases are dysfunctions of each individual's physiological functioning; they are due to varied causes, and they demand treatment approaches as different from one another as are the individuals.

So while it may be convenient to group together common signs and symptoms and call them "diseases," that isn't the way to address what's making us sick. It is not the way to think about medical care in the face of a changing pattern of health problems as we live longer lives—but lives that are increasingly limited and burdened by subpar health. We need a new model of care that will personalize treatment to the individual's particular genetic makeup, environment, lifestyle, and diet. That is what functional medicine does.

Grounded in a systems-based understanding of the way the body functions, functional medicine provides the tools we need to change the messages our genes receive so we can shape our own pattern of health. In empowering us to address the chronic illnesses that are the health issue of our time, it is revolutionizing medical practice and changing the face of health care.

CHAPTER 1

The Disease Delusion and the Chronic-Illness Conundrum

Y ou would like Peter. Everyone does. At thirty-six, he is living a picture-perfect existence—married to the love of his life, father of two boys ages six and eight, owner of a lovely home in a suburb everyone always describes as posh, a highly successful software engineer at the top of his profession and at the top of his game. If Peter weren't such an all-around good guy, it would be easy to resent him. But he *is* an all-around good guy—bright, caring, gracious, generous, and to all appearances happy and thriving.

Not quite. The outward signs are only part of the story. Behind the trim, fit-looking exterior, Peter suffers from high blood pressure, headaches, and fatigue. He spends his weekends catching up on sleep, when what he really wants to do is participate in activities with his sons and take his wife out on the town. The headaches, he says, come on every afternoon, and by the time Peter arrives home at the end of the day, he feels exhausted.

Of course, he has seen his doctor about all this. The tests showed significantly elevated blood pressure, and the doctor prescribed an antihypertensive medication. When it failed to lower Peter's blood pressure sufficiently, a second companion medication was prescribed; as the doctor said, "We've got to bring down those numbers."

The numbers came down all right, but the second medication—or the combination of the first and second—brought on erectile dysfunction, and for some time, Peter has been on what he calls "a slippery slope," trying to find the right combination of drugs to manage his blood pressure *and* enable him to maintain a vigorous physical relationship with his wife. No luck so far, but the doctor, a guy Peter went to college with, is "sure we'll find it." Meanwhile, the headaches, fatigue, and sexual dysfunction continue, and now a pall of depression is settling in as well.

Yet there's nothing medically wrong with Peter. Other than the blood pressure—definitely something to be dealt with, although not terribly unusual in an ambitious individual in a high-powered environment—he has no health issues. He can't remember the last time he had a cold. A former varsity athlete in track, he can still run one hundred meters in about twenty seconds. He passed his stress EKG with flying colors, and except for the headaches, he has been a stranger to bodily pain and discomfort—"blessedly," as he says. So why does he feel so lousy? Why is he plagued with this steady level of low energy, no energy, no hunger to do anything but sleep?

Catherine is sixty-four years old, and you would like her too. Outgoing, funny, even sassy, she just celebrated her fortieth wedding anniversary at a big party thrown by her two children and their spouses and attended by friends, relatives, and her five grandchildren. For more than twenty years Catherine has worked in the financial controller's office of a large company downtown. It's a good place to work, with pretty good benefits. Some time ago Catherine opted for a point-of-service health insurance plan: the company pays 20 percent of the premiums, while she pays for the remainder out of her bimonthly paycheck. The plan covers only Catherine's own needs; her husband, Ted, four years older, is on Medicare.

But Catherine sees doctors frequently. She is bothered by a bit of arthritis in her hands and knees and has slightly elevated blood pressure. She is postmenopausal—like her mother, she went through menopause early—and since her mother suffered from osteoporosis and Catherine herself has what her primary care physician calls "not great" bone density, she is on an osteoporosis management plan.

For these three conditions—arthritis, high blood pressure,

osteoporosis—Catherine currently takes six different drugs. She regularly sees a rheumatologist, a cardiologist, and a gynecologist in addition to her primary care physician, and an endocrinologist consults with her gynecologist about her osteoporosis program.

And Catherine feels diminished. Sometimes it's hard to get up out of a chair. She reminds herself to be careful going down steps. The arthritis comes in painfully sharp episodes that bring her life to a halt. If she gets a flare-up at work, she simply has to stop what she's doing. She hears herself reciting her ailments to Ted or to friends her own age—and listening to their complaints in turn—and wondering who these old, sick people are.

Yet, like Peter, Catherine is not sick. She has no disease that can be zapped by a drug or cut out of her. And although she is nearly twice Peter's age, she is not an old woman, either. True, her doctor frequently tells her that her various conditions are simply "part of growing older," while also advising Catherine to "lose some weight." She would love to shed five pounds, but she also insists that she is basically a vigorous woman, able to put in ten-, twelve-, even fourteen-hour days when the quarterly financial report is due, and still be ready for a brisk walk with Ted at the drop of a hat, although she's somewhat slowed down by her deteriorating knees. Now she worries: Will the knees just get worse? Is she looking at surgery up ahead? Are her bones going to break—as her mother's did? Will the high blood pressure translate into a stroke someday? Will the flare-ups of pain grow worse? Could they become more frequent? Might they become permanent? One doctor tells her to keep moving. Another tells her to take it easy.

Catherine expects to retire in two years, when she will qualify for full Social Security. Ted will retire then too; at the age of seventy, he'll get the maximum monthly benefit. Both of them have pensions from work and some savings in the bank—not a fortune but enough for the two of them to enjoy what they used to think of as a third age of life. Now they're not so sure. Catherine wonders if she will spend her third age in doctors' offices and at the pharmacy, and if she'll watch her nest egg go for co-pays and supplemental coverage over and above Medicare. Mostly, she wonders if she will grow old stuck in a chair, held there by pain or weakness or fear—or all three.

Granted that you don't personally know these two likable people. Yet the odds are that you find their situations recognizable, if not familiar. Neither of them belongs in a hospital bed. Neither of them has a disease as such. Neither of them is unable to carry out most of life's responsibilities and pleasures, although both are somewhat limited in doing some things. That's it, really: they are limited. And there's no real end in sight. What's going on?

We all know that we're living longer—that's certainly good news. The bad news, however, is that we don't seem to be doing the longer living very well. Far too many of us spend far too much of our longer lives like Peter and Catherine—not wholly sick but not wholly well. Rather, we're suspended between the two states, between good days when everything feels okay and bad days when nothing does. It's a difference that's hard to split; the limitation is always potentially there. It hovers over us, disabling or debilitating us physically, mentally, emotionally.

Chronic diseases—those persistent or recurring illnesses or conditions that don't go away and that in fact grow progressively worse— are keeping us from enjoying our extended longevity to the fullest. When these diseases are not killing us before our time, they are burdening our lives with pain, discomfort, or limitations that undermine the living of life and rob us of the quality of life.

And the incidence of such illnesses seems to be on the rise. Look around. People are either on meds like Peter, or excusing themselves from an activity as Catherine occasionally feels she must do, or complaining endlessly because of their arthritis, asthma, high blood pressure, acid reflux, gout, fibromyalgia, or chronic fatigue syndrome. Or so it seems.

In fact, chronic illness *is* becoming more prevalent—and at an ever faster rate. The quarter century from 1985 to 2010 saw dramatic increases in the number of people diagnosed with diabetes, cardiovascular disease, and chronic obstructive pulmonary disease. More people suffered strokes and depression. More of us experienced bone loss from osteoporosis, failure of muscle strength, kidney and liver ailments, and macular degeneration and degraded vision. The incidence of autism in children and dementia in adults increased alarmingly. Today, almost half of adult Americans—133 million of us—suffer from at least one chronic illness. Among Medicare beneficiaries sixty-five and older, the statistics are worse: more than half are being treated for multiple chronic conditions—diabetes *and* hypertension *and* heart disease, to take one common example.

It all comes at a high price. The Centers for Disease Control (CDC) estimate that managing these illnesses accounts for some 78 percent of the nation's health expenditures. Health-care spending for a person with one chronic condition is almost three times greater than spending for someone without a chronic condition. Spending is seventeen times greater for someone with five or more conditions. A 2011 study by the World Economic Forum projects that by the year 2030, the cost of chronic illness treatment worldwide will exceed $47 trillion. That represents the kind of economic impact that can bring countries to their knees.

In addition to what we spend, there's what we lose. Chronic diseases are the main cause of absenteeism from work and of lowered productivity on the job. The CDC ascribes seven out of ten American deaths to chronic diseases, with heart disease, cancer, and stroke accounting for more than half of all deaths each year. Worldwide—for this is a global epidemic—these illnesses rob us of more years of life than all the infectious diseases combined everywhere, except in sub-Saharan Africa.

But of course, the cost to the individual sufferer is ultimately immeasurable. How do you quantify that burden—the pain, discomfort, encroaching disability and dysfunction, the shame of feeling yourself a burden to those you love, the sorrow of losing the quality of your life?

Actually, a study published at the end of 2012 tried to do that very thing, examining diseases attributable to sixty-seven risk factors in order to define what it called the global burden of disease. The study, covering the years 1990 to 2010, used a measure called the disability-adjusted life year, or DALY. The DALY combines the years of life lost because of premature mortality and the years lost because they were lived in a state of subpar health, both due to these risk factors. The study results paint a startling new picture of the nature of disease globally.

For so much of world history, the burden of disease was to be found in the risks of infectious diseases in children, which caused rampant infant mortality and early childhood deaths. Now, the study showed, the risks are at the other end of life—in what the study called the "years lived with chronic disease." These are the non-infectious diseases that put a brake on living, sapping an individual's vitality on the way to his or her premature death. Indeed, the dramatic reduction in mortality among infants and children under the age of six—grounds for celebration and gratitude—has been answered by an even more dramatic rise in mortality from chronic illness. If you're looking for the health headline for our time, this is it.

The study also told us why the rise has been so dramatic—not that we didn't already know. It's the way we live. In the twenty-year period the study covered, from 1990 to 2010, the greatest increase in disability—that is, in limiting our lives—came from heart disease, stroke, depression, and metabolic diseases like diabetes, all of them directly related to environment, diet, and such lifestyle behaviors as exercise. Ischemic heart disease, as it is called—that is, heart disease due to hardened arteries that reduce the blood supply to the heart—which was the fourth-ranked disability in 1990, rose a whopping 29 percent to assume the dubious top rank by 2010, while the incidence of stroke increased 19 percent and depression 37 percent. Diabetes, meanwhile, has become a global epidemic, with China and India at the epicenter of its growth. These are the afflictions of our era, and they are killing us slowly.

Whereas our forebears were bedeviled by contagions that science has now virtually put an end to, we are plagued by illnesses we have to battle constantly. It means that where health and well-being are concerned, we are in a whole new ball game, and we confront a whole new set of challenges. That is the conundrum of chronic illness.

It is a dilemma with many horns. The challenges we confront touch upon the health infrastructure and delivery system; our current medical strategy for treating chronic illness and the training and education of those who execute the strategy; even our understanding of chronic illness, of its origins and causes, and of the individual's role in addressing it. It's a lot to deal with.

THE GLOBAL HEALTH SYSTEM

It is axiomatic that this rising burden of chronic illness sets up a very direct set of challenges to health-care systems around the world. The problem is that our health-care systems are in no way ready for the challenges.

Yes, we have now a sophisticated medical infrastructure, honed to the sharpness of a weapon, to address infectious diseases and acute care. You go to a doctor's office or enter a hospital or clinic sick or injured, and you exit cured—your body stitched together, your malady diagnosed, prescription in hand. Everything about the infrastructure—the training of physicians and other health professionals, therapeutic processes and procedures, hospital and clinic organization, not to mention insurance and reimbursement—is geared to curing a contagious illness that derives from a single cause or remediating an acute injury or medical event like a heart attack or stroke. Unfortunately, this pill-for-an-ill system is in no way suited to addressing the chronic illnesses that are today's health reality.

Neither is the clinical education of the physicians and other health-care professionals charged with delivering and administering cure and care. Medical schools in the United States and around the world do a superb job training physicians to be experts in crisis care, but they offer little education in how to manage chronic illness. This disconnect is measurable: The management of chronic illness constitutes nearly 80 percent of our health-care expenditures but occupies close to zero time in the training of physicians.

What's more, our current approach to chronic illness—palliating its effects, episode by episode—mandates a different paradigm of health-care delivery from the one we now have, the paradigm developed to provide acute care in a crisis. Lacking a single, easily identifiable beginning and end, chronic illness as we now deal with it will require long-term management—actually, self-management by the patients themselves. Yet today's health-care infrastructure, geared to the acute care of infectious illness or health emergency, just isn't set up for that. It doesn't have the tools such long-term self-management demands as an absolute prerequisite of success. Granted, many medical schools have begun to think in fresh ways about training and to make changes in both course work and practicum experience. And there are some schools—notably, Bastyr University in Seattle, Washington—that are dedicated to the kind of medicine that is clinically applicable to the management of chronic illness. (Full disclosure: I was a founding trustee of and professor at Bastyr.) These developments are very welcome, yet they serve to etch in even sharper relief the disconnect between the health care we have and the health care we need.

THE DISCONNECT

At the heart of the disconnect is the fundamental medical fact that an infectious disease can be traced to a single cause or agent. That fact became the basis of a now well-defined process for developing drugs that could address the identifiable cause or agent and thus cure the disease. It also gave rise to the now humongous pharmaceutical industry that carries out the process.

Remember high school biology and learning about all those metabolic processes going on in our bodies—the zillions of biochemical reactions happening all the time within our cells, step by step by step? Put very simply, think of a disease as caused by an overly active step in one of the metabolic processes going on in the body—a single step that has gone out of sync or out of control. If you can find or create a substance that will interfere with that overly active step—block it, inhibit it, alter it in some way—you more or less transform the effect of the disease and reduce its symptoms. That's precisely what drugs do.

Back in the day—it's worth remembering that the therapeutic use of antibiotics dates only to 1940—drugs were made from natural sources like medicinal plants or, in the case of antibiotics like penicillin, which was derived from a naturally occurring blue mold, were the products of bacterial and fungal metabolism. These naturally derived compounds were pitted against the specific metabolic process known as cell wall synthesis, a process unique to the bacteria that cause infectious diseases; tellingly, the process was not found in animal cells. This lucky distinction between bacterial and human cell metabolism made the antibiotics both safe to use and highly selective in their action—naturally so. And they did just what the doctor ordered: They literally altered the cause of the illness, more or less morphing it out of existence.

Flushed with success, particularly given the role antibiotics played in saving lives on the battlefields of World War II, the pharmaceutical industry turned its attention to realms beyond infectious disease—to the kinds of infirmities suffered by those diagnosed with chronic illnesses. For these illnesses, scientists knew they would not find a specific bug causing a specific infection. Instead, their aim was to identify the particular biological process related to the *dominant symptom* of the particular chronic illness—whether pain or inflammation or a specific misstep in a metabolic activity associated with the disease—so they could then develop a drug that would modify the effects of this process, blocking or altering the misstep in the complex web of metabolism.

A different kind of development process evolved to create these drugs, and it profoundly reshaped the pharmaceutical industry. The process begins with what is known as high-throughput screening, in which chemists evaluate exactly how tens of thousands of chemicals synthesized in the lab influence the metabolic activity being targeted.

The smaller the amount of chemical required to interfere with a particular step in the metabolic process, the more active the chemical is considered to be—and the more effective the drug. Next, those compounds identified as most active are screened for safety across a range of different models. A substance showing both high activity and acceptable safety in this screening is then tested in humans, and if it passes those tests, it goes onto the market. That is, your doctor can prescribe it to you as a short-term therapy to cure an acute illness caused by the specific misstep in a particular metabolic process for which the drug was developed.

And where chronic illness is concerned, there's the rub. For today's rising burden of chronic illness cannot be attributed to alteration in a single step in the complex metabolic web. Rather, the diseases and conditions we call chronic derive from a variety of causes, each expressed in its own symptom or set of symptoms. And because the drugs for the illnesses treat only the dominant symptoms—that is, the effects, not the ultimate cause—you don't really get over a chronic illness, no matter how often you pelt it with drugs or how many kinds of drugs you pelt it with. Instead, it either persists or recurs; in fact, it actually gets worse over time. The outcome of the treatment isn't a return to good health but rather increasing disability and a diminished quality of life.

You see what the problem is. You tell your doctor you feel tired and you sort of ache all over. Pressed for specific details, you report that you haven't been sleeping well, can't concentrate, have no energy, and just feel wiped out. Trained in a pharmaceutical strategy that seeks one cause to explain one disease that can be treated with one drug, the doctor is stymied at best; how can he or she help you, the poor suffering patient?

Eager to alleviate your multiple symptoms, your doctor typically prescribes multiple drugs. What else is a doctor to do? There is no drug for the specific cause of the patient's complaints—for the reason that the cause, which is complex and multifaceted, doesn't lend itself to being cured by a single drug. But thanks to a booming pharmaceutical industry, there are lots of drugs for the various symptoms.

So, for example, a patient with type 2 diabetes might be prescribed one drug to treat the fatigue she feels, another to suppress her appetite, something else to deal with the headaches, and yet another treatment for her blurred vision. Someone with arthritis might take a range of anti-inflammatory medications in combination with pain-killers to alleviate the discomfort. Unlike antibiotics that address the cause of a specific infectious disease, the therapies prescribed for these chronic illness sufferers treat the effects of their disease, not its multiple causes.

It's called polypharmacy—simultaneously taking a number of different drugs to treat a range of symptoms of an ailment. Of course, if you suffer from more than one ailment—from diabetes *and* arthritis, for example—the polypharmacy multiplies even further. It's why Catherine is taking six drugs for her three recognizable complaints; her well-meaning doctors are stemming the impact of her arthritis, cardiovascular weakness, and possible osteoporosis—camouflaging them to a sufficient extent that she can get on with her life—without ever tackling the origins of the impacts.

What happens as a result? One outcome is that the disease or diseases will continue to progress over time. As this happens, the symptoms become more severe and more medications are required to alleviate them. In effect, these patients become lifetime consumers of medications that were expressly designed—and approved by regulators—to be used for a limited time only so they could get on with their lives.

But so far from getting on with their lives, patients may actually be undermining their lives as they continue to take the medications, for they become increasingly susceptible to adverse drug reactions. "Adverse reaction" may sound like a minor irritation, but in fact, ADRs are a leading cause of death in the United States. Remember Vioxx, the anti-arthritis drug pulled from the market when it was implicated in potentially tens of thousands of deaths? And Avandia, the antidiabetic implicated in heart attacks and left on the market only under the most stringent restrictions?

Perhaps the most striking example of all was that uncovered by the Women's Health Initiative study, initiated by the National Institutes of Health in 1991, on the use of hormone replacement therapy, HRT, to treat the ill effects of menopause. It had been assumed for more than fifty years that the use of estrogens and synthetic progesterone replacement therapy by menopausal women was good for their bones, breast health, heart, and brain as well as being a salve that could assuage night sweats, hot flashes, and the mood swings and depressive symptoms associated with the onset of menopause. Millions of women took this combination of drugs for several decades, quite naturally assuming that the drugs had been thoroughly tested and found to be safe for long-term use.

Their assumption was wrong. No long-term outcome studies had ever been done on HRT until the Women's Health Initiative study, the results of which were so alarming that the study directors felt morally bound to announce them early, before all the data were in. The study found that for many women, the particular combination of equine estrogens (Premarin, from pregnant mares) and synthetic progesterone not only did not improve heart and brain function but actually increased the risk of both heart disease and dementia.

How could this happen? Vioxx, Avandia, and the Premarin-progesterone combination had all passed rigorous safety testing in different assays and in animal models, not to mention undergoing a range of human tests in double-blind, placebo-controlled trials to receive the seal of approval of the Food and Drug Administration. How can drugs that have passed muster in the toughest safety tests on earth turn out to be so tragically unsafe?

I have alluded to one reason already: the safety testing is based on the use of these drugs for a limited duration, not for the course of a lifetime. What appears safe in a short-term study may, over the long term, begin to show very different effects, especially when the drug is taken by so many different people with very different genetic profiles, different lifestyles, and different causes of their disease. It looks very much as if a law of unintended consequences may apply to any drug used by many people over many more years than the studies evaluated in the approval process.

There's another possible reason for ADRs. Remember how drugs work: they interfere with—they block or inhibit—certain overly active metabolic steps associated with the symptoms of the disease. Anti-inflammatory drugs, for example, inhibit the effects of key enzymes that cause tissue to swell and send alarm signals to your brain. Anti-ulcer drugs block the production of stomach acid. Drugs that treat high blood pressure either block the hormones that regulate the complex process for controlling blood pressure or prevent their release. Drugs that treat depression inhibit the normal regulation of certain neurotransmitters in the brain. The problem is that the specific biological target a drug blocks because it is related to a disease state in one place in the body may be important for normal functioning in other places within the body. To put it very simplistically, the inflammation that is causing symptoms of severe pain because it is out of control over here in one part of the body is a normal, essential housekeeping process over there in another part of the body. Obviously, if a patient continues to take an anti-inflammatory drug over a long period of time, that can adversely affect the "distant" normal housekeeping and induce a dangerous situation seemingly unrelated to the original problem.

That is indeed what happens. As with Peter, your blood pressure may be going down, but keeping it down knocks out your sexual potency. Your ulcer may be under control, thanks to your antiulcer drug, but it may be causing anemia. Or your arthritis pain may now be manageable due to the powerful anti-inflammatories you're taking, but those same anti-inflammatories may be contributing to your risk for kidney disease. And who knows what other impacts blocking those specific enzymes may have elsewhere in your body's systems? In fact, in many cases, we know all too well. It is why your doctor tells you to go easy on over-the-counter ibuprofen or naproxen, not to mention acetaminophen. Long-term use of the former can lead to gastric bleeding, heart attack, and stroke, while the excessive use of the analgesic acetaminophen can damage the liver irreversibly.

This does not mean that there is no value in taking specific medications to manage the symptoms of chronic illness. It suggests, however, that it is best to use fewer medications, at the lowest dose able to manage the condition, and for the shortest time possible. It also means that the disease is very likely still there—and getting worse.

ACCEPTING THE INEVITABLE?

So there's the dilemma—part of the dilemma anyway. We have a health-care system equipped and ready to cure the occasional acute disease, and our health-care horizon is packed with the chronic suffering of people like Peter and Catherine. The short-term drugs being applied as a long-term remedy to this suffering hold the potential for scary adverse impacts and treat only the effects of an ailment, which continues to progress in severity over time. Our health system and the understanding of disease on which it is based aren't working for the health reality of today, which is chronic illness.

Yet the most commonly voiced response to this dilemma is that it is inevitable. The longer we live, the more chronic ailments we will get and the more severe they will become as we age. Accept it.

Well, no. Not if we don't have to. And we don't.

Let me tell you about my great-grandfather. He pursued a number of careers in his life of ninety-six years: dentist, jeweler, rancher, antiques dealer, and, in a kind of near-career, marathon canasta player. He was married to my great-grandmother for sixty-five years, and after her death, he enjoyed a fifteen-year relationship with a woman he traveled seventy miles by bus to visit. On Thanksgiving of his ninety-sixth year, after six hours of playing cards with his children, grandchildren, and great-grandchildren, he announced that having seen us all grow up, and having outlived two wonderful women partners, he would be moving on soon, and he wanted us to know that. Two weeks later, he died in his sleep.

That some of his physical powers had diminished somewhat in his last years was undeniable, but he never lost his zest for living and never stopped reaping the joy of life. He had no reason to; he wasn't sick or infirm or particularly disabled in body, mind, or spirit. It seemed to me he lived the maximum life span at the optimum level of health and well-being that his genetic potential enabled. Wouldn't it be great if everybody could?

Everybody can. And they can for a reason articulated most succinctly and powerfully, in my view, by Dr. James Fries, a professor of medicine at the Stanford University School of Medicine. Very early on in his career, Fries became interested in the question of why people get more chronic illnesses as they age, especially since there is no evidence that aging in and of itself is the cause of any disease. In a watershed 1980 paper in the *New England Journal of Medicine*, Fries described the reserve of function in the body's organs that, in youth, is well above what is needed for average everyday living. It's like a savings account of extra biological capability that we can draw on when we need to—say, when we confront trauma, injury, or illness. At a moment of stress, for example, the heart and lungs can increase their response three to four times above what is needed for functioning at rest. Once the stress is over, both organ functions return to normal baseline with no adverse consequences.

This is true for every organ system, by the way—for liver function and its ability to let us tolerate toxins, drugs, and alcohol; for kidney function and its ability to control blood pressure; for muscle function as it relates to endurance; for immune function and our resistance to infection; for brain function as it relates to memory and cognitive function. Each system has its own reserve that equips it to bounce back from an exceptional response to an exceptional need.

As we age, however, we lose organ reserve. There's simply less in the account—less for Catherine than for Peter—which means there is diminished function to draw on in times of need and less ability of the organ to bounce back. The rate of speed at which we lose this reserve is what more or less shapes our individual process of biological aging, and it has been well proved that people lose organ reserve at different rates and therefore age differently. We all know fifty-year-olds who are biologically seventy. They feel old, look old, act old. And it's true: based on their loss of organ reserve, they *are* old. It is also possible to be chronologically seventy with the biological age of the average fifty-year-old; we probably know people like that as well—although we may not like them very much.

What Fries taught us in his paper, however, is that our biological age is correlated with our individual risk of chronic illness. While our average life expectancy has nearly doubled over the course of a century, we are spending a lot of that extended life span at risk for chronic illness or disabled by it. In other words, we spend a lot of that time drawing down, using up, and thereby losing organ reserve, thus speeding up our own biological aging.

So if we could reduce the loss of organ reserve as we grow older, thus slowing our biological aging and, since the two are correlated, the amount of unnecessary chronic illness we experience, we could not just increase average life expectancy but also lengthen our time of vigor and shorten our time of infirmity or disability. Fries used the phrase "compression of morbidity." He meant we could squeeze down the time between the onset of disability and the moment of death by lengthening the time *before* the onset of disability. We could, in short, stay younger longer.

How do we do it? Fries's idea was to make it happen by implementing the particular lifestyle behaviors and ensuring the particular kind of environment that would enable the individual to retain organ reserve as long as possible. It's the way we live, in other words, that can maximize our time of vigor and compress the period of chronic illness and senescence to a very short period at the end of life.

When Fries first postulated in 1980 that lifestyle and environment could minimize the rate of loss of organ reserve and compress morbidity, he received no small amount of criticism on the grounds that he had no "proof" for the hypothesis. Eighteen years later, he offered the proof. His 1998 follow-up article in the *New England Journal of Medicine* showed the results of a study of 1,741 university alumni. They underwent baseline health surveys in 1962 when their average age was forty-three and were then examined annually starting in 1986. The results of the study confirmed Fries's hypothesis: those university alums showing high-risk lifestyle behavior and environment at the baseline in 1962 and at the first annual checkup in 1986 experienced twice the cumulative disability—the biological aging—of those with low risk. For the latter, lower-risk group, the onset of the first disability was postponed *more than five years* beyond the onset of infirmity experienced by those showing greater health risks in their forties. That's a lot of years. And it confirms that it isn't your chronological age but your biological age that counts.

GENETIC INHERITANCE

Well, I hear you saying, but what about genes? Your DNA is your DNA, and you can't fight your genetic inheritance. No, you can't, but "inherited" does not mean "inevitable." Certainly, genes are important in influencing our health, but there is simply no such thing as chronic-disease genes, as was once generally assumed. What we have are genes that encode our uniqueness in how we respond to the circumstances of our environment and to our own individual behaviors.

The term for it is "genetic expression." Our genes get messages from our interactions with our environment and with how we choose to behave, and they translate those messages into cellular instructions; these instructions are what then control our health and disease patterns. You might say our environment and our behaviors talk to our genes, and what they say can change the way our book of life is read in the process of genetic expression—that is, through the translation our genes make.

What does it mean? For one thing, it means we are not hardwired to come down with the diseases that undermined the later years of our parents or grandparents. Your mother and father both gasped their way through an asthmatic old age and you figure you will too? Not if that gene encoded for asthma gets a totally different message. Your doctor tells you you're in danger of succumbing to the hereditary heart disease that killed your father? You have time to deactivate that fatal legacy by changing the messages your genes receive. Catherine is not doomed to become a brittle-boned old lady just because that's what happened to her mother. She can make changes to her lifestyle, her diet, and her exercise habits and thereby bring the needle back from osteoporosis.

Do you know about the BRCA gene, the feared mutation that prompts so many women found to possess it to submit to radical double mastectomy to save their lives? It is actually a prime example of this reality about changing the message our genes receive. Before 1940, the incidence of breast cancer developing in women with the BRCA mutation was 24 percent. By 2013, the incidence was greater than 85 percent. What changed to cause that extraordinary leap in the occurrence of the disease from this mutation? Not the gene; genes can't and don't change. It was the environment influencing the gene's expression that changed: diet, exercise, other lifestyle behaviors. Alter the environment and you alter the way genes express themselves in response—and the health outcome. It all depends on the message the gene receives.

The bottom line is that genetic inheritance is not fate. Your lifetime health was not predetermined at your conception. On the contrary: you have the opportunity—and the power—to shape your own pattern of health and longevity. It's what personalized health management is all about.

A NEW MODEL—AND A PIONEER WITH PROOF

So chronic illness, the rising global burden that our current health systems are inadequately equipped to address, is not the inevitable circumstance of old age or the predetermined outcome of our genetic history. Rather, it occurs at the intersection of the information encoded in our genes and the messages transmitted to our genes from our environment and our behavior. This is a revolutionary change in our understanding of the origins and causes of the chronic ailments that afflict so many of us. It is forcing us to take a revolutionary approach to the way we treat these diseases. Clearly, our health as we grow older is much more under our control than previously assumed. The information encoded in our genes doesn't tell us how we are going to get sick; it enlightens us about how we should live to maximize our health over a longer life span.

We need a new health model to deal with that fact, and fortunately, one is emerging. Based on the realization that genes don't cause chronic illness and most drugs don't cure them, it is providing clinical proof that when we address chronic illness through environmental and lifestyle factors, positive health outcomes result.

The person who really brought this to everyone's attention is Dr. Dean Ornish. I first met Dr. Ornish in 1982 in San Francisco; I had taken a sabbatical from teaching to become a research director at the Linus Pauling Institute of Science and Medicine in Palo Alto. Some years before, Dr. Ornish had initiated his landmark clinical study of people diagnosed with—some of them suffering quite substantially from—existing cardiovascular disease. The study went on for five years—sufficient time to produce truly reliable results. Participants agreed to eat a diet of minimally processed whole grains, vegetables, fruits, and low-fat animal products, and to practice stress reduction exercises and yoga. A matched control group would not follow these behaviors. Because so many of the study participants had serious heart problems, the program regimen was considered by many to pose a very high risk. Of course, Dr. Ornish and his team were aware of the risks and were prepared for the challenges of administering the study. Detractors—and there were a number of them within the world of medicine—nevertheless felt that the study would at best produce ambiguous results and at worst do harm to the participants.

The results, published in the 1990s, proved all the detractors dead wrong. Using the sophisticated diagnostic tool known as positron emission tomography (PET), which measures the amount of plaque in the major arteries that serve the heart, the Ornish program resulted in modest regression of existing plaque after five years of participation in the program, whereas the matched group of patients who did not engage in the program experienced progression of their disease over the same period of time. A follow-up study three years later reported a relative reduction of nearly 8 percent in the amount of plaque in the arteries of the group complying with the program versus a nearly 12 percent average worsening of plaque in the group of nonparticipating matched patients. The Ornish group's conclusion was simply put: "More regression of coronary atherosclerosis occurred after five years than after one year in the experimental group. In contrast, in the control group, coronary atherosclerosis continued to progress and more than twice as many cardiac events occurred."

It was a groundbreaking study—in the way it was designed and executed, in its duration, and of course in its impressive results. It put to rest the long-standing criticism that no well-controlled clinical trial offered data to support the hypothesis that an aggressive intervention in lifestyle and nutrition could have a positive influence on heart health in people with the disease.* On the contrary. The Ornish study showed that changing lifestyle behaviors improved health and maintaining the changed behavior improved health even more. In essence, it proved the role of lifestyle and environment in determining genetic expression and influencing health status. How do we know that's what it proved? I'll put it this way: there's an app for that.

ASSESSING HEALTH STATUS: BIOMARKERS

What do I mean when I use the word "health"? One answer is that it's biological age. More generally, it is a state of optimal physical and physiological function—the maximum functional organ reserve possible at any particular time. The good news is that today's medical technologies provide us with important new tools for measuring function and therefore for assessing not just the absence of disease but the presence of health.

For example, did your last annual checkup include an electrocardiogram: an EKG? If so, that display of your heartbeat provides a good check for the presence of heart disease. But it is possible to have

---

* Ornish and his colleagues followed the heart study by applying the same program to men with prostate cancer, with equally potent results, proving yet again that aggressive compliance with a personalized lifestyle medicine program trumps drug treatment when it comes to chronic illness.

a normal heartbeat as recorded in an EKG, get a clean bill of heart health from your doctor, and suffer a heart attack on the way out of the doctor's office. It has happened—more than once.

That is why doctors often use another tool in addition to the EKG—the cardiac stress test. You hop up on the treadmill and walk or jog or run while the treadmill moves at different speeds and is inclined upward and downward to different grades of steepness. This challenges the heart, and the testing technology can then measure its ability and the ability of the blood vessels to accommodate the increased demands put upon them. The result is much closer to a measurement of the biological age of the organs than what a resting EKG test can provide.

Something similar is used in testing for diabetes. The standard test measures the amount of glucose in the blood after an overnight fast; an elevated level is a hallmark of the disease. But it is possible for a person in the early stages of diabetes to produce a normal result on the fasting blood sugar test. A more telling measure is to determine how well the body can metabolize glucose; this can be done through an oral glucose tolerance test (OGTT). Like the cardiac stress test, the OGTT is a challenge that can help measure organ reserve. The subject drinks a solution containing a specified amount of sugar. The level of glucose in the subject's blood is then monitored periodically over the next three to six hours. During this time, of course, the stress of the sugar load is challenging the subject's ability to properly metabolize it. Difficulty in handling the load—in metabolizing the sugar—will indicate a reduced organ reserve, and the test will read as abnormal. Yet it is not unusual for a person with a normal fasting blood glucose level to have an abnormal OGTT.

This ability to evaluate the actual functional reserve is crucial to curing chronic illness. Chronic conditions, after all, start with subtle changes in function that can precede the diagnosis of a disease by decades. If there were some way to assess these subtle functional changes early—before a disease develops—we would be able to monitor and track our functional health status. There *is* a way— through biomarkers—and it is fueling a major shake-up in medicine.

Biomarkers are indicators of our functional health status. They reflect how our genes are being expressed in terms of our own unique lifestyle and the various conditions and circumstances to which our personal environment exposes us. Blood pressure, percentage of body fat, the level of glucose or triglycerides or cholesterol in our blood, the way that cholesterol is packaged in LDL or HDL forms: these are just some of the more common biomarkers, all of them signals that indicate how our genes are being translated into physiological, physical, and mental functions—gauges of our genetic expression. When we undergo stress, get an infection, eat nothing but supersized junk foods on vacation, confront trauma, or are exposed to toxins, our genetic expression changes in response. Of course it does: our environmental circumstances are disrupted, so our interactions with the environment necessarily change in response, and the message to our genes is different from the message they would receive when our bodies are in a state of peace. The change in genetic expression also shifts the pattern of biomarkers, and the shift in turn indicates that our health status is disturbed in response to the present environment. But because we each possess different genetic information, we will each experience disturbances in our health status in a different way.

Let's say your genes are stimulated by the threat of an infection floating around in your environment—a cold or flu, for example. Your genetic expression shifts into gear, mobilizing your body's response to that threat by activating your immune system. In the short term, this response is highly beneficial: you avoid getting sick or you get less sick than you might. But over the longer term, such a change in genetic expression can turn what was beneficial into something downright injurious to the specific tissues and cell functioning that keep getting involved. That injury is what we call chronic illness.

It means, among other things, that chronic illness isn't something you "contract," the word we tend to use for getting an illness; you don't catch a chronic illness the way a fielder in baseball nabs a line drive smack into the pocket of his glove.

In the purest sense of the word, in fact, there are no real diseases. This is why I say disease is a delusion. Rather, the individual's unique genetic makeup responding over time to a perceived threat alters the functioning of specific tissues, and that "injury," like a banked fire that burns slowly, becomes a sustained, low-grade impairment. We call it a disease or illness, and if it goes on for a while, we call it a chronic illness. But it's really our genes responding to messages from our diet, our environment, and our lifestyle behaviors. Through their changing levels in the body, biomarkers show us just how the genes are responding to specific environmental threats.

But here's the headline. In addition to the many well-known examples of biomarkers—cholesterol, blood pressure, triglycerides, or glucose in the blood—there are also literally hundreds of new biomarker candidates that can help to pinpoint changes in a person's health well before disease develops. There's a biomarker for assessing a woman's risk for uterine cancer using the Pap test. The prostate-specific antigen (PSA) biomarker test evaluates a man's risk of prostate cancer,* while the levels of hemoglobin A1c in the blood as a marker for diabetes have become routine over the past twenty years. One of the new biomarkers in the blood that we'll meet again later is high-sensitivity C-reactive protein: hs-CRP. This biomarker is an indicator of chronic inflammation and, especially when combined with a companion biomarker in the blood, homocysteine, can alert us to a person's early risk of heart disease, arthritis, diabetes, or dementia, four of the five major chronic illnesses.

What is crucially important, of course, is that these biomarkers are the smoke signaling the fire of altered health status and suggesting there just may be a chronic illness lurking up ahead. Sniffed out early enough, they provide time to take steps to avert the potential chronic illness or alter its progression.

There are, to be sure, certain factors in the environment—like a famine or an infectious epidemic—that send such a strong message to the genes that everyone's health is affected, regardless of genetic

---

* There is ongoing controversy over the clinical specificity of the PSA test in defining cancer risk; my view is that the evidence strongly indicates that rapidly rising PSA levels *over time* are a strong indicator of prostate cancer.

history, and biomarkers will record the fact. But with most of the environmental factors and lifestyle behaviors we experience on a daily basis—like smoking or eating a diet high in saturated fats—the influence on genetic expression will vary from person to person.

What the Ornish study demonstrated was that biomarkers register the shifts in an individual's genetic expression as the individual's environmental factors and lifestyle behaviors change. In those participants who followed the program and changed their diet and exercise levels, the biomarkers signaled improved heart function; in those who did not follow the program, the biomarkers of heart disease were still there and the heart function of those people regressed. Among other implications, this means that biomarkers are the key to shaping the kind of personalized approach to curing chronic illness that this book is about.

The Ornish study is foundational to the development of today's emerging new approach to the management of chronic illness, and Dean Ornish himself is one of the principal pioneers of this burgeoning revolution in lifestyle medicine. Whether they're aware of it or not, millions of people down the generations will have reason to be grateful to him.

THE PERSONAL TOUCH

The Ornish study offered proof of the gene-environment connection to chronic illness. Since the study, there have been considerable additional advances in understanding how the connection applies to those chronic illnesses that together account for the bulk of healthcare expenditures today—heart disease, arthritis, dementia, cancer, and type 2 diabetes—as well as the common secondary effects of type 2 diabetes: chronic kidney disease, stroke, liver disease, neuropathy, and loss of eyesight.

So we can say there has been progress indeed in our understanding of the chronic-illness conundrum—the essential first step in changing our approach to dealing with the rising global burden of chronic illness. One final challenge remains, however, and that is the recognition that in order to maximize the health outcomes of any new approach, it must be individualized—that is, personalized to the health status and specific health profile of the individual and, in great measure, managed by the individual over the long haul.

Why are a personalized approach and individualized self-management so important? First of all, we know from current clinical studies that a one-size-fits-all approach is inherently a hit-or-miss proposition. In any clinical study evaluating any medical protocol, there is always a group of participants who respond well and a group that either does not respond or experiences an adverse outcome. Take a look at the published data for overall drug effectiveness in managing some key chronic illnesses:

- Alzheimer's disease: 30 percent effective
- Anti-inflammatories: 80 percent effective
- Asthma: 80 percent effective
- Cardiac disease: 60 percent effective
- Depression: 62 percent effective
- Diabetes: 57 percent effective
- Migraine: 52 percent effective
- Rheumatoid arthritis: 50 percent effective
- Cancer: 30 percent effective

Surprised? Wondering how the rate of effectiveness can be so relatively low after all the clinical trials and the years of use of these drugs? It is because we typically overlook the nonresponders in a clinical trial for regulatory approval of a drug as long as the trial is large enough that the outcomes of the responders demonstrate statistical significance against the outcomes of nonresponders. To a very great extent, therefore, when you take a medication prescribed by your doctor, you're putting your faith in a remedy that has worked for a lot of people and has not worked for a lot of others. Cross your fingers, wear a rabbit's foot, and pray that it works for you.

No wonder one of the pharmaceutical industry's highest-ranking and most respected scientists, Dr. Allen Roses, onetime global vice president of genetics at GlaxoSmithKline, said back in 2003 that "most prescription medicines do not work on most people" who take them. Roses went on: "The vast majority of drugs—more than 90 percent—only work in 30 to 50 percent of the people." It is why doctors routinely use a trial-and-error approach to drug therapy—that is, if one drug doesn't work, try another.

The problem is compounded with polypharmacy—an individual using several drugs together in order to address the different symptoms arising from a range of causative factors. The issue here is the way the various drugs may interact with one another in the individual. There is "cross talk" among drugs; one medication may adversely influence another. An individual taking a number of different drugs simultaneously, whether he or she knows it or not, is involuntarily enrolled in an uncontrolled experiment, for it is almost certain that no study has ever been done to demonstrate the safety and effectiveness of the particular combination of medications that individual is taking. Ideally, such a review should be done—to assess not just the potential adverse reactions from combining the drugs but also the effectiveness of the combination, or its lack of effectiveness, in the individual.

I first came across the term "patient empowerment" a number of years ago, through Dr. Halsted Holman, a professor at the Stanford University School of Medicine. Holman articulated and advocated four principles of personalized and self-managed medicine that my decades of experience tell me are the right approach to both preventing and managing chronic illness. Here they are:

- There is no complete cure for chronic illness unless the cause of the individual's own disease is discovered and successfully managed; individualized management over time is essential.
- For effective treatment of chronic illness, the individual must engage continually in different approaches to his or her health.
- The individual knows the most about his or her own condition and about the effects of certain therapies and must apply that knowledge in shaping a self-management program.

- To achieve success, the individual and the individual's health professionals must share knowledge and divide authority.

In the next chapter, we'll learn how the revolution in genomics is pointing the world of medicine precisely in the direction those principles embody. And we'll see how the amazing discoveries of the genomics revolution can be harnessed to meet the global challenge we confront in the rising burden of chronic illness.

CHAPTER 2

The Biological Breakthrough That Is Changing Everything

Conventional wisdom has long held that our health is 70 percent heredity and 30 percent everything else. The breakthrough discovery at the heart of the functional medicine revolution flips that ratio on its head. This pulls the rug out from under genetic determinism and sends it on its way. Our genes are not our fate; no disease or dysfunction—or particular strength or level of longevity, for that matter—is foreordained.

Like the physiological discoveries of the late nineteenth century, today's biological breakthrough has fundamentally altered our understanding of how the human organism works and will change medical practice fundamentally and thoroughly. The word "breakthrough," however, seems to connote in many people's minds a stunning revelation that comes out of left field and, in an instant, makes everything clear. Science doesn't actually work that way. Remember the scientific method, which you probably first learned about back in elementary school, with its painstaking process of observation, hypothesis, experiment, testing, modifying, retesting, and retesting again and again and again? That's how science works, and the breakthrough understanding of the relationship between our genes and chronic disease happened in just that way, building on the work of scientists from decades—even centuries—ago.* In fact, it is still happening; the story continues to unfold as the research presses on.

---

* In fact, some medical historians suggest that the real origins of today's genomic revolution can be found in the Yellow Emperor's Inner Canon of China and the work of Hippocrates of Greece, both circa 500 BCE, and in the principles of Ayurvedic medicine formulated in India in the first and second centuries CE.

But to begin the story, let's go back to the latter part of the nineteenth century. As a biochemist, I have always thought that if time travel really were possible and if I were given my choice of an era to be transported back to, this is the one I would choose. Florence Nightingale, dispatched to the Crimean War in 1854, had found that more soldiers were dying of infectious disease than in battle and had commenced a methodical statistical analysis of British servicemen that fingered poor hygiene and sanitation as the culprits. She was perhaps the first epidemiologist, and her advocacy of sanitary living conditions would be felt worldwide. Charles Darwin had returned from his epic voyage on the *Beagle* and in 1859 had published *On the Origin of Species*, laying out the process of natural selection and explicating the theory of evolution. Gregor Mendel had published his experiments on inherited traits in peas in 1865. In France, Louis Pasteur was setting forth the principles of what would become known as microbiology, while in Germany, Robert Koch was discovering the bacterial origin of disease. What a time of discovery that was!

If I could choose the place to be transported to, I think I would ask for London, where all of these discoveries were being discussed and debated—in a language I understand!—by some of the finest minds of all time. The biologist Thomas Huxley was a prominent spokesman for Darwin's theory of evolution, while his fellow biologist, William Bateson, translator of Gregor Mendel's work on inheritance and the man credited with coining the word "genetics," disagreed, refusing to accept the evolution argument. Archibald Edward Garrod, later Sir Archibald, the son of one of Queen Victoria's personal physicians and himself a biochemist who discovered genetic diseases of infancy, is credited with having integrated Mendelian genetics and Darwinian natural selection into medical thinking. The Huxleys, the Batesons, and the Garrods regularly dined together, discussing their discoveries and arguing about natural selection and genetic inheritance. Can you imagine how energetic those dinner conversations must have been?

Out of this time of great discovery and debate came the two dominant concepts that shaped medical thinking from that time to

our own: that our species evolves through the process of natural selection, and that we inherit dominant and recessive characteristics
through our genes. Thread the two concepts together, filter them
through the lens of medical practice and its need to apply remedies,
and our perception of health and disease comes down to the notion
that some people are born with fit genes and therefore flourish, while
others are born with disease-producing genes and therefore get sick.
Under this rubric, medical practice becomes focused on saving the
less lucky among us from the inheritance of the disease-producing
genes over which we have little control.

By the early twentieth century, further work had found that our
genetic characteristics are carried on our chromosomes, of which
humans have twenty-three pairs. One half of each pair of chromosomes is provided by the biological mother through her egg, the
other half by the biological father through his sperm. So half our
genes come from each parent. Actually, as we'll see shortly, some
additional genetic material, mitochondrial DNA, is contributed only
by the mother. Nevertheless, the overall perception held: our genetic
inheritance, lucky or unlucky, comes from both parents in pretty
much a fifty-fifty split. If that inheritance produces diseases in us, we
have only our lineage to blame.

The perception was reinforced by Garrod's discovery in the early
twentieth century that a number of diseases found in infancy—
specifically, phenylketonuria (PKU), sickle-cell anemia, Tay-Sachs
disease, and Gaucher's disease—were defined by dominant genetic
characteristics on a single gene. The idea that one characteristic from
one gene could so dramatically affect a life fed right into the idea
that your lifetime pattern of health and disease was preordained at
conception. The embryo that would become you was already coded
with the diseases that would afflict you; whether those diseases were
disastrous or benign was the luck of the draw. If it wasn't your "fault"
that you weren't among the fittest—it was *natural* selection, after all—
there was also little you could do about it; it was the hand you had
been dealt. The term for it is "genetic determinism," and it left a lot
of people feeling doomed to suffer the same chronic diseases their

parents suffered because those diseases were inscribed on at least one half of their genome.

Against such diseases, it's little wonder that the therapeutic model was based on the perception that medicine existed to do battle with disease. Health-care providers fighting a bad-luck genome were seen as heroic soldiers on the front lines of combat, striving to win the war on smallpox or diphtheria or cancer, or to overcome each individual's genetically determined flaws and weaknesses through whatever therapeutic measures might be required—whatever it might take to get the job done. When all you have is a hammer, everything is a nail. And the model did indeed hit the nail on the head many times over many years, achieving great victories in the treatment of acute disease with aggressive, short-term interventions. But as we have seen, it did little to manage chronic diseases safely and cost-effectively.

In truth, there had long been studies that modulated the armor-like purity of both dominant shapers of medical thinking—the luck-of-the-draw survival of the fittest and the genetic determinism that you were stuck with the hand you had drawn. Some researchers came up with findings that suggested we are not locked into our genes and there is not just one single track—or rather, two parental tracks—along which genetic information arrives to influence our patterns of health and disease.

By the late twentieth century, serious doubt had been cast on the rigidly fifty-fifty split between maternal and paternal genetic inheritance. Much of the doubt was propelled by the finding of that additional genetic material, the mitochondrial DNA contributed solely by the mother. Mitochondria are the energy powerhouses of the cell, the place in which food-derived molecules are transformed into cellular energy. In the male, mitochondria are in the tail of the sperm, and since the tail drops off once an egg is fertilized, none of those mitochondria get incorporated into the embryo. In short, mitochondria come from Mom; that is, the genetics of our cellular energy centers are connected particularly closely to our mothers, with no contribution to this particular function from fathers. So if we're 50 percent our fathers, it looks like we're slightly more than

50 percent our mothers—and the slightly more than 50 percent affects a pretty important function.

Half a century later, in the mid-1960s, a young faculty member at Boston University, Lynn Margulis,* propounded what she called the endosymbiotic theory of the mitochondrion. Margulis held that mitochondria were originally bacteria that millions of years ago had infected a host pre-human cell, had then adapted to being there, and have remained there ever since thanks to a mutually beneficial symbiosis: the cells provide a harmonious residence, and the bacteria/ mitochondria pay rent by producing energy for the cells. It is certainly true that the structure of mitochondrial DNA is very much like that of bacteria and that the genetics of mitochondrial DNA trace back farther than human cells—two facts that seem to support Margulis's theory.

For Margulis, these findings of internal symbiosis, called endosymbiosis, confirmed her advocacy of the Gaia hypothesis, which suggests that the competitive, survival-of-the-fittest concept of evolution is "incomplete," in Margulis's word. To complete it, the Gaia hypothesis suggests that it is cooperation rather than competition—networking rather than the struggle of the unfit against the fit—that is the true driving force of evolution. Or perhaps it is that cooperation eventually derives from the competition, the struggle of unfit against fit finally settling into network as each adapts to the naturally selecting "best" of the other. In this view, evolution is a self-regulating symbiosis between organisms and their environmental surroundings, and it is this self-regulation that keeps life on the planet ticking over, even as conditions change.

That is just what had happened with those ancient bacteria that had come to attack a human cell; they had stayed on and adapted until they had become integral contributors to the evolution of that cell, morphing into mitochondria that enabled humans to use energy better than organisms without mitochondria. To Margulis, that fact

---

* Margulis was named the distinguished university professor of geosciences at the University of Massachusetts in 1988, a post she still held at the time of her death in 2011. She was elected to the National Academy of Sciences in 1983 and was awarded the National Medal of Science in 1999.

supported the idea of symbiotic harmony, not combat, as the "success factor" in shaping evolution.

What does this idea of self-regulating symbiosis tell us about our genetic inheritance? Simply put, it tells us that we're carrying genetic information that doesn't just derive from Mom and Dad and isn't split evenly between them. Our mitochondrial DNA is carrying genetic information that dates from millions of years ago and derives from these ancient bacteria; it is capable of adapting, it is sensitive to environmental influences, and it can affect our health.

Suppose, for example, that your mother and father are the two liveliest and most energetic people you know, yet you're constantly exhausted. If you didn't inherit the fatigue gene from their chromosomes, maybe you got it from the way your mitochondrial DNA interacts with your environment or with your particular lifestyle. So while your exhaustion wasn't genetically predetermined, it's there nonetheless, but because it is susceptible to factors of your environment and your behavior, you can change it by changing those factors. And that is something we humans have the power to do.

This thinking was a shot across the bow of the notion that our health is predetermined by our genes, and as the twentieth century proceeded and the twenty-first got under way, other discoveries further challenged the primacy of genetic determinism. Where chronic diseases in particular were concerned, the concept was found to be not exclusively true. In fact, it began to look like only some 30 percent of the common chronic diseases resulted from genetic inheritance, while 70 percent were shown to come from something else—namely, from the influence of environment on genetic expression.

Then along came the mapping of the human genome, the core scientific event of our era, to really illumine for us this relationship between environment—the resources and faculties we draw on in our daily lives and our habits of behavior vis-à-vis these resources and faculties—and genetic expression. The result has been a profound change in what we know about disease and how we think about medicine.

THE HUMAN GENOME PROJECT: A NEW BOOK OF REVELATION

The mapping of the human genome was initiated in 1990 under the direction of Dr. Francis Collins with $3 billion in U.S. government funding. Eight years later, a private group, Celera, headed by Dr. Craig Venter, announced it would compete with the government-sponsored research, using a different approach that ultimately cost 10 percent of what taxpayers had paid. But it was thanks to both groups that the first-draft sequencing, as it was called—that is, the decoding of the human genome—was successfully completed in 2000. And although the results of the project would not be finalized until 2003, the moment was marked in 2000 by an announcement in the Rose Garden of the White House joining representatives of both groups and presided over, appropriately, by the president of the United States, Bill Clinton.

The achievement represented one of the largest international science collaborations in history. It was the culmination of efforts begun back in 1953 when James Watson and Francis Crick discovered the structure of DNA—the iconic double helix of genetic code locked in two spiraling chains of nucleic acids coiled around a single axis. From Watson and Crick to the White House Rose Garden in just under forty years represents a truly extraordinary milestone in our understanding of the chemical nature of our book of life, and the research this culmination set in motion continues to yield insight after insight to this day.

It started by shattering assumptions. Scientists had assumed that the mapping would confirm, first, that humans had many more genes than other species and, second, that all human genomes were fundamentally similar to one another. So where common diseases were concerned—in particular, chronic diseases—the genetic variants causing the diseases must also be common. It would mean an easy path ahead for medicine. All that had to happen was for research to find the common genetic root, and it would be a snap to generate a universal treatment—the pill or injection that would do the trick.

Medical researchers and practitioners held their breath waiting for the mapping project to give them the go-ahead to find, develop, and administer these cures.

It didn't happen. The research told a far different story, and that is the breakthrough that is changing everything. It is changing our notions of genetic determinism, demonstrating that we are not fated to suffer the same diseases or disorders as our parents. It is showing us how our genetic expression works and the factors that can influence it. It is even showing us how our genetic expression can be changed by mechanisms outside or unrelated to our underlying DNA.

Let's take it a step at a time.

THERE'S MORE TO THE STORY OF EVOLUTION THAN WE THOUGHT

First, at the start of the project, there was that assumption that the human genome would comprise nearly 100,000 genes, many more than other species. After all, we humans are both bigger and more complex than most other organisms, and if you think of our genes as the stories that make up our book of life, then it seemed logical that what was "written" in our chromosomes—our genetic code—would also be relatively more complex, with a greater number of genes than the average squirrel or the tree the squirrel lives in.

We were in for a surprise. The total number of genes in the human genome is approximately 25,000—fewer than are found in a number of plants. The genome of the pinot grape, for example, has nearly 30,000 genes—making us seem perhaps less complex than the wines we drink.

There were other surprises in store. As the deciphering went on, we learned that the human genome is about 96 percent identical to that of the chimpanzee, a finding that focused scientific scrutiny like a laser on that 4 percent difference. The reason? Chimps don't get cancer, don't experience autism, don't get heart attacks. Finding out why not could offer clues to why we do.

Within the human species, the deciphering showed that while

your genes and mine are very similar in the larger sense—again, as the stories that make up our book of life—there are small differences between us in the individual words that encode the stories. These differences, it turns out, can be significant. The difference of just a single nucleotide—in effect, a single letter in a single word of a single gene—can influence our susceptibility to disease. The difference might, for example, make me, with a particular nucleotide in a specific position in the particular gene, less susceptible to a particular disease than you, whose corresponding gene has a different nucleotide at that position. On the other hand, where another disease is concerned, I might be more susceptible than you, because of that very same nucleotide in that very same position in that very same gene. There are more than 3 million of these variants in humans; they are called single nucleotide polymorphisms, SNPs—routinely pronounced "snips"—and they are evidence that while we may have a mere 25,000 genes, there is plenty of variation in their construction.

What do these 3 million SNPs have to do with our patterns of health and disease? It is the way they influence specific functions that is so crucial. Take the example of one SNP, methylenetetrahydrofolate reducatase polymorphism—MTHFR polymorphism for short. Yes, even in its short form, the name is over the top, but the importance of this SNP cannot be overestimated. It turns out to be extremely influential in controlling the metabolism of the important B vitamin known as folic acid. Folic acid is pivotal to numerous functions of the heart, brain, blood cells, and immune system as well as being an essential component of fetal development. People who carry the variant SNPs of the MTHFR gene—and whose metabolizing of folic acid is therefore modified in some way—have been found to have higher risk of depression, heart disease, and dementia. Many are unable to function normally *unless* they get a higher dietary intake of folic acid—or its relative, 5-methyltetrahydrofolate—from food or from a nutritional supplement. This discovery of nutrient-dependent SNPs has spawned the new field of nutrigenomics, which is aimed at determining the correct intake of specific nutrients that will meet the genetically determined needs of the individual. With

3 million SNPs already identified, and with a goodly number of them no doubt nutrient-dependent, nutrigenomics would seem fertile territory indeed for empowering us to take some control over managing our own health.

Certainly, the idea that nutritional therapy should be tailored to individual needs is not new. Back in 1950, renowned biochemist Dr. Roger Williams of the University of Texas had a famous paper in *The Lancet* entitled "The Concept of Genetotrophic Disease." In it, Williams suggested that the recommended dietary allowance (RDA) levels of nutrients established by the Food and Drug Administration were essentially useless because, as Williams proposed, the nutrient needs of individuals differ far more substantively from person to person than the RDAs took into account. I was in a seminar with Dr. Williams in 1974 when he delivered his classic statement that "nutrition is for real people; statistical humans are of little interest." He meant by this that while most medical and nutritional training focuses on the so-called 70-kilogram human—a 155-pound male accepted as statistically average—there is in fact no such thing as a statistically average person. (Well, maybe a few men qualify.) But there's something fundamentally flawed in making the 70-kilogram human male the focus of tens of thousands of published research studies because the results of such studies simply won't be germane to the vast bulk of us, who are as individual as snowflakes. To Williams, applying the rule of the statistical average to the needs of the individual is therefore a path to failure in treatment because it is based on this flaw of understanding.

It means that if you toss back a multivitamin at breakfast, you're probably not doing yourself any harm, but you may not be providing yourself with the levels of specific nutrients that you need for optimal function—and if you think you are, you are laboring under a delusion. On the other hand, there may well be specific genomic reasons for you to be complementing or supplementing your intake of one or another nutrient in that multivitamin, but in an amount and for a purpose that can make a difference to *your* health, not that of the 70-kilogram fantasy. The completion of the Human Genome Project and additional studies on SNPs have proved Roger Williams right.

So was Dr. Linus Pauling, the only person to have been awarded two individual Nobel Prizes in different fields. His landmark paper in the journal *Science* in 1949 concerned the cause of sickle-cell anemia, a disease well known to be genetically linked. It was in this 1949 paper that Pauling first used the term "molecular disease" in describing how the genes of the person with sickle-cell trait created a form of hemoglobin in the blood cells that was just slightly different from normal hemoglobin. This small change in the structure of hemoglobin, Pauling contended, was what had so huge an impact on the individual's health.

Pauling advanced this concept further in 1968 in another article in *Science*, this one entitled "Orthomolecular Psychiatry," proposing that certain forms of mental illness were the result of an alteration in the metabolism, which in some cases could be a result of insufficient nutrient intake—that the people suffering these forms of illness were not getting the nutrients they needed to meet their genetically determined requirements for proper brain function.

Pauling made up the word "orthomolecular," based on the Greek prefix *ortho*, for "upright" or "correct," using it in the general sense to describe a medicine that would mix and match substances native to human physiology—vitamins, minerals, nutrients, hormones, metabolites, and cellular building blocks—to the right levels for an individual's optimal health and function. It was an early instance of a kind of medicine that contrasted sharply with the standard allopathic approach. Allopathic medicine uses drugs that are not native to the human body to block, inhibit, antagonize, or alter specific physiological functions. Pauling was convinced that the more scientists learned about the origin of chronic diseases and about the relationship between genes and environment, the more medicine would focus on adjusting the balance of substances associated with healthy metabolic function through orthomolecular therapy, and the less it would depend upon allopathic substances to alter physiological functions.

Again, the Human Genome Project and the research it has inspired have proved Pauling correct, although he did not live to see the genomic revolution confirm his thinking. Among people with the MTHR SNP who suffered from depression but who had become resistant to antidepressant drugs, oral administration of therapeutic levels of the active form of folic acid, 5-methyltetrahydrofolate, resulted in successful management of the depression, just as Pauling had suggested in 1968.

Imagine the implications.

THE GENETIC ORIGINS OF CHRONIC ILLNESS

Researchers were at first stumped by the lower than expected number of genes in the human genome, along with the greater than anticipated diversity of human function. In exploding the assumption that we had a lot of common genetic variants, the first-draft sequencing also put the kibosh on the notion that these common variants were the roots of chronic disease—and therefore also killed the idea that it would be possible to develop a drug to put each chronic disease out of business. The high number of SNPs in the human genome pretty much put that hope out of business instead.

What's in the gap? What's between the relatively low number of genes and the relatively high number of variants—and what does it all have to do with chronic disease? That has been a topic of intense scrutiny since the publication of the Human Genome Project's results. And what all the scientific detective work that has unfolded over the years made clear is that although the human genome has fewer genes than expected, it has the largest amount of what was originally called "junk DNA" of any organism, plant or animal, on the planet.

Junk DNA takes up more than half the real estate in the human genome. We called it junk because we thought, incorrectly as it turns out, that it was just the remnants of ancient infections that were simply floating around uselessly in the genome—like tiny, worthless shards of ancient pottery at an archaeological site.

In fact, however, while not part of the specific coding of our genes—it is called noncoding DNA—what we used to think of as junk DNA actually contains the information that controls the expression of our genes. Think of it as the executive function of the genome, regulating the changing expression of our genes and determining how genetic characteristics function in each of us. The "junk DNA" label yielded to the term "promoter regions" within the human genome, and so far from being junk, the promoters are absolutely central because what they control is the translation of our genotype into our phenotype. Genotype is our genetic makeup, the potential of various traits to develop in us; phenotype is what happens when our genotype interacts with the environment, realizing the potential of particular traits and thereby giving rise to observable characteristics in the way we look, act, feel, and perform. Our genes represent many possible phenotypes. What makes the difference is how the genes are expressed. What controls that process is information encoded in the promoter regions.

This also goes a long way toward explaining that 4 percent difference between us and chimps; in fact, the difference is qualitative, not quantitative. For while it is true that the genes of the chimpanzee are more than 96 percent the same as human genes, the information encoded in the promoter regions of the human genome is far more complex than what is encoded in the chimpanzee genome. It is this complexity of humans versus all other plants and animals that is the great differentiator, and the complexity is determined by the sophistication of the genetic messages contained in the promoter regions of our genome—messages that control how genes express themselves and that can be influenced by such factors as environment, lifestyle, and diet. Recent discoveries on the rapid evolution of animals in the Cambrian period 500 million years ago suggest that this was when changes began in the promoter regions of the genome, rather than just in the genes per se, that eventually would lead to the differentiating complexity of the human genome—the complexity that divides us from chimps. So the clue as to why chimps don't get cancer or suffer autism is in the complexity of our genetic expression versus theirs, a complexity susceptible to changes in environmental factors and one that can take us to wholly different disease and health patterns—and wholly different health outcomes—from those of all other species.

This is a whole new ball game of understanding. If our genetic expression can be changed, we're not hardwired for disease. If signals from the environment can change genetic expression—if they can be converted by processes in the cell to inform the promoter regions that translate genotype into phenotype—then we have the power to affect our genetic expression, and thus our health, by changing the environmental factors sending the signals.

Apply the new understanding to chronic disease and you can see how profound it is, for it implies that there is no specific gene for a specific chronic disease. Rather, there are families of genes that may be susceptible to expressing a particular chronic disease process *if* the genes are exposed to factors that regulate their expression to create the phenotype of that disease. It sounds circular, I know, but put it to work explaining the global epidemic of obesity, for instance, and you can see how powerful it is. It tells us that there is no one specific gene that causes obesity. Instead, there is a family of genes that, when exposed to specific environmental and lifestyle factors, can be modified in their expression to turn on the storage of fat. What pushes that expression-changing button in one person, however, may be very different from what pushes it in another and thereby sends that person into obesity, as we'll see in greater detail in Chapter 10.

This new understanding demands a new health-care paradigm; it constitutes the scientific basis for altering the way we think about and deliver medical therapies. If we cannot change our genes—and we cannot—we can nevertheless change the messages that our genes receive from the environment that regulates genetic expression. It means that what we are talking about is health care that is personally tailored to the individual. The more we know about the factors that modulate genetic expression in the individual, the more effective the program we can design to optimize that individual's health and maximize his or her organ reserve. I call it personalized lifestyle medicine.

HOW TO CHANGE GENETIC EXPRESSION: CHANGE THE MESSAGE THE ENVIRONMENT TRANSMITS

Can we really control our genetic expression? After all, isn't it true that a number of diseases of infancy are closely linked to genetic inheritance? Absolutely. That is why fetal screening looks for such genetic disorders as Down syndrome if certain family or individual risk factors are present. But what we have learned is that most of these genetic diseases can vary in severity from mild to extreme. In the case of the sickle-cell trait, which is certainly genetically linked, it has been found that if those with a mild version of the trait take certain drugs—namely, hydroxyurea and sodium butyrate—this alters the genetic expression of the trait and reduces the risk of the disease. The same holds true for phenylketonuria, one of the most common genetically linked diseases of infancy. Historically, children born with PKU risked retardation and early death. It is now known that both can be avoided if the child in his or her early years is fed a controlled diet low in the amino acid phenylalanine. In both these cases, the genes that are traits for both Down syndrome and PKU have not been changed—they can't be. But the environment the genes are exposed to has been altered, and the result has been significantly reduced risk that the diseases will take hold and flourish. Simply put, the environment is sending a different message, and the genes are expressing themselves differently in response.

We are also seeing results in applying this principle to autism, the incidence of which is growing dramatically throughout the world's developing countries. Fifty years ago, what we today define as autism was found in one child out of more than 8,000. The Centers for Disease Control and Prevention (CDC) now report that this once rare disorder affects one out of 50 children in the United States, a prevalence as of 2012 of 2 percent, up from 1.6 percent in 2007—an increase so stunning it raises the question: Are more children being affected or are more children with autism being detected? The likely answer is that both phenomena are at work, but the dominant reality is a real increase in prevalence—and not only in the United States but in other industrialized countries as well. The CDC and the American Academy of Pediatrics find it sufficiently disquieting that they jointly released an "Autism ALARM" over what they judge to have been a tenfold increase in incidence of autism over the last decade of the twentieth century and the first decade of the twenty-first.

Of course, everyone—scientists above all—want to know why. What is the explanation for the stunning growth of this disorder, and what is the cause of it? A determined scientific search for the gene that codes for autism is well under way. Dr. James Watson—the Nobel laureate of double-helix fame—established a research group at his Cold Spring Harbor Laboratory on Long Island, New York, that is searching for the genetic bases of autism and schizophrenia. Around the world, many other prominent geneticists are doing the same. Already, this extensive genetic screening has found more than three hundred genes with some relationship to autism, but not one of them is strong enough to be termed the autism gene.

In the meantime, many scientists and health-care providers are leaning to the view articulated by Dr. Michael Stone, a remarkable family physician in Ashland, Oregon, who has had significant clinical experience with autism. Stone told participants at a medical meeting in 2013 that "once you know one child with autism, you know one child with autism." In other words, because autism presents in so many ways and with such different severities, there is no one gene causing a single disease called autism. In fact, autism is more appropriately termed autistic spectrum disorder, ASD, and the origin of the disorder is likely to differ from child to child. For parents and caregivers of children on the spectrum, what it comes down to is the recognition that a range of environmental factors interacting with multiple genetic susceptibilities is likely to have caused autism in their child, and by changing the child's diet, environment, and therapies, they can alter the genetic expression of characteristics that are termed autism.

THE AUTISM DILEMMA AND THE LIFESTYLE MEDICINE APPROACH TO ASD

Dr. Bernard Rimland, trained as an experimental psychologist, was the father of a son, Mark, born with infantile autism in 1956, when the condition was very rare. Rimland dedicated the remainder of his life to trying to better understand the origin and treatment of the condition. He wrote the classic *Infantile Autism: The Syndrome and Its Implications for a Neural Theory of Behavior*, published in 1964, which debunked the then-dominant theory of the origin of autism advanced by University of Chicago professor Bruno Bettelheim. The legendary Bettelheim, the well-known, highly regarded child psychologist, had theorized that autism was the result of a traumatized and loveless childhood, a theory now almost universally discredited, thanks primarily to Rimland's work.

In 1967, Rimland founded the Autism Research Institute in San Diego, California, to conduct scientific studies and advance the frontier of knowledge on autism. The institute's first task was to mobilize a group of researchers and clinicians to begin accumulating a database of clinical case studies by organizing the parents of autistic children to become sources of information. More than 26,000 parents responded, supplying a wealth of information to the database. It was this more than anything else that concentrated the focus of doctors, parents, and researchers on the need to act aggressively and to broaden the scope of their collaboration in order to find a successful approach for managing what was becoming an epidemic.

I met Dr. Rimland in 1973 and am proud to consider myself one of his students. He was a man of charm, wit, determination, and intelligence, with a bigger-than-life personality that drew people to him. Rimland served as the primary technical director on autism for the 1988 movie *Rain Man*; his son, Mark, who had become an accomplished artist, was one of the models for the character portrayed by Dustin Hoffman, and Hoffman interviewed Mark as part of his preparation for playing the role. Dr. Rimland died at the age of seventy-eight in 2006.

One of the leaders in the group of researchers and physicians he gathered about him was Dr. Sidney MacDonald Baker. A onetime professor at the Yale Medical School, Baker worked extensively on difficult pediatric medical cases. He is the kind of physician medical professionals think of as a doctor's doctor. Once physicians meet him and get to know how he approaches patient management, they want him to become their personal physician. In the early 1990s, in collaboration with Dr. Rimland and many other forward-looking physicians, researchers, and patient advocates, Baker was instrumental in founding the Defeat Autism Now organization—DAN. Over the past twenty years this organization has focused on the development of successful approaches to the management of autistic spectrum disorders. DAN doctors recognize that autistic spectrum disorder is not a simple, genetically determined disorder but rather a complex constellation of conditions resulting from the unique interaction of a child's genetic constitution with specific environmental damage that can occur at conception, in utero, or more frequently in infancy.

So matters stood on autism in the first decade of the twenty-first century. While early psychological explanations for the disease had been dismissed and most doctors and researchers agreed that the multiple expressions of the disorder probably meant multiple causes, a few innovators in the field were actively pursuing assertive new approaches to treatment. Against this background, a most remarkable medical detective story unfolded.

In 1998, Dr. Andrew Wakefield, an academic pediatric gastroenterologist affiliated with the prestigious Royal Free Hospital in London, published a paper, with his associates, that set the world of medicine whirling. The paper, in the February 28 issue of *The Lancet*, identified a problem with the digestive system of children as strongly associated with autism-like conditions. The paper described an enlargement of the lymph glands of the intestines as suggestive of a connection between autism and the alteration of immune function in the digestive tract. The most controversial assertion in the paper was that the onset of the autistic symptoms and the presumed alteration in the immune system of the children was associated with vaccination for mumps, measles, and rubella, the MMR vaccine.

Wakefield's suggestion that the principal environmental trigger was the MMR vaccination ignited a high-profile and often heated debate between those who support childhood vaccination and those who do not. After a number of years of controversy, *The Lancet* appointed an independent group of experts to carry out an inquiry into the research—that is, to evaluate the data and results. The inquiry prompted a retraction published in *The Lancet*'s March 6, 2004 issue; the paper's assertion that vaccination was the cause of the onset of the autistic symptoms was withdrawn, the inquiry panel having concluded that Wakefield's data supporting this association had been falsified. Dr. Wakefield was defrocked and left his position at the Royal Free Hospital and School of Medicine.

Putting aside the specific question of immunization and the ethical concerns over his research, Dr. Wakefield did open up a major area of investigation—namely, the possibility of a connection between intestinal immune activation and autism. It is a field of research that has taken the medical field from the notion that autism is strongly genetically linked to the present view that the environmental influence on genetic expression plays a major role in the origin of the disease.

The question is: What are the major environmental factors that we should be concerned about vis-à-vis autism? One key area in which evidence is accumulating is that of specific allergy-producing foods. Among these are gluten-containing grains and cow's milk proteins, which are often introduced into a child's diet at a time that the immune system has not yet developed tolerance for them. Obviously, the evidence in no way suggests that all cases of autism are due to exposure to wheat or cow's milk, but it raises the issue that autism might be seen as a condition in which the child's immune function has been altered because of specific exposures to which the child is intolerant, and that such alterations have induced altered gene expression in the brain that translates to behavior we call autistic.

This major change in thinking about the origin of a chronic condition was the model that Dr. Baker and his colleagues had in mind when they formed DAN in the 1990s; it would shape the way they looked for a solution to the autism epidemic. It is also the conclusion articulated by Dr. R. F. Tuchman at the Miami Children's Hospital Dan Marino Center, who has written widely in the field of autism. In the *Revista de Neurologia* in 2013, Dr. Tuchman asserted the likelihood that "there are risk genes and early environmental risk factors for autistic spectrum disorders that contribute to an altered trajectory of brain and behavioral development." Clearly, we are at a major turning in the road in how we think about not just conditions like autism, but the whole family of chronic diseases.

Exemplifying this new pathway forward is the pioneering work of Dr. S. Jill James, a distinguished pediatrics researcher based in Arkansas. Dr. James and her colleagues have focused on better understanding the connection between specific genes and environmental factors associated with autism. For example, her team has identified specific genetic characteristics that reduce a child's ability to properly metabolize folic acid, so critical for brain function. The team's studies have found that in a child carrying that particular impaired ability, cow's milk protein, gluten, and other allergenic substances can help alter brain function and development.

How that happens is complicated, but it distills down to a very important takeaway for the management of autism. It's the lesson that was expressed most powerfully by Sidney Baker in the late 1990s in defining his approach: "Take away the things that are a problem and provide the things that are missing." In short, eliminate those things in the child's environment that are causing alteration in his or her nervous system function, and add back the things the child needs more of—the active form of folic acid, 5-methyl tetrahydrofolate; or methylcobalamine, the active form of vitamin B12. This is a very different strategy from relying on medications to manage the child's autistic symptoms.

It is historically noteworthy that it was back in 1988 that Bernard Rimland, in reviewing the clinical experiences reported by parents of autistic children, first offered observational data from many parents of the positive effect of providing supplemental amounts of vitamin B6, folic acid, and vitamin B12 to their autistic children. The detailed work of Dr. James and her colleagues has now identified exactly how this approach might be valuable to certain autistic children with specific genetic susceptibilities.

The work continues, offering new ideas and fresh opportunities for parents with autistic children to improve their children's brain function and behavior. Above all, the new work is changing the conversation—and thereby changing people's perception of autism. In this regard, one of the most exciting approaches is that of Dr. Martha Herbert of Harvard and Massachusetts General Hospital. Dr. Herbert is a remarkably talented researcher and autism activist, and in her 2012 book, *The Autism Revolution: Whole-Body Strategies for Making Life All It Can Be*, she sets out a strategic approach to the disorder that takes advantage of all the recent revolutionary discoveries on the relationship of genes and environment in autism. Dr. Herbert dismisses the one-size-fits-all assumption about autism and its treatment, replacing it with an analysis of the specific factors that might contribute to the disorder given specific genetic susceptibilities. The book is an exemplar of the new medicine, coupling genomic understanding with personalized lifestyle intervention.

GENETIC DETERMINISM AND ALZHEIMER'S DISEASE

The same logic that for too long has governed our perception of autism as genetically controlled holds true for our perception of Alzheimer's dementia—namely, that it is inherited. While it is true that certain forms of early-onset Alzheimer's disease are strongly linked to genetic inheritance, these constitute less than 5 percent of all diagnosed cases. The later-age form of the disease, typically affecting people over the age of sixty, is far more common and is not strongly linked to any specific genetic inheritance factor; rather, like autism, it is a product of the interaction of certain genes with environmental and lifestyle factors.

One of the genetic markers for Alzheimer's disease that has gotten a lot of press is the ApoE4 gene. People who have this gene from their mother, their father, or both have been found to have increased risk for both Alzheimer's and heart disease. To know that you carry this gene has been understood by many as the mark of an inescapable fate; naturally, a lot of people would rather not know they face a disaster they can do nothing about.

But that is not the full story—or the true story—of the ApoE4 gene, as ongoing research has shown. It is now recognized that this gene does not create Alzheimer's disease by itself; rather, it describes a susceptibility to the disease that the individual's choices of lifestyle and diet can affect. Simply put, a person with the ApoE4 gene is highly susceptible to the dangerous effects of a diet high in saturated fats and sugar and of a sedentary lifestyle. So the ApoE4 gene isn't telling the individual who carries it that he or she will die of Alzheimer's. On the contrary, it is saying instead, "Go out and design your lifestyle behavior and your diet in ways that reduce your risk for Alzheimer's and heart disease." It's a warning, a lesson, and a directional signal all in one.

Increasingly, this understanding is being confirmed in the many different approaches to Alzheimer's research. Neuroscientists like Dr. Dale Bredesen of UCLA[*] have looked at the Alzheimer's disease–producing processes in animals and have identified more than thirty different causes of the disease, all of them related to lifestyle, diet, and environmental factors. Dr. Bredesen, a dedicated physician researcher who has long worked on neurodegenerative diseases and is now a leading Alzheimer's researcher, has said that the more he finds out about the disease, the more convinced he is that we will never find a single drug to treat it, so varied is its origin from person to person. As Bredesen reminds us, more than $5 billion has been spent on developing Alzheimer's drugs thus far in the twenty-first century, and not one of the drugs has proved successful in safely and effectively treating the disease.

---

[*] Augustus Rose Professor, Director of the Mary S. Easton Center for Alzheimer's Disease Research, and Director of Neurodegenerative Disease Research at the David Geffen School of Medicine UCLA.

That is why Dr. Bredesen has designed a clinical study that examines what happens at the intersection of an individual's genetic uniqueness and his or her environment. The study involves early-stage Alzheimer's disease patients and is evaluating the use of a new drug under controlled conditions of diet, lifestyle, and environmental conditions. The aim is to manage all of the more than thirty identified factors associated with the development of Alzheimer's to prove that its solution will never come from one drug.

Bredesen's ideas about the origin of the disease are shared by a fellow Alzheimer's disease clinical research expert, Dr. Suzanne Craft. Dr. Craft, a neuropsychologist, and her research team have identified what she has termed "diabetes of the brain" or "type 3 diabetes" as the origin of Alzheimer's in certain individuals. Specifically, people whose diets encourage poor control of blood sugar have been found to experience a particularly high incidence of Alzheimer's disease. The conclusion is that all those desserts and refined white-starch foods over many years create imbalances in brain metabolism that are linked to Alzheimer's disease. Craft's research shows that intervention in the form of a diet low in sugars and refined starches improves brain function in Alzheimer's patients. "Our results suggest," Craft wrote in a 2011 study published in *Archives of Neurology*, "that diet may be a powerful environmental factor that modulates Alzheimer's disease risk through its effects on central nervous system concentrations of $A\beta42$, lipoproteins, oxidative stress, and insulin."

So far, Dr. Craft's suggestion is just that: an indication of a fact, if not yet completely proved. Yet all of these new paths of inquiry and research in the field of Alzheimer's have something very important to say to people who have the ApoE4 gene. They affirm the biological breakthrough that is changing everything: the recognition that genes in and of themselves don't control the appearance of later-age Alzheimer's disease; the environment in which the genes are expressed does. Among the major factors related to the risk of Alzheimer's disease uncovered by these new paths of inquiry and research are these:

1. ApoE4 gene and a diet high in saturated fats
2. Chronic inflammation
3. Elevated level of homocysteine in the blood
4. Insulin resistance and type 3 diabetes
5. Poor tolerance for exercise—that is, the person tires quickly and cannot sustain the activity
6. Lack of brain stimulation
7. Exposure to toxic substances

All of these risk factors for Alzheimer's disease are in our control. Each can be modified. Change your diet, change various factors of your lifestyle, and in effect you are treating the cause of the underlying alteration in physiology that is associated with the development of Alzheimer's disease. Such diet and lifestyle changes are precisely the type of clinical interventions that Bredesen and other neurology specialists are now recommending for people with early-stage memory loss and cognitive impairment.

Medicine is changing. Haltingly, perhaps, and unevenly, it is incorporating the breakthrough discoveries of the era and learning how to personalize the management of chronic disease. With Alzheimer's as with autism and the other debilitations we dread, our genetic inheritance tells us more about how we should live than about the chronic disease we are doomed to suffer. We are not doomed at all.

The breakthroughs that are bringing about this changed approach to chronic disease management tell an amazing story, but the story is not complete until we understand perhaps its most amazing subplot—epigenetics.

EPIGENETICS: THE GENETIC WILD CARD

One more time: the revolution that is changing health care is the recognition that our genes do not hardwire us for chronic disease but instead offer a menu of what we can be under differing environmental conditions. This is empowering. It means that at any age, we have the choice about what information to send to our genes from our environment, diet, and lifestyle.

Let's be clear. When I use the word "environment," I am not just talking about trees and streams, although our natural surroundings, like our physically constructed surroundings, are certainly part of the environment. What I am referring to is all the things present in our lives that we draw on to satisfy our needs and desires—hand creams and toothpaste, nail polish and hair gel; the fabrics we wear; the stuff we buy for cleaning our house; whether we heat up dinner in a BPA plastic dish in the microwave or start the meal from scratch by handpicking ingredients at the farmers' market. In other words, our environment comprises all the assets and amenities, comforts and conveniences, practices and arrangements we employ in the choices we make about behavior.

When I use the word "diet," I mean an individual's way of eating—kinds of foods, amount of food, diversity of food, even personal taste. In short, given what is available for this individual to eat, what are his or her choices, tastes, habits, likes and dislikes, and approach when it comes to food and drink?

Given all those environmental factors and available ways of eating, what choices does the individual make in terms of behavior, habits, and way of living? That's what I mean by "lifestyle"—the totality of actions, functions, and kinds of conduct that define how an individual operates in his or her daily life.

On all three of these planes, what we do sends messages to our genes, but empowering as that is, it sets up an important question. If all the cells in our body have the same genes, then how are they able to differentiate their function? Surely we need to know how that works if we're going to send the right message to the right genes?

Heart cells, for example, must function in a specific way to keep the heart pumping. That means those cells express only heart-related information from the genome's book of life. Ditto liver cells, muscle cells, brain cells: Each cell must function in a specific way, and it is therefore required to express only selective genomic communications. In order to be sure that any change we make in environment, diet, or lifestyle gets transmitted to the right cells, we need to know how this works.

The first step in telling us how came from the science of developmental biology and specifically from the so-called father of this field of science, Edinburgh University professor of animal genetics Conrad Waddington, who died in 1975 at the age of seventy. A renaissance figure in biology who made fundamental contributions to paleontology, genetics, embryology, systems biology, and the new field of developmental biology, Waddington was almost equally talented in the arts and somehow found time to indulge his passions for painting and writing poetry.

In a period of amazing scientific creativity in the late 1930s, he coined the term "developmental epigenetics" to describe how animals develop from a fertilized egg to a fully formed organism. The Greek prefix *epi* signifies something over and above, so epigenetics refers to things that reside above the control of the expression of the genome—in the epigenome. In today's terms, we might say that the genes are the computer hardware and the epigenetic controlling factors are the software that tells the computer hardware how to perform. In coining the term in those pre-computer days, Waddington was giving a name to his understanding that the environment in which the fertilized egg develops influences the organism, and that environmental stress during the period of development can change the way the organism will end up functioning. In this as in many things, Waddington was ahead of his time, since his ideas on epigenetics came well before there was universal understanding of the importance of genes in controlling development.

In fact, not until the latter part of the twentieth century was it recognized that in the development of an embryo, only certain genes are expressed in certain cells; that's how a single genome message gets differentiated into multiple cellular functions. Exactly how this works was not well understood until the start of the twenty-first century, but it was accepted that Waddington's epigenetics was the mechanism of the differentiation. In essence, epigenetics is the genome's gatekeeper, regulating which genes are expressed in which parts of the body at any given time.

Full understanding of the epigenetic mechanism—and of how it relates to the origin of chronic disease—had to await the completion of the Human Genome Project in 2000. A most unexpected discovery, by Drs. Randy Jirtle and Robert Waterland at the Department of Radiation Oncology at the Duke University Medical Center, is what shed the clarifying light on the subject. The two were engaged in a study of the influence of maternal nutrition on fetal development when they came upon an earlier observation by British molecular biologists Robin Holliday and John Pugh. In 1975, Holliday and Pugh had found that methyl groups attached to the genome silenced the expression of certain genes so they could not be read. These methyl groups are composed of chemical units comprising a carbon atom with three hydrogen atoms "fastened" to it, and they are made in the body out of some of those same B vitamins mentioned previously— folic acid and B12—along with B6, choline, and betaine.

Jirtle and Waterland decided to explore the impact of high supplemental doses of these gene-silencing nutrients on the developing fetus of a pregnant agouti mouse. Their aim was to find out whether changing the nutritional environment could stimulate the epigenetic mechanism to influence fetal outcome; specifically, they wanted to see what *particular* genetic expression might be silenced by the methyl groups. The agouti mice they used for the study were excellent test animals—genetically well scrutinized and inbred to get fat, contract diabetes and cancer, and die young. Their fur color was always tan.

The first unexpected outcome from the study was that the offspring born to the pregnant mice supplemented with the methyl nutrient were not tan but had mottled fur. Even more interestingly, these offspring did not get fat, did not contract diabetes or cancer, did not die young like their mothers. They had the same genes as their parents, but the expression of their genes had been altered by the methyl nutrient supplement to result in agoutis that lived 30 percent longer than their parents and without the chronic disease bred into those parents. Some lines of genetic expression had indeed been muted.

Jirtle and Waterland published their findings in the 2003 issue of *Molecular and Cellular Biology* and won awards for the enormous impact the findings had on the field of nutrition and for giving birth to the field of nutritional epigenetics. Beyond this, their discoveries have profoundly affected medicine and the understanding of how environment and lifestyle exposures can imprint the epigenome and control the expression of our book of life. As I write this, more than 3,000 subsequent research papers on environmental epigenetics have been undertaken as a result of the agouti mouse study, and researchers around the world continue to confirm the significance of the work.

I've had the chance to talk with Dr. Jirtle frequently over the years; he is the first to point out the obvious, which is that humans are not agouti mice. It is a long way from a mouse to human fetal development, but the power of the original finding is that epigenetics is a process shared across all animal species, and since nutrition and other environmental factors can influence this process, what happens in the epigenome can directly affect health and disease patterns in an individual.

And what can happen there ranges well beyond simply silencing genes. While some environmental factors can blot out parts of the record in our epigenome, others are like sticky Post-it notes that emphasize a particular part of the record, saying, "Read here." Still others can actually switch chromosomes around. In less time than it takes to say deoxyribonucleic acid, we've gone from thinking of ourselves as genetically predetermined and pretty well fated for certain illnesses to having a whole new console of buttons to turn on and off to affect our health patterns and life span.

That's an essential realization, because forecasts about the health of children being born today are truly alarming. Indications are that specific chronic diseases are rising in prevalence in this group much faster than would have been expected in traditional models of disease prevalence. The first evidence of this alarming trend came in 2005 in a study in the *New England Journal of Medicine* suggesting that, given certain chronic disease problems now appearing in children in the United States, it is possible that the current generation of children will be the first in history to have a shorter life span than their parents.

How is this possible? We spend more per person on health care than any other country in the world. We talk about health, write about health, go to the gym to improve our health, worry about our health constantly. Could it be that twenty-first-century environmental factors are altering our epigenetic mechanism so that our functional health is declining? Could this help explain the rising incidence of such childhood health problems as asthma, allergy, autism, attention disorders, hyperactivity, type 2 diabetes, autoimmune arthritis, and obesity?

This question becomes even more significant when we take into account the work of Drs. Moshe Szyf and Michael Meaney of McGill University. McGill is the very institution, of course, where Dr. Hans Selye coined the term "stress" to define environmental factors that alter the flight-or-fight arousal system; the word has since become the most used—and perhaps the most useful—English word in medicine. Drs. Szyf and Meaney have taken our understanding of stress to a whole new level of understanding, determining that an individual's social environment influences his or her epigenetic makeup and, as a result, changes both the physiological and behavioral response to stress. It is particularly the case with young children. In a sense, what the Szyf-Meaney work tells us is that traumatic events can imprint the genome with epigenetic marks that alter the way we respond to stress over a long period of time.

What does this mean to children born and raised in conditions of fear, anger, and violence? I have had the opportunity to ask the question of Dr. Szyf himself; not surprisingly, he says that one of his greatest fears is what is happening to children born where such conditions are the norm during the pregnancy of their mothers and throughout their childhood. His fear, quite simply, is that the epigenetic marks left by such exposure not only will adversely affect the mental and physical health of the current generation but may be transmissible to the next generation as well, as recent animal studies have suggested. The studies define a whole new field, transgenerational epigenetics, exploring whether and how characteristics can be passed down to the next generation by epigenetic inheritance, not via traditional genetics.

Transgenerational epigenetics studies may also show how and why chronic disease patterns may change much faster than one would expect—that is, if your expectation is that the only way to create change in offspring is through genetic natural selection over millions of years. Rather, epigenetics indicates that there are two ways that the health of a population can change over time. The first is the traditional inheritance of a disease-producing gene like that of sickle-cell anemia or phenylketonuria. The second is epigenetic in origin and can occur much more rapidly through the epigenetic response to a change in the environment. Animal studies, like those by Dr. Michael Skinner of Washington State University, have shown that exposure to environmental toxins can result in epigenetic changes transmissible to the next generation and can create increased incidence of chronic disease. More and more, we are seeing that nutrition, social stress, and environmental toxins can all influence the epigenome and alter gene expression patterns—thus increasing the risk of chronic disease.

The good news is that we can correct the influences that are altering our genetic expression and putting us at risk for chronic disease. That is the great lesson of the biological breakthrough represented in the mapping of the human genome and in the explosion of research it set off—that the translation process from genotype to phenotype is complex and dynamic as our genome responds to messages received from the environment. Therefore, to the extent that we can change the messages, we can also shape the response—and thereby affect our health outcomes.

How can we change the messages? By changing what is in our environment, what substances we take into our bodies, and what we do with our bodies for exercise and a sense of well-being. By making changes that take away the things that are a problem and that provide the things that are missing, we may indeed improve our health outcome.

This is all within our power. Modifying, altering, or radically redoing environment, diet, and lifestyle is entirely within the reach of every individual. How do we harness the understanding of the stunning biological breakthroughs of our era to make the changes that can prevent or reverse the chronic diseases that steal our organic reserve, vitality, and longevity? As the next chapter shows, the answer is personal.

CHAPTER 3

The Functional Medicine Revolution: Winning the Battle with Chronic Illness

There's a Greek island in the middle of the Aegean Sea called Ikaria. It's a small island, not even a hundred square miles in area, with a population only slightly in excess of 8,000 souls. It is mountainous—most inhabitants live near the coast—but the slopes of the hills and ravines, though steep, are covered in lush green vegetation. Fishing and the production of a strong red wine are the residents' main occupations.

Ikaria also tends to be crawling with scientists. That is because it is one of those pockets of healthy longevity, dubbed "blue zones" by researcher Dan Buettner in his book of that title, in which everything conspires to keep people free of disease well into advanced old age. Ikarians routinely live well into their nineties, and the island boasts a disproportionate number of centenarians. But the point isn't the Ikarians' longevity; it's their good health and vitality. Ikarians somehow manage to avoid the chronic illnesses that plague the rest of the world and to remain physically and mentally sound and active until, at very advanced ages, they die. The scientists come here to find out why, and the answers stare them in the face.

Start with the Ikarian diet of fresh fish and plant-based, unprocessed foods packed with nutrients; clean water; local olive oil; herbal tea; and of course red wine. Add in the fresh air, the fact that the primary means of locomotion is walking—up and down the hills—and the easy access to swimming in warm salt water. Ikarians sleep late and like to nap each day, as a way to refresh themselves from their daily labor in the vineyards. And their island is a community, its people united by ties of culture and faith, by the impulse to render mutual aid and emotional support, and by peer pressure to do your part.

To the scientists examining Ikaria's off-the-charts longevity, the explanation for the population's remarkable good health is to be found in those mutually enhancing behaviors in all the factors that affect our physiological processes, from nutrition to exercise, from sleep to emotional support. And of course, it sounds idyllic—a pure and simple life on a sun-splashed island in the middle of an azure sea.

But what is particularly telling about Ikaria is that when its residents move to other places and necessarily adopt a different lifestyle, they start having chronic illnesses just like everyone else. In other words, it is not genes that protect the Ikarians from chronic illness but the message they send to their genes through their lifestyle and environment. Change the message, and Ikarians too succumb to the same debilitating conditions that burden the rest of us.

That is why Ikaria is so clearly a jumping-off point for the battle with chronic illness. To win the battle, we will have to change the messages our lifestyle and diet and environment are sending to our genes. We will have to create our own Ikarias in our own way. That is what the functional medicine revolution is all about.

PRESENTING WITH SYMPTOMS

Remember Peter and Catherine from Chapter 1? Peter at thirty-six and Catherine at sixty-four each suffered from a range of symptoms, each symptom diagnosed as exemplifying a decline in function, each treated with a pill—in Catherine's case, each treated with two pills, doled out by a battery of specialists.

Now meet Joe. He has a zillion things wrong with him. As they say in the medicine game, he "presents with" a variety of health complaints. To begin with, he has high blood pressure. Like his father and grandfather before him, he has prostate problems and suffers, often excruciatingly, from gout. Joe also complains of a persistent ringing in his ears, even when absolute silence reigns; the medical term for this is tinnitus. As if that weren't enough, he periodically experiences nocturnal leg cramps—spasms that knot up his calves and thighs, wake him from sleep, or keep him from falling asleep.

He has seen and been treated by several different specialists, all of whom provided diagnoses from within their expertise. As a result, he is now taking a medication for his elevated blood pressure and another for his leg cramps, both prescribed by an internist; a medication for his enlarged prostate, prescribed by a urologist; a medication for his gout, prescribed by a rheumatologist; and a sleeping pill prescribed by his primary-care physician—not to mention a white-noise machine he runs at night at the suggestion of an audiologist he went to see for his tinnitus. In other words, he has been assessed by expert medical practitioners as suffering from six distinct conditions, each separate from the other, and each therefore requiring its distinct and separate prescription drug or engineered remedy.

The problem is that Joe still feels lousy. Although he gets some minimal relief from the medications, the symptoms related to each of his presenting complaints persist. His quality of life remains compromised: his leg cramps and foot pain are chronic, the gout sporadically brings his life to a halt, he rarely sleeps through the night, and he simply feels, in his words, "bone-weary."

Ditto for Peter and Catherine.

The reason is that all three of these individuals are being treated for symptoms, not cured of their chronic conditions. Their suffering is being palliated—at least temporarily—but the underlying causes of their sufferings have not been addressed; in fact, they have not even been identified. The focus has been on what ails Peter and Catherine and Joe, not on what is wrong with their health. And here's the truth of the matter: Given today's operating model of medical practice, it couldn't be otherwise.

NAME THE DISEASE, PRESCRIBE THE CURE

The operating model of medicine you and I grew up with derives, as we saw in the preceding chapter, from the acute-care practice that developed in the wake of the bacteriological revolution. Its focus is disease; its modus operandi is for the practitioner, typically a specialist in a particular area of the body, to find and identify the pathology—that is, diagnose the disease—and then write a prescription or schedule a surgery to zap it.

The specialist practitioners—all highly educated, intelligent, and compassionate—attending to Peter, Catherine, and Joe learned their professions under the banner of this acute-care model. They were taught an organ-centric view of the diseases they were being trained to chase, identify, and treat—a view of the body as a collection of organ systems, the major ones being:

- Gastrointestinal system
- Nervous system
- Immune system
- Musculoskeletal system
- Cardiovascular system
- Eye, ear, nose, and throat system
- Reproductive system—one male, one female
- Dermatological system
- Hematological system

Sound familiar? Of course. These are not only the major organ systems in our body; they are also the major medical specialties. That's logical: If that's what the body is—that is, a collection of separate organ systems—then that is how medical practice will be structured: that is, as separate anatomical divisions corresponding to the major organ systems.

And of course, that is in fact standard operating procedure in the acute-care model that has come to define medical practice today: a doctor becomes expert in a particular organ system and treats a problem in that system as a disease independent of anything else that may be bothering you. The "anything else" is the business of another doctor in another specialty. It's why Joe sees five different doctors—plus an audiologist—each trained in a specific organ, each focusing solely on that organ.

True, the specialists seeing Joe know that he has other complaints that don't concern the organ system that is their area of expertise. They're likely to see such complaints as ancillary if not secondary to Joe's main disease, the one in their area of expertise, and they may well describe these other complaints as comorbidities or adjacent morbidities—that is, conditions existing simultaneously with but independently of what they consider the main problem—the organ system in which they have expertise.

So each specialist will continue to prescribe a course of therapy for Joe aimed at fixing what's broken in his or her particular specialty, where "broken" is defined as something different from the healthy version of that organ or tissue. And each will probably shake his or her head at the bum deal Joe is getting from those other ancillary maladies the specialist can do nothing about.

This is the operating model of medical practice that would indeed work if Joe had heart disease, cancer, rheumatoid arthritis, kidney failure, or some other disastrous condition for which a causative pathology can indeed be identified—something "broken" in a particular organ or tissue that the specialist could fix with surgery or a prescribed course of treatment.

But Joe doesn't have such a condition, and the model doesn't work for him. There is no single pathology behind his multiple complaints, nor behind the multiple complaints of Peter and Catherine and the rest of us who may be suffering from depression, dementia, chronic fatigue syndrome, fibromyalgia, high blood pressure, muscle weakness, irritable bowel syndrome, sleep disturbances, chronic pain syndrome, autistic spectrum disorder, or any of the chronic illnesses that dog our footsteps in the twenty-first century. Instead, we experience signs and symptoms of reduced function in a number of organs and tissues. Reduced function is no picnic, so we seek relief in treatments that blunt the signs and symptoms, diminishing their effects and quieting them down—at least for a while.

Unfortunately, the genomic revolution has taught us that if we just keep blunting these signs and symptoms without addressing their underlying causes, those causes later do indeed become a pathology that will manifest itself as an acute disease. That is precisely what is happening to our three favorite patients. The prescriptions doled out to Peter, Catherine, and Joe are not improving their health. All three of them still feel sick. All three of them are continuing to lose function and to feel their mobility, their energy, their lives curbed and constrained. The sad truth is that the pills they keep swallowing may actually be undermining their health, and all three patients may be setting themselves up for worse health to come later in life.

This too is logical. Since the underlying causes of their afflictions are not being addressed, the genes of all three individuals continue to struggle to respond, as they were long ago programmed to do, not just to whatever in their environment was originally making them sick but also to the onslaught of drugs that are now part of that environment. In time, the struggle itself becomes the usual state of the body's functions. I think of it as "friendly fire," being injured by your own side in a fight, with an eventual result best expressed by another martial term—"collateral damage." Thus do chronic illnesses—unattended to, their symptoms dulled by palliatives—progress into acute disease.

What can we see ahead for Peter and Catherine and Joe? It doesn't look good. Joe is still a high-risk candidate for an early heart attack or stroke. Peter is on a path that could well lead to kidney disease or heart disease—or both. And Catherine is a candidate for later-stage bone fracture, rheumatoid arthritis, and the nation's number one killer, heart disease. And by the time the three arrive at these likely eventualities, their resources for a real recovery and the life span left to enjoy it will be significantly diminished.

Yet this organ-centric, acute-care model of medical practice, one that works brilliantly for infectious diseases and emergencies, is the operating template that still prevails today. Perfected throughout most of the twentieth century, it operates as a highly efficient system achieving high throughput in churning out solutions for discernible organic causes or medical emergencies. To achieve those efficiencies, practitioners have perforce regressed to the mean; deviations from the average are outliers, and an operating model geared to acute care and medical emergencies must of necessity treat the average, not the individual. That is the only way it can be effective at all.

Yet that is also why the model is out of date, out of sync, and just simply insufficient for today's health reality. For as we know, the medical challenge facing us now is chronic illness, not acute care, and the science behind chronic illness calls for a focus not on the average but on the individual. Precisely because every one of us is, in fact, an outlier, an operating model that treats us as average can't possibly be effective. If you are one of the concerned, caring doctors attending to Peter, Catherine, and Joe, looking for something "broken" that you can repair, and you have only a few minutes, in the current operating medical model, to come up with a diagnosis and scribble a standard-ized solution for it on your main medical tool—your prescription pad—you are perforce going to regress to the mean, surrender to the average, and fall back to a "safe" solution that will bring some relief and, you hope, do minimal harm.

Such an operating model is of limited power at best, helpless at worst in the face of symptoms that cut across multiple organ systems. And clearly, that means the model is also not efficient—not if you define efficiency as achieving maximum outcome with minimum wasted effort or expense. Peter, Catherine, and Joe are certainly not getting improved outcomes, yet as we know, the cost of provid-ing those outcomes is off the charts. Unfortunately, that is a perfect description of health care today: fortunes spent globally on disease care while the incidence, pervasiveness, and life-limiting impact of chronic illness rises steadily.

So the prevailing health-care model simply doesn't work for most of the health challenges that confront us, and its costs are way too high. That is not a good equation. It underscores that the model is inappropriate for dealing with the chronic illnesses that dominate today's medical landscape.

What the model is, is easy—mostly because it's been in place for so long. And alas, we all know why it stays in place. Partly, it's inertia. Partly, put it down to third-party insurers and huge pharmaceutical companies that have invested heavily in the model and have managed it down to a fine art—absolutely formulaic, predictable, prescriptive. The protocols have been developed and refined; the reimbursement system is geared to the model in place based on the organ-centric view of medical training and practice. Changing it all would be disruptive.

Doctors are victims of this operating model too. Over forty years as a medical researcher and educator, I have always been impressed by the intelligence, capabilities, and sheer dedication to helping people shown by the medical students my associates and I have taught. But it seems to me that over time, these dedicated individuals are worn down by the current operating model. The requirement to spend no more than something like six minutes with a patient—fifteen at the absolute outside limit—and the demand for a by-the-numbers "standard of care" eventually replace their ability to think and act in the best interests of their patients. Their practice becomes routine, their patients all begin to look like named diagnoses, and their treatments become choices they check off on a list of standardized solutions. No wonder MDs are leaving the profession in droves. All that time and training and effort—and all that brainpower and compassion—should be put to work innovating individual care for patients, not just writing a scrip for their latest complaint.

But the most compelling reason for a new operating model is the science we've been reviewing in the previous chapters. It is the genomic revolution that is making the functional medicine revolution necessary. Our understanding of why and how the interactions among our environment, lifestyle, and genetic predispositions can alter our physiology and erode our function is what requires us to find a new approach to treatment, one that can reverse the dysfunctions that are making us feel sick. That is precisely what the functional medicine operating system does.

Make no mistake: I am in no way suggesting we jettison the acute-care operating model. If you have a heart attack, contract an infectious disease, are injured, or suffer a medical emergency, acute care is precisely what you need, and the efficient, effective system in place to provide it can be stretched to heroic lengths to return you to health. We need to hold on to that system. But given its unsuitability for today's dominant medical challenge, we need to supplement and complement it with a new approach to assessing, preventing, and treating complex chronic disease.

It is already beginning to happen.

PATIENT-CENTERED, SCIENCE-BASED

Let me tell you about the Pima Indians. A once-powerful Native American tribe now concentrated on a reservation in central Arizona, the Pima today suffer one of the highest rates of diabetes in the United States. The reason has long been ascribed to ethnicity, it being assumed that the Pima people were simply born with diabetogenic genes, genes preprogrammed for diabetes. In other words, Pima babies are dealt a bad genetic hand at birth and just have to expect to inherit diabetes.

It's a nifty assumption that provides a nice, neat answer. But it's dead wrong. The fact is, diabetes was not seen in Pima Indians until the 1940s. By then, they had been living on the reservation for about two generations and their traditional tribal diet had been entirely replaced with refined carbohydrates, sugars, and fats.

So Pima genes were not preprogrammed for diabetes; rather, the genes had collided with a totally new reality of "nutrition." In fact, if Pima genes had evolved to be anything in particular, it was thrifty. They developed that way millennia ago in response to what has historically been the Pima's greatest survival risk: starvation. Native to one of the most hostile places on earth, the desert of the American Southwest, the Pima from time immemorial have faced an environment in which water and food were often scarce. Over many thousands of years, therefore, their genes were naturally selected for characteristics that would allow individuals to survive through periods of low calorie intake. That's what I mean when I describe Pima genes as "thrifty"; they are able to hold on tightly to every calorie—an obvious advantage for responding physiologically to the reality of periodic starvation.

Then came life on the reservation and a new, untraditional certainty that starvation could always be avoided. How? Just drive on over to the reservation grocery store and treat yourself to excess empty calories in the form of processed foods, soft drinks, and alcohol. Shazam! What was once a genetic advantage has become a genetic liability. The genes are not diseased; the environment feeding the genes is diseased.

I relate this sad story because it is the perfect framework for understanding the functional medicine approach. Specifically, it tells us why functional medicine looks not at the disease—assumed to be isolated in a single organ system—but at the patient. In the case of the Pima, the patient is a defined people with an identifiable biochemical individuality. Only by looking at what may have changed in the patient's physiological processes, and therefore at the lifelong interactions between those processes and the environment—only by examining Pima genetics, lifestyle, and environment all together—could we learn the truth of their health problems. And only that truth can point the way to the restoration of health for the Pima people.

That's what functional medicine does with each individual patient. It is a way of looking at a patient's health in terms of his or her genetic uniqueness and how that uniqueness interacts with environment and behavior. That means that doctors who practice functional medicine are not so much trying to figure out a diagnosis as they are seeking to understand the complex web of interactions in the patient's history, physiology, and lifestyle. In the totality of those interactions, the functional medicine practitioner can pinpoint the ones that can lead to illness. Then and only then can the practitioner and patient together design ways to change the interactions and prevent or reverse the illness.

A SYSTEMS APPROACH

To do this, functional medicine takes a systems approach to the body. We've already spoken of the network of organ systems in the body—immune, nervous, endocrine, cardiovascular, etc.—but here the important word is "network"; in other words, all these systems are linked. Therefore, as we know, an event in one system can affect something else in another system; we even know that an improvement in one system may adversely affect something else in another system. As we've seen, an anti-inflammatory that diminishes pain in your musculoskeletal system may at the same time be causing serious harm in your gastrointestinal system, so although your arthritis may feel better, you've suddenly got a miserably painful ulcer. Or take the case of statins, which are known to lower the risk of heart attack and stroke but have also been shown to increase the risk of dementia and diabetes. Why? Because while they affect the cardiovascular system, they also affect the nervous and endocrine systems; the effect in one case is benign, in the other case adverse.

It therefore stands to reason that we should look at the body's systems in relation to one another, and we should look at the components of each system in the same way—not as isolated "silos" that never touch or communicate with one another, but as parts of an overall system that operate together, as physiological processes that cut across all organ systems.

Using the systems approach, functional medicine practitioners don't stop looking if they can't find a specific defective organ that can be "repaired" through acute care. They keep on going, exploring the entire physiological network to find the place or places where genetic expression has been altered by environmental factors. What they are looking for are imbalances—either within the different components of a physiological system or between systems. These imbalances exist in the actual mechanism of health—in the way the environmental inputs into your physiology are processed through your unique genetic predispositions. Find and address the physiological process that is out of balance, the theory goes, and you finally deal with chronic ill health. That's how to make your symptoms go away.

But functional medicine isn't concerned solely with health *problems*; it isn't looking at the connection between your outside world and your inside physiology just to rid your body of its health problem. Rather, its systems approach is a way of finding the proper match between your genetic uniqueness and your environment, lifestyle, and behavior so you can realize all the potential positive vitality of your genes and top up your organ reserve till it overflows. Functional medicine is out to extend your life span and fill your health span to the brim.

Two things have to take place before that can happen. First, you need to identify the imbalances in your own individual physiology, and second, you need to design a personalized program that will rid your body of its health problems and let you realize your unique genetic potential.

THE PHYSIOLOGICAL CORE: WHEN AN IMBALANCE OCCURS

There are seven core physiological processes that affect all of the body's organ systems, and imbalances can occur in any and all of them. These imbalances are the source—the origin—of most chronic illness. They are at the heart of our being sick.

How do they happen?

Your environment and your behavior send messages to your body in various ways—through your diet, from your surroundings (air, shelter, landscape), in the exercise you do or fail to do, from stress or trauma—and these inputs are processed through your unique genetic predisposition. Somewhere, something in those interactions malfunctions. Given that your genes are responding all the time to the messages they receive from your interactions, constantly translating the messages into cellular instructions, it's not unlikely that a particular input may evoke a particular response that throws off the balance in one of your core physiological processes. It's not impossible that some mismatch just might occur between external and internal, between the world out there and the genetic uniqueness within. Such an imbalance gives rise to symptoms of ill health.

That is why functional medicine pays attention to the full expression of dysfunction. How else can it find the imbalances and restore equilibrium between physiological processes and environmental inputs?

The next seven chapters of this book will focus on the core physiological processes, explaining how each process works and the possible effects of clinical imbalances in each. All seven of the process chapters start with a questionnaire; if you answer yes to five or more of the questions asked, chances are good that you have an imbalance in that particular process. Keep track of your yes answers if you can, and keep track of those processes in which you note an imbalance. You'll see why in Part 3 of the book. By the way, all seven questionnaires appear again in Part 3, and it's there that you'll start putting to practical and personal use what your questionnaire answers tell you.

Here are the seven core processes:

1. *Assimilation and Elimination.* The functions involved in digesting, absorbing, and using nutrients and then excreting the waste products constitute a complex, multistage physiological process. Clearly, nutrition is only as valuable as the ability of the nutrients to be digested and assimilated, and a kind of physiological teamwork between the two halves of the process—digestion-assimilation and elimination-excretion—is critically important to maintain health throughout the body.

The process of breaking big food molecules down so the body can make proper use of them begins in the mouth and continues in the stomach and in the small and large intestines. It goes through several stages as important vitamins and minerals as well as other plant-derived nutrients are released for absorption and assimilated throughout the body. The waste products from cellular activity then need to be eliminated either in the stool or in the urine passing through the kidneys. The slightest imbalance in any stage of this process can lead to serious disorders.

2. *Detoxification.* We humans have always lived in a less than perfect environment. One way or another, we are exposed to a range of toxic substances in the air, in our water and food, often in the

materials that shelter us, from intestinal bacteria and cellular metabolism. That is why, over several million years, our bodies evolved the highly sophisticated physiological processes we call detoxification. These processes, occurring primarily in the liver, where most of the detox machinery resides, convert toxic substances into nontoxic by-products, and eliminate them via the kidney and intestines, which have some additional detoxification abilities as well.

It is interesting that a huge chunk of each individual's genetic inheritance is connected to controlling the detoxification function—an indication of just how important this process is to human health. In fact, a deficiency in detoxification ability is considered something like the canary in the mine—a signal of exposure to a potentially toxic substance that the body cannot adequately detoxify. It typically results in ever-worsening chronic illness.

3. *Defense.* I mean by this the various processes that stand guard to protect us from infection and cellular injury. Each day we confront such foreigners as bacteria and viruses that would love to find a place to live in our body. It is the responsibility of our immune system, acting as cellular defender, to seek and destroy these uninvited guests whose presence could create acute infection or give rise to a range of chronic illnesses. We also need defensive action in recognizing and eliminating old and dead cells within our body; if not eliminated, this accumulating debris can have a serious adverse effect, so its elimination is another job for the immune system.

4. *Cellular Communications.* Our cells continually sense and respond to the environment and send physiological messages back and forth from one region of the body to another; that's the cellular communications process. A number of systems are involved in this process, which we'll learn more about in Chapter 7. But basically, the nervous system connects the brain to all the regions of the body. Hormones, neurotransmitters, and a range of special-purpose messengers—inflammatory messengers, growth and repair messengers, and more—bind themselves to a specific receptor on the surface of cells with which they are communicating and influence the physiological function of that organ. Within each cell there are also

specific communication systems—the kinase regulatory network and nuclear transcription factors, for example—that carry messages from outside the cell to the genes within the cell, thereby also changing the cell's physiological function. Altered function anywhere along any of these communication mechanisms—and the resulting functional changes in physiology—give rise to signs and symptoms associated with numerous chronic disorders.

5. *Cellular Transport*. Substances have to get from one part of the body to another. The nutrition our digestive system has assimilated, to take just one example, needs to get to our cells. How? That's the job of the transport process. Basically, it works through the circulatory system, pumped by the heart, through the lungs, and via the lymphatic system, also called the glandular system, which constantly refreshes the blood. Altered function in any of these transport functions will clearly result in a range of disorders. In the circulatory system, it is the cause of cardiovascular disease, which continues to be the most prevalent and most destructive chronic illness in the nation, if not the world.

6. *Energy*. Sometimes termed "bioenergetics," the processes that convert food to energy and manage the use of energy are carried out within an organelle of the cell called the mitochondrion. (An organelle is a structure that functions within each cell as organs do within the whole body.) It's in the mitochondria that food molecules that result from the assimilation process—glucose, amino acids, fatty acids—combine with oxygen to be broken down into energy and the waste products carbon dioxide, water, and urea. Alteration in the mitochondrial function typically underlies many of the chronic health problems associated with pain and fatigue.

7. *Structure*. How can we keep the body's building blocks healthy so that structure supports function properly? We used to think that the human skeleton and the connective tissue gluing the bones together via ligaments and tendons were like the steel girders of a building or the frame of a house. Once they were constructed, thus did they stand, having no influence on daily life within the structure and unaffected by it.

We now know that this is not correct. For one thing, our skeleton is remodeled every five to seven years. For another, our bones and connective tissue constantly affect our function, and precisely because proper structure defines proper physiological function, structure also defines our health or disease. Change the structure, and function is altered too. This means that posture, muscle tone, skeletal health, and the integrity of our connective tissue are essential to defining our health. A loss of skeletal health, for example, doesn't just translate into an increased risk of bone fracture; it increases the risk of a range of chronic illnesses as well.

Where all of this converges—genes, external messages from environment and behavior, and possible imbalances in one or more of the seven physiological processes—is where functional medicine finds its operating model. It looks like this:

FIGURE 1: THE FUNCTIONAL MEDICINE OPERATING SYSTEM

The four factors you can modify to affect the seven core physiological processes that determine your health.

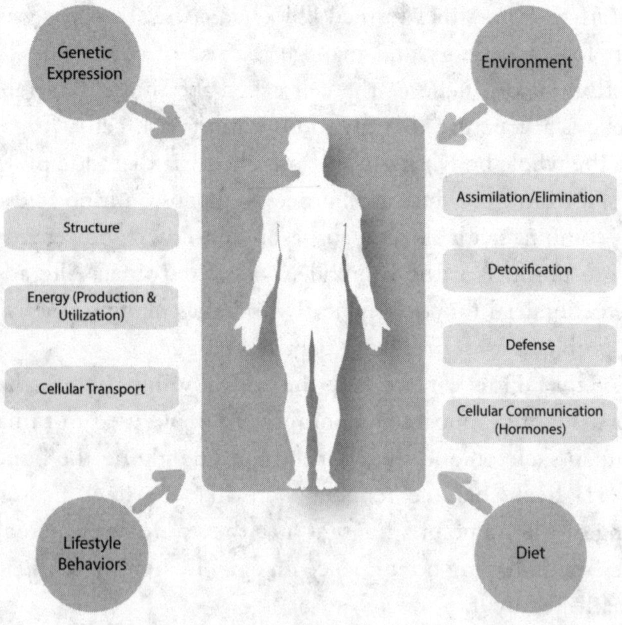

Genetic Expression

Environment

Structure

Assimilation/Elimination

Energy (Production & Utilization)

Detoxification

Cellular Transport

Defense

Cellular Communication (Hormones)

Lifestyle Behaviors

Diet

FINDING THE IMBALANCE

The detective work that finds the core clinical imbalances is step one toward developing a personalized program to correct or end them. The detection process isn't always easy. No two individuals will manifest the same imbalance in the same way. Since no one organ owns a physiological system or controls a physiological process, since imbalances represent dysfunctions that cut across all physiological processes, and because the interconnections among systems may be hard to unravel, the origin of any chronic illness is going to be complex.

But in a way, that is precisely the point: One underlying cause may manifest itself in multiple disorders that don't look anything like one another. Have you heard of the drug Cymbalta? Chances are that if you ever watch the evening news, you've seen the ads for it. Originally approved by regulators for use in the treatment of depression, it was soon recognized as useful for the treatment of chronic inflammatory pain from certain types of arthritis. How can that be? Depression and arthritis are two very different diseases that are treated by two very different subspecialties of medicine—depression by psychiatrists and arthritis by rheumatologists. How can the same drug be used for such different diagnoses?

The answer is simply that depression and arthritis share core clinical imbalances. They are not, in fact, independent; the chronic inflammation of arthritis and the communications disturbance of depression are connected through the cross talk between the immune system and the endocrine system. An imbalance in the physiological process of defense becomes an imbalance in the physiological process of communications—and vice versa, of course. A drug that affects one also affects the other.

Actually, there is even more to it than that. A supersystem is at work here, and there is a name for what it involves— psychoneuroimmunology. Remember the lyrics of the old song about bones—"the heel bone's connected to the foot bone, the foot bone's connected to the leg bone," etc.? In the case of this physiological supersystem, the nervous system is connected to the endocrine system is connected to the immune system. All talk together across common shared pathways. We know this because the receptors for messages of each one of those systems are found on the cells of the other two systems. The three systems thereby operate as a team, and the team's mission is to translate outside messages to inside function.

Naturally, therefore, a drug developed to treat one system will affect the other two. What we used to think of as unexpected adverse side effects are not unexpected at all; we just didn't understand the interrelations among the systems. Now that we do—and now that we have given the name psychoneuroimmunology to the interrelations—there's no mystery at all to the fact that Cymbalta, which blocks a certain process in the nervous system related to depression, also reduces the pain of arthritis. The two responses are literally on the same wavelength.

So while it may seem comforting to receive a diagnosis from a specialist—you have arthritis, or you have depression—that is only a starting point for understanding the shared mechanisms that underlie that manifestation of illness. In functional medicine, such a diagnosis is but the first step toward finding out how to manage the condition effectively. Solving a health problem comes not from naming it but from understanding the physiological disturbances that have resulted in the changed function we refer to as disease. How does functional medicine undertake that task?

THE FUNCTIONAL MEDICINE TOOLKIT: ASSESSMENT

Certainly, identifying core clinical imbalances greatly simplifies the story of our health and is the groundwork for designing the right personalized program for the individual's lifelong health. Where does it begin?

The first step is to retell the patient's story. By "retell," I mean that the functional medicine practitioner seeks to elicit that story in a new way—not just as the symptoms that have impelled you to seek medical help but rather as a narrative of the physical and social environment in which you live, your diet, how you think about your own health, any factors that make you feel worse or better, the things you believe help you recover from illness or make you sick. The aim here is for the practitioner doing the identifying work to understand the antecedents of your health problem.

The practitioner will then want to know what may have triggered the specific illness or the particular symptoms you're complaining about. For chronic ailments in particular, a number of precipitating events may have been at work, all interacting to trigger the health problem.

Many other factors may contribute to a health problem, and the functional medicine practitioner will be keen to determine these mediators, as they are called—events or factors or even beliefs and emotions that produce symptoms or bring about the kind of behavior we associate with being sick. Mediators can be anything from hormones to thousands of other messenger molecules that communicate from one part of the body to the other. Doctors often analyze these as biomarkers that can identify physiological imbalances that may be early signs of later disease.

With this understanding of antecedents, triggers, and mediators as background, the functional medicine practitioner will want to know about a range of lifestyle factors—your patterns of sleep and habits of relaxation, your routines of exercise or movement or sports activity, your typical nutrition and hydration, any points of stress and your resilience from same, and the personal relationships and networks of friends and acquaintances on whom you rely or with whom you routinely interact.

All of this information is essential as an organizing principle for finding and tracking your core clinical imbalances. And that's where the practitioner's next key tool kicks in—functional biomarkers. As we saw in Chapter 1, biomarkers measure characteristics that are known to be associated with specific physiological processes and that can thus signal health or disease. Cholesterol in the blood, for example, is a biomarker for determining the potential risk of heart disease and stroke. It does not provide a diagnosis; it informs us about the potential status of cardiovascular function. If the count is elevated, it means the individual's liver is making too much cholesterol. Numerous antecedents, triggers, and mediators may be influencing that fact—genetic makeup, stress, smoking, a poor-quality diet with too little fiber, vitamin and mineral deficiencies, excessive saturated fat intake, and lack of exercise. The biomarker doesn't tell us how the elevated cholesterol happened, just that it is there and is knocking a core physiological process off balance—a marker of ill health that needs to be addressed. Take a look at how some key biomarkers signal a potential imbalance in a core process that may one day lead to a chronic medical condition:

KEY BIOMARKERS FOR TRACKING CORE CLINICAL IMBALANCES

Biomarker	Imbalance Indicated	Medical Condition
Hemoglobin A1c	Communication	Type 2 diabetes
Hs-CRP	Defense	Inflammation
Homocysteine	Communication	CVD and Alzheimer's
Transglutaminase	Defense	Celiac disease
HDL	Transport	CVD
GGT	Detoxification	Diabetes
Ferretin	Assimilation	CVD/inflammation

JOE, REDUX

Naturally, applying the functional medicine model to a practitioner's operating system significantly changes how medicine is practiced. Joe found this out in spades when he came to the Functional Medicine Clinical Research Center in Gig Harbor, Washington, some years ago. Remember his presenting health complaints? They included elevated blood pressure, gout, tinnitus, prostate problems, and nocturnal leg cramps that resulted in sleep disturbance. He had been treated by several different specialists, each of whom focused on disease diagnoses within his or her expertise. Joe had been taking separate medications for all his health problems—plus sleep aids—under the assumption that each of these conditions was separate from the others.

He still felt awful, his symptoms were still there, and Joe was living a narrowed life with compromised mobility.

At the research center, he received a very different kind of assessment. Based on the functional medicine systems approach, the assessment tried to determine how all of Joe's presenting symptoms might be interconnected to one another and therefore to an imbalance in one or more of his core physiological processes—and it took a hard look at his genetic history, through the paternal line, of gout and prostate-related issues. What the new assessment found was that there were imbalances in both his communication and detoxification processes; these disturbances, the researchers determined, were what underlay Joe's multiple and diverse symptoms.

A personalized health-management program was put together to address these imbalances. The approach was to treat the cause of the imbalances that resulted in his complex symptoms and not just the effects.

It started with a diet on which Joe would eat substantial amounts of cruciferous vegetables—which contain substances particularly effective in improving the body's detoxification function—and of vegetable protein from legumes. The diet also reduced Joe's normal intake of animal protein. Joe, no kale-lover, wasn't thrilled, but he was determined.

In addition to the foods to embrace and those to eschew, he was advised to take some nutritional supplements. One, containing 300 milligrams of indole-3 carbinol, one of the active substances derived from cruciferous vegetables, was aimed at providing added support for his detoxification process. Another supplement contained 200 milligrams of a magnesium compound that is effective in supporting cellular communications. He was also given an antioxidant nutritional supplement containing 50 milligrams of coenzyme Q10, 500 milligrams of N-acetylcysteine, and 500 milligrams of lipoic acid to improve his cellular integrity. Joe was also advised to drink five glasses of water throughout the day to further improve detoxification.

What happened? It took three weeks for Joe to feel a diminution in all of his symptoms. Within three months, he was able to stop taking all the drugs the specialists had prescribed for him—except for a low-dose medication for lowering his blood pressure.

Needless to say, Joe feels great. If he still hasn't developed a taste for kale, he finds he is partial to cauliflower, radishes, and—of all things—brussels sprouts.

THE FUNCTIONAL MEDICINE TOOLKIT: CURING CHRONIC ILLNESS

Not surprisingly, Joe and others like him see the improvement in their health outcomes as heaven-sent, brilliant, and altogether wonderful. Yet one doesn't have to have been "cured" to see that such improvements will ultimately rival in magnitude the advances in global health that resulted from the bacteriological revolution of the late nineteenth and early twentieth centuries. Certainly, the results presage a new form of health care that will personalize the therapeutic approach to chronic illness using a strategy focused on genes and environment.

The tools of this new form of health care will include diet, supplemental nutrition, exercise, lifestyle and behavior therapies, and environmental modification as well as traditional pharmaceutical drugs. Nutraceuticals and phytochemicals—specific nutrients and plant-derived substances used in therapeutic doses to remedy imbalances in the seven core physiological processes, like those Joe takes to bolster his detox process—will hold an important place in the new toolkit of therapies. Medical foods, defined by the FDA as foods that contain a specific composition of nutrients identified as necessary for a particular disease state, will also play a role. Today, medical foods have been formulated for type 2 diabetes, inflammatory arthritis, inflammatory bowel disease, kidney disease, cardiovascular diseases, and such genetic diseases as PKU. All of these tools—and others as well—may be part of the toolkit you'll use as you go through the next chapters and begin to develop your own personalized plan.

Remember Ikaria? There in the middle of the Aegean, the communal lifestyle and inherited culture of a defined community result in extending the life span and health span of the community as a whole. Now imagine what the benefits can be when the trajectory is absolutely individual, when the messages from your environment and lifestyle speak directly and pointedly to your unique genetic potential. It's time now to learn how to target those messages to create your own Ikaria, to unlock your unique genetic potential and restore healthy balance to your own core physiological processes.

It starts in the gut.

PART TWO

THE SEVEN CORE PHYSIOLOGICAL PROCESSES

You've seen how the global rise of chronic illness makes a new model of medical care necessary and how the genomic revolution makes the new model possible. Now Part 2 shows how the model must work. Taking a systems approach to the body, the chapters that follow examine the seven core physiological processes that define how we function:

- Assimilation and elimination
- Detoxification
- Defense
- Cellular communications
- Cellular transport
- Energy
- Structure

In these seven chapters, you'll learn how each core process functions and how all interconnect to create your health pattern. A self-assessment questionnaire is provided for each core process. The questionnaires offer a frame of reference that will help you think about any process imbalances you may have. Later, in Part 3, you'll use these self-assessments as tools for zeroing in on your process imbalances and for understanding your own health pattern and how to shape it.

CHAPTER 4

Assimilation and Elimination

1. Do you alternate between constipation and urgency?
2. Do you get indigestion?
3. Does your stool have an oily appearance?
4. Do you suffer from frequent intestinal gas or bloating?
5. Is stomach or intestinal pain a regular occurrence?
6. Do you ever get gastric reflux? Do you get it frequently?
7. Are headaches a common occurrence?
8. Are you allergic or sensitive to many foods?
9. After eating, do you find you experience joint or muscle pain?
10. Do you have bad breath?
11. Are you depressed? Subject to mood swings?
12. Do you have trouble keeping your weight under control even though you watch your diet?
13. Is your blood sugar elevated?
14. Do you suffer from kidney stones?
15. Is your blood pressure higher than it should be?

I experienced no small amount of anxiety just thinking about sitting down to write this chapter. To me, it is particularly important that I make clear to you, the reader, the understanding gained through recent scientific discoveries about our system of digestion and assimilation. It is so central to the functional medicine revolution that my self-imposed pressure to do justice to the explanation tied my stomach in knots for days as I approached my task.

And that, I realized, is precisely the point the chapter needs to bring home—namely, that it is no accident that anxiety has twisted my stomach into knots. Nor is it just a figure of speech. It is a medical fact, and the reason for it is the reality of the interconnections we've been talking about, more or less in the abstract, in the previous chapters and what those interconnections mean for a new way to approach chronic illness. The gastrointestinal system that carries out our functions of digestion and assimilation of food is connected to our nervous system, and both are linked through cells of the immune system. When you get butterflies in your stomach because the exam you're taking counts for half the grade toward your professional license, or if you feel the urgent need for a rush call to the lavatory just seconds before a key presentation to your boss, it's because your nervous system, now going into overdrive, has kicked off rhythmic muscle contractions in the intestines and has activated the more than 50 percent of the body's whole immune system that is clustered around the gastrointestinal tract, stimulating substances that in turn send an alarm you feel right smack in your gut.

That's why the gut is the starting point for an awful lot of chronic illnesses that seem to have nothing to do with the stomach; it's the launch pad for numerous symptoms affecting parts of the body far distant from the gastrointestinal area. And vice versa. A glitch in the process of assimilation and elimination can make you sick, and because of the interconnections with the body's nerves and immune mechanisms, all sorts of things can cause such a glitch.

So let's begin by taking a look at this part of our physiology and at the process that takes place there.

THE PROCESS OF ASSIMILATION AND ELIMINATION

The intestinal tract in the adult human is some twenty-five to thirty feet long. That's about midway between the longer intestinal tract of the cow and the shorter intestinal tract of the tiger. Herbivores like cows have long digestive systems because it is harder to absorb nutrients from plant foods than from animal foods; the herbivore tract needs more room to carry out the process than does the intestinal tract of a carnivore like the tiger. Since we humans are omnivores, we split the difference.

Food provides protein, carbohydrate, and fats—the nutrients from which we derive our cellular energy and construct the building blocks of our body. But for these nutrients to be used by the body they must be broken down through the process of digestion, and the waste products must then be excreted. The process begins in the mouth, where an enzyme called amylase, secreted in saliva, starts to break down carbs; it continues in the stomach, where other enzymes and acid released by specialized cells in the stomach lining start the breakdown of the large protein molecules into their smaller amino acid building blocks. The next step down the digestive system is through the duodenum, where bile is added to break down fats till they are absorbable. From here, the partially digested food, called the chyme, travels into the small and large intestines. The intestines are inhabited by many different types of bacteria, collectively known as enteric microflora; "enteric" simply means having to do with the intestines, and "microflora" are the many bacteria that make their home in our intestinal tract.

There are zillions of these enteric microflora—more in a single ounce of stool than there are stars in the known universe. In fact, there are many more bacterial cells in the intestinal tract than there are human cells in the whole body. These bacterial cells are very small compared with human cells, but their contribution to the overall health of the person can be quite significant.

For one thing, enteric microflora belong to one of three families of bacteria—symbiotic, commensal, or parasitic. Symbiotic bacteria enjoy a mutually beneficial relationship with us, commensal bacteria live in harmony with our bodies in relationships in which one of us benefits but neither is harmed, and parasitic bacteria get a free ride in our bodies and do us no good at all; in fact, their metabolism generates caustic substances that can harm us. Each of these families of enteric bacteria has its own preferential food to be metabolized. For example, the friendly bacteria in the intestinal tract—members of the symbiotic or commensal families—prefer certain fibers known as fructans, which come from plant foods. A diet too low in fiber can cause these friendly bacteria to die of starvation and be replaced by parasitic bacteria. The result can be such digestive complaints as irritable bowel syndrome, esophageal reflux, and chronic constipation. (One antidote is probiotics; another is specific kinds of fibers that support the growth of the friendly bacteria.)

As the digested food travels down the intestinal tract, its nutrients are constantly absorbed at different "stops" along the way. A disturbance in the process anywhere along this journey may reduce the absorption of specific nutrients, and that in turn can cause specific nutritional deficiencies—even when the overall diet contains adequate levels of the nutrients. We've seen this in patients taking certain antacid medications to manage their gastric reflux and acid stomach symptoms. A number of these patients develop a form of anemia and experience the kind of low energy associated with deficiencies in vitamin B12 and iron. Since adequate stomach acid secretion from the stomach lining is necessary for the absorption of vitamin B12 and iron, suppressing acid secretion, as these antacids tend to do, can have these unintended adverse effects.

Once our food nutrients have been absorbed and converted to energy, the body needs to eliminate the waste products. The relevant organs in the elimination process are the intestinal tract and the kidneys and urinary bladder, which eliminate waste via urine and stool; the skin, which eliminates waste through perspiration; and the lungs, which exhale carbon dioxide and water vapor. Any glitch in the proper process of elimination can contribute to a range of chronic illnesses, and, because the system of assimilation and elimination is integrally linked with the immune system and the nervous system, the messages transmitted among these interconnected systems can reach to every part of the body, affecting our well-being in myriad ways. Figure 2 shows the anatomy through which the assimilation–elimination process works.

THE IMMUNE CONNECTION

If the whole of the intestinal tract were flattened out, its surface area would be about the size of a doubles tennis court. That surface is

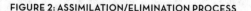

FIGURE 2: ASSIMILATION/ELIMINATION PROCESS

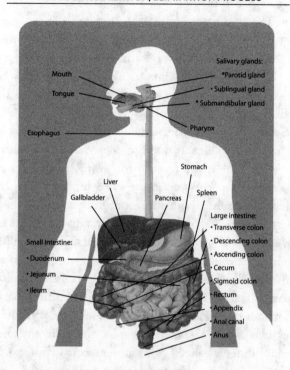

lined with millions of tiny folds called microvilli, and it is through the microvilli that nutrients are absorbed across the intestinal lining, transported from the inside of the tract to the rest of the body via specific transport processes in the intestinal cells.

On the other side of this lining sits the immune system of the intestinal tract, a system comprising more than half of the total immune system in the body as a whole. It is there not because there wasn't any other place to put it, but because that's where it has to be to defend the body from what might happen over a lifetime of ingesting nearly twenty-five tons of food items—"foreigners" to our body brought inside us from the external environment. Just keep in mind the assertion articulated by Linus Pauling that if you get the structure right the function will follow; the structure of the immune system of the gastrointestinal tract is what it is and where it is because of the importance of the function it must perform.

And its function is to serve as gatekeeper at the gastrointestinal barrier, ever alert to the arrival of foreign substances absorbed from our food that may be in some way harmful to our physiological functioning. The gastrointestinal immune system is precisely where it is so it can catch these substances before they create havoc in the body and can then process them into harmlessness.

It does this job by monitoring the metabolic substances produced by the enteric microflora. If the immune system senses that such a substance is harmful, it will react by increasing the number of alarm cells. When that happens, you feel it—as pain, or bloating, or diarrhea perhaps, or intestinal inflammation. But as those alarm cells hit the bloodstream and radiate outward, you might also feel it in places far removed from the gastrointestinal tract. Headache, joint pain, bad breath, muscle pain, skin and vision problems, even mood swings— symptoms that seem far away in every respect from the intestinal tract—may in fact be kicked off by the intestinal immune system. In fact, some of the toxic microflora in the gut can actually convert hormones like estrogen and testosterone into different forms that then produce different effects from those normally produced by the body's natural hormones. No wonder mood swings are so confusing.

We now understand how all this happens. We owe it to the fact that the gut has its own nervous system. Dubbed "the second brain," a term first coined by Columbia University research gastroenterologist Michael Gershon, this enteric nervous system consists of billions of neurons and is filled with the same kinds of neurotransmitters found in the brain in our skulls.

This "second brain" secretes messengers that communicate back and forth between the gut and the brain. Some of these messengers are hormones—cholecystokinins, ghrelins, secretins, gastrins, somatostatins, and more—produced by endocrine glands and sent forth into the bloodstream, while others are neurotransmitters released directly from nerve terminals in the brain's central nervous system. One of the best known of these messenger substances is the hormone serotonin, known as the mood-elevating neurotransmitter. It may calm the brain, but the majority of the serotonin produced in the body comes from the gut, so that meddling with serotonin may also mean meddling with the gut. As it turns out, that's exactly what happens with the class of pharmaceutical antidepressants known as selective serotonin reuptake inhibitors, or SSRIs, which increase serotonin levels in the nervous system. It has now been found that excessive serotonin availability is associated with increased risk of bone loss. Does this mean that these SSRI antidepressants are interacting with gastrointestinal function? The answer is yes; in fact, it has been reported that the use of SSRIs alters the important role that serotonin produced by the gut plays in influencing the balance between bone loss and bone formation. It also confirms the connection between the intestinal system and the nervous system.

Meanwhile, other messengers operate in other regions throughout the length of the gastrointestinal system. While serotonin affects mood, the hormone ghrelin, for example, affects appetite. Gastrointestinal inhibitory peptide influences insulin secretion and therefore blood sugar. Compared with ghrelin, cholecystokinin affects appetite in exactly the opposite way. Glucagon-like peptide 1, or GLP-1, regulates insulin secretion and also seems to influence the feeling of satiety in the brain. And so on, with other messengers affecting bone density, cardiovascular function, inflammatory responses, and more. The bottom line is simply that the channels of communication between the gut and the rest of the body—and certainly between the gut and the brain—teem with information flying back and forth, up and down, every which way, all profoundly influencing our physiology and our health.

A MATTER OF TASTE

Research into the connection between the brain and our process of assimilation and elimination is ongoing, and it is fascinating. A case in point is the work begun some time ago at the Monell Chemical Senses Center in Philadelphia by research neurologist Alan Hirsch. Hirsch's work focused on understanding taste and smell and their relationship to human perception. At one point, he and his research group zeroed in on the effect of various nutrients on smell and taste—specifically on how nutrients influenced acuity, the keenness or sharpness of an individual's smell and taste. A key finding was that zinc and a specific fat known as phosphatidylcholine, abbreviated PC, were effective in preserving taste and smell. Further study suggested that people who lose acuity of taste and smell may regain both with supplemental doses of these two nutrients. Some people have been reported to have regained the sense of taste and smell after such supplemental doses.

Later research went even further, finding a connection between the loss of taste and smell and early problems of the nervous system—specifically, with the particular nervous system problems that often presage Alzheimer's and other neurological diseases; it meant that loss of taste and smell acuity could be used as a functional marker for aspects of nervous system function or dysfunction.

Taste, not surprisingly, starts on the tongue, where there are specific receptors for specific tastes—sweet, salty, bitter, sour, and a new taste termed "umami," the taste activated by monosodium glutamate (MSG). What we perceive as taste sensations are the interactions of specific foods we eat with the taste receptors on our tongue. But not just on the tongue.

In the case of the bitter taste, for example, the surface receptors on specialized cells called L cells in the small intestine turn out to be identical to the bitter taste receptors on the tongue. In essence, our digestive system also "tastes" our food when the specific taste sensation—in this case, bitter—alters the gene expression of the L cell and its function. But this digestive system "tasting" sets up another reaction altogether. Here's what happens.

When what we think of as a bitter-tasting substance is exposed to the L cells, it causes them to secrete the messenger mentioned a moment ago, glucagon-like peptide 1, into the bloodstream. GLP-1 is what is known as an integrin hormone; that means that it passes signals between a cell and its surroundings. In the case of GLP-1, that signaling stimulates the action of insulin, helping to control blood sugar levels after eating.

The bottom line of all this? Bitter-tasting foods can stimulate the L cells to release GLP-1 and in turn help to manage blood sugar and insulin levels. And indeed, certain foods that contain specific bitter substances have been shown to reduce blood sugar after eating. Bitter melon (*Mormordica charantia*), common hops, prickly pear cactus, and cow plant all do just that. Interestingly, all of them have historically been used by indigenous cultures to treat what we now call diabetes. But the discovery of how GLP-1 secretion improves blood sugar has also prompted the development of a class of medications for diabetes aimed at stimulating the release of insulin; one such is Byetta (exenetide), which increases GLP-1 activity.

In other words, what we eat and what we like to taste are significant in determining how our gastrointestinal system produces and secretes a stunning range of messenger substances affecting a stunning range of physiological functions—and our pattern of health and disease. In so many ways, food really is information, and it talks all the time to the genes regulating our core physiological processes.

Interestingly, we owe the start of our understanding of all this to a starfish off the coast of Sicily.

THE THORN IN THE STARFISH AND THE GUT-BRAIN CONNECTION

The man studying the starfish, the man who would teach us how the intestinal system influences so many health conditions, was Ilya I. Mechnikov, a Russian-born biologist, zoologist, and physician awarded the Nobel Prize in Physiology or Medicine in 1908. Mechnikov would spend the bulk of his career as director of the prestigious Pasteur Institute in France, but it was in the late 1800s, while he was working at his own laboratory in Messina, Italy, that he made his most famous discovery. He was studying starfish larvae, and when he happened to insert a thorn into one larva, he observed a crowd of strange cells racing to the point of insertion and gathering there. Literally as Mechnikov watched, the cells engulfed and destroyed whatever tried to make its way in through that point of injury. Mechnikov dubbed these engulfing-and-destroying cells phagocytes, and he concluded that they live inside an organism for the precise purpose of ingesting—and thereby killing—what might be harmful to the organism.

We call this phenomenon innate immunity, and one of the things it explains is the cruel world in which we humans protect our physiology from infection. Simply put, there are these specialized white blood cells inside us that are on a constant search-and-destroy mission to recognize, chemically kill, and then consume foreign cells that enter the body. It's what equips us to do battle against foreign invaders and potential cancer cells.

But Mechnikov's observation about cellular immunity also explains how balance is maintained in the process of assimilation and elimination. In his 1907 book, *The Prolongation of Life: Optimistic Studies*, Mechnikov asserts the important role of healthy intestinal microflora in achieving good health. The good health depends, he wrote, on a kind of peaceful coexistence among all the symbiotic bacteria in the intestinal tract—our own cells and tissue and all the microorganisms that live there as well—and phagocytes are key to keeping that peace. A disturbance of the peace—a microbial imbalance, known as dysbiosis—would equally disturb our good health. In a sense, the combination of Pasteur's work on the origins of infectious disease and Mechnikov's discovery of cellular immunity resulted in the recognition that the bacteria in the intestinal tract could be friends or foes. Too many foes anywhere in the process of assimilation-elimination would cause the gut to release various toxins that would range throughout the body, even as far as the brain.

That is why Mechnikov was an early advocate of yogurt in the diet. He saw it as a way to increase the number of friendly bacteria in the intestines and strengthen their effectiveness in preventing disease throughout the body and therefore in prolonging life. He saw intestinal health as integral to overall health.

What is interesting is that Mechnikov based this understanding, which would come to dominate medical thinking, on observation—coupled, of course, with his knowledge, experience, and sheer genius. What he did not know at the time, however, was exactly how it worked, how the gut produced and secreted messenger hormones and neurotransmitters that carry information throughout the body, from the gut to the brain and back again. But he sensed that the gastrointestinal system is in direct contact with the outside world—namely, with what we eat—and that the direct interaction between the microflora that live within our guts and what we ingest is central to our health. From there, it was an easy step to understanding that by changing the factors of that environment—that is, by eating more yogurt—we could influence the balance in the assimilation-elimination process and improve our health.

In truth, when Mechnikov first articulated his phagocytic theory, many prominent biologists, including Pasteur, were skeptical. In time, however, Pasteur summoned Mechnikov to be his deputy and successor at the Pasteur Institute, thereby awarding the theory his imprimatur. The 1908 Nobel sealed the deal, and the notion that many conditions of ill health, including those affecting the brain, could be treated by focusing on the gut became accepted medical wisdom for years to come—until a gruesome medical scandal subverted this wisdom and set back the course of medical progress in this area for eight decades.

TRAGEDY, SCANDAL, AND RETROGRESSION

Back in the 1920s, the largest mental hospital in the United States was the New Jersey State Hospital in Trenton, under the direction of Dr. Henry Cotton, a well-known psychiatrist. In an extreme and somewhat twisted version of Mechnikov's theory of intestinal health as integral to overall health, Cotton held that insanity was fundamentally a toxic disorder resulting from chronic infections in the intestines and other parts of the body. His "cure" for the insanity was the surgical removal of parts of the body believed to be infected—including teeth, tonsils, sinuses, stomachs, and portions of the intestines.

Although his methods were controversial, Cotton had had exceptional training, was well connected in the world of psychiatry, and held a prestigious post. Moreover, it must be pointed out that from 1915 to 1925, surgery was the standard therapy, in all major hospitals and medical schools throughout the country, for the presumed "chronic infection" that caused mental dysfunction. So as Andrew Scull relates in his riveting 2007 book, *Madhouse: A Tragic Tale of Megalomania and Modern Medicine*, Cotton wasn't stopped until it was found that he had falsified data on outcomes.

When the ax fell on Cotton, however, it didn't fall so much on the procedure as on the whole idea of the gastrointestinal connection to mental illness. In fact, his fall from grace was hard enough to shatter not just his reputation but the entire concept of chronic intestinal infection—dysbiosis. For nearly eighty years, no one dared even discuss gastrointestinal toxicity at any major medical center or meeting out of fear of reprisal from the medical establishment.

Nearly a century later, we understand that the blanket condemnation of Cotton and everything connected with him, while perhaps understandable given the barbarity of his methods, threw out the baby with the bathwater. Indeed, by taking our eye off the connection between gut and brain, the distaste for Cotton may actually have slowed our ability to address the real imbalances in our assimilation-elimination process. Today, we once again recognize and have investigated the association between the intestinal tract and brain function, and we see how very profound it is in its impact on our health. Few connections exemplify that association as clearly as the connection between celiac disease and dementia.

THE GUT-BRAIN CONNECTION: CELIAC DISEASE AND DEMENTIA

You've probably heard of celiac disease. It is a really unpleasant disorder in which the lining of the small intestine is damaged by a family of proteins, called gluten, found in cereal grains, and it has long been recognized that a genetic susceptibility to that grain protein is the cause of the disease. Its symptoms, apart from pain and discomfort, may include chronic constipation and bloody diarrhea, fatigue, in children a failure to thrive, autoimmune disease, and a high incidence of dementia.

Traditionally, the dementia was considered a disease adjacency or comorbidity—just a statistical happenstance. But the discoveries that have shown us the links connecting the gut, immune system, and nervous system have changed that story. We now see a cause-and-effect relationship between celiac disease and dementia that starts with the activation of the intestinal immune system and ends with the triggering of brain inflammation. Here's how it happens.

The gastrointestinal system of a person with the genetic suscepti-bility to gluten reacts to its presence in food as to a hostile foreigner. That reaction activates inflammatory messenger molecules that travel through the bloodstream from the gastrointestinal immune system to the liver. Ten percent of the cells that make up the liver are called Kupffer cells—after the scientist who first observed them. Kupffer cells are specialized immune cells, and although they reside only in the liver, they are derived from the same lineage of cells as the gas-trointestinal immune system cells.

So when the inflammatory messenger molecules from the gut arrive in the liver, they stimulate their relatives, the Kupffer cells, to release messengers from their genes. These messengers in turn activate an inflammatory response in white blood cells that are also part of that same immune cell lineage. These white blood cells then travel to the blood-brain barrier, where they trigger an inflammatory response in cells in the brain called microglial cells, which are—you guessed it—*also* relatives of the gastrointestinal immune cells, the Kupffer cells in the liver, and the circulating white blood cells. In fact, the microglial cells *are* the brain's immune system and, when activated, they produce their own inflammatory messengers.

But these messengers sent from the brain's immune system con-stitute an inflammatory response that causes collateral damage to the neurons in the brain. The result? Certain types of brain function—specifically, the functions of memory and cognition—suffer losses, causing the clinical outcome we know as dementia. It is a classic example of the gut connected to the liver, connected to the immune system, connected to the brain. What we understand from it through the lens of our twenty-first-century focus on systems biology is not to treat the brain dysfunction with a drug—and there are numerous medications for doing so—but rather to treat the immune inflammatory response of the gut. Eliminating gluten from the diet to normalize gastrointestinal function is certainly a more sensible first step than throwing more medications at all those physiological messengers.

HOLES IN THE BARRIER

This treatment model—addressing the assimilation-elimination process of the body as a way of treating chronic illnesses that may have their origin there—extends also to the management of other neurological diseases. A number of clinical studies have demonstrated improvement in neurological function in patients with multiple sclerosis (MS), who were put on a gluten-free diet plan. A good friend and colleague, neurologist David Perlmutter, in his superb book, *Grain Brain*, has described his pioneering work in treating various neurological conditions with a gluten-free diet.

The question is how the hostile foreign substances manage to get into the blood from the gut in the first place. Didn't we say that there's an intestinal immune system that puts up a barrier prohibiting the absorption of immune-activating substances? Has something somehow been poking holes in the barrier?

The answer is yes, and the term for it is endotoxemia. It means that toxic substances produced in the intestinal tract are indeed leaking through the barrier into the blood. Research gastroenterologists call it "leaky gut syndrome," and they have confirmed that it primarily occurs after the consumption of foods high in fat and sugar or from ingesting other caustic chemical or food substances. The leaks allow the entry of substances the barrier normally prohibits. These substances spill through into the intestines, where the intestinal immune system sees them as foreigners, takes defensive action, and turns up the dial on the genes that control the production of inflammatory messengers.

But just what is poking holes in the barrier? What is responsible for this loss of integrity in the mucosal barrier? Researchers believe it is exposure to caustic substances—possibly from food allergens, infectious bacteria, viruses or yeast, drugs and alcohol, or harsh chemicals. Whatever the precise cause, this loss of integrity in the barrier that normally prohibits access to the intestinal immune system stirs such diverse chronic symptoms as sinus problems, joint pain, headaches, skin problems like eczema, and anxiety. Just how bad the symptoms get will depend on just how leaky the barrier has become and just how many endotoxins get absorbed into the blood.

WHAT TO DO?

Back in 1990 when I and my close friends and medical colleagues, David Jones, Leo Galland, Sidney Baker, Joseph Pizzorno, Graham Reedy, and J. Alexander Bralley, were first talking about the clinical applications of functional medicine, we all agreed that addressing an imbalance in the assimilation-elimination process would be among the most important.* At my suggestion, we even developed an acronym for the functional medicine approach to what we call gastrointestinal restoration. We named it the Four R Program, and over the subsequent decades, it has been tested, refined, and taught to more than a hundred thousand health practitioners around the world.

The Four Rs stand for:

- Remove
- Replace
- Reinoculate
- Repair

Here's how it works.

---

* This may not have been a totally original assessment. It is of historical interest that the naturopathic medical approach to chronic illness, born out of the Mechnikov model of gastrointestinal health, can be summarized as "Start with the gut."

Step One: Remove

Simply put, get rid of all food allergens or food substances producing sensitivities. Start by evaluating the reaction to gluten in grain products; to casein protein in dairy products; and to soy products, citrus products, peanuts, eggs, and shellfish—all classic producers of immune response. Be careful also to reduce exposure to moldy foods and fermented foods.

Step Two: Replace

If the stool contains undigested food materials or fat, that is a telltale sign that the enzymes normally released during the digestive process may not be adequate for proper function. Take a digestive enzyme supplement before meals to improve digestion and absorption. A pancreatin digestive enzyme tablet that can break down protein, carbohydrate, and fats may help in improving assimilation when taken along with meals.

Step Three: Reinoculate

Add a prebiotic and probiotic supplement to the daily regimen. Probiotic organisms of the *Bifidobacterium bifidum* and *Lactobacillus acidophilus* strains have been proved to be safe and effective for improving digestive function, but do start slowly with these supplements, and increase the dose over two to three weeks. The ideal daily dose consists of 3 grams per day of the prebiotic and a 2 billion probiotic count. The ideal probiotics dose is considerably higher than one can get in a standard serving of yogurt, so it may be more convenient to take in a therapeutic tablet or powdered delivery form.

Step Four: Repair

Take a supplement of the nutrients that can support the healing of the intestinal mucosal barrier. The most important of these are zinc (15 milligrams), pantothenic acid (vitamin B5, 500 milligrams), omega-3 fish oils (2 to 3 grams), and the amino acids L-glutamine (5 grams) and magnesium (200 milligrams), along with a B-complex nutritional supplement.

Let's be clear: The Four R Program isn't for the odd stomach upset; nor is it a maintenance program. It addresses a fundamental imbalance in the core physiological process of assimilation-elimination. For a researcher like myself, nothing brings me up short quite as abruptly or quite as formidably as getting the opportunity to understand what this means in personal terms, as happened to me some years ago in Denmark.

I was there to deliver a lecture at the Copenhagen Hospital and Medical School about the gastrointestinal restoration program. After the lecture, a woman approached me, introduced herself as Ilsa G., the head surgical nurse in the hospital's gastroenterology department, and began to tell me about her daughter—I'll call her Margret. By the age of fifteen, Margret had a history of inflammatory bowel disease that had left her malnourished and slow to develop. She had undergone several surgeries for the condition, but her health was so uncertain that she could not leave the house or attend school. Instead, she was tutored at home, where she lived a limited, isolated life.

Ilsa somehow heard about the Four R Program and wondered if it might be worth trying with Margret. She asked her boss, head of gastroenterology at the hospital, what he thought. He hadn't heard anything about it, but he thought it sounded "strange" and didn't recommend it because Margret's condition was, as he put it, so "unstable."

It was at this point in the conversation that something happened that for me was transformative. Ilsa turned to a statuesque young woman standing just a bit behind her and introduced her as Margret, now eighteen. Despite what her boss "recommended," Ilsa had decided to implement the Four R Program for Margret. From the start, the intestinal flares subsided and Margret was able to eat. She gained weight, grew seven inches, and had her first menstrual period. During the second year of the program, Margret was able to withdraw from all the multiple medications she had taken for years. Now, said Ilsa, "as you can see, the results speak for themselves."

But Margret had something to say as well. In superb English, she told me that for her, most important was the trip she had taken the previous summer—she and a bunch of friends, traveling around

Europe, backpacks on their backs, wandering wherever the fancy took them—and, said Margret, "I had no problems.

"Thank you," she added, "for your program that saved my life."

I don't know if you can imagine how it feels to hear something like that. My only rather feeble response was to thank her for sharing her story and to wish her the best in her life.

Sometimes, we scientists need reminding that the end result of our research is the real lives of real people.

So, yes, the core process of assimilation-elimination can be central to the health of the entire human organism. Co-equal in importance is our process of detoxification, without which we would be in a constant state of toxicity while our health and our longevity would be in perpetual jeopardy.

CHAPTER 4 TAKEAWAY

1. The digestive system is also the center of the immune system.
2. The digestive system, nervous system, immune system, and hormone-producing endocrine system all function together in an interconnected way.
3. Nutritional deficiency can result from poor digestion or ineffective or incomplete assimilation of nutrients.
4. The digestive system is inhabited by several hundred different species of bacteria and microbiota that influence health and disease patterns.
5. Specific foods affect the secretion of substances from the digestive system and in so doing can influence the risk of various chronic diseases.
6. The Four R Program represents a clinically proven approach to managing complex health problems associated with imbalances of the assimilation-elimination process.

CHAPTER 5

Detoxification

1. Are you sensitive to fragrances and odors?
2. What about food—any sensitivities?
3. Sensitive to particular medications?
4. To alcohol?
5. Do you get a bad reaction from monosodium glutamate in food?
6. Do you have sensitivity to caffeine?
7. Have you ever been sick from exposure to chemicals?
8. Does cigarette smoke bother you or make you sick?
9. Are you sensitive to smog or air pollution?
10. Do you sometimes wake up in the morning feeling as if you've been drugged?
11. Ever have unexplained skin rashes?
12. Do you ever experience brain fog?
13. Do you feel a tingling in your hands or feet?
14. Is there consistent ringing in your ears?
15. Do you experience unexplained muscle pain?

The office coffeepot keeps perking all day long. Alan allows himself half a cup when he arrives at eight o'clock in the morning, and it wires him for the rest of the day. Sue, in the next cubicle, drinks cup after cup all day long and remains as calm and unruffled as a stone statue of the Buddha.

On the other hand, Sue's head hurts on the rare occasions when

she indulges her passion for chocolate. Alan can eat a ton of chocolate, but a single glass of red wine will send him to bed with a
crashing headache; he'll occasionally drink a glass of white wine but
mostly just avoids the grape.

His wife, Barbara, can eat and drink anything without feeling the
slightest effect, but after Alan sprayed the house to get rid of the mos-
quitoes that fly in because the kids don't close the screen door tightly,
Barb's whole body was suddenly covered in red welts. It took a trip to
the emergency room and a hit of steroids to calm the reaction.

While they were in the ER, a man was brought in on a gurney
suffering even more than Barb. His affliction? An adverse reaction to
acetaminophen, of all things; the guy had taken your basic over-the-
counter Tylenol, and next thing he knew, he was flat on his back in
an ambulance. Yet the physician attending to Barb told them the ER
got more visits for this than for an adverse reaction to any other drug.

Why? What's going on? Why do our bodies respond to different
things in the environment in these ways—and why are the responses
so individual and so varied? The answers are to be found in the core
process we call detoxification. The process is kicked off by the natural physiological reaction of all organisms to reject "foreign" things
that may be toxic—that is, things the organism senses don't belong
to it and may be harmful to it in some way. The term for such things
is xenobiotics—from the Greek *xenos*, meaning "stranger," and *bios*,
meaning "life." What makes the process tough to figure out is that
what seems foreign and toxic to one organism may not seem so to
another organism, which is why Alan and Sue have such drastically
different physical reactions to a simple substance like coffee. What
we can say, however, is that each individual's personal detoxification
response to one or another specific substance is tied to both the individual's genetic heritage and his or her lifestyle and diet.

THE PROCESS

Scientists have known at least since the middle of the nineteenth
century that organisms throughout evolutionary history have been

exposed to toxic substances in their environments and have developed ways to protect themselves from these toxic exposures. In the middle of the twentieth century, the question being asked—and the big push in laboratories everywhere—was about the process itself. Exactly what was it that protected organisms like us against toxic exposure? In 1955, Dr. Bernard Brodie, the founder and head of the Laboratory of Chemical Pharmacology at the National Institutes of Health, together with two of his students, Julius Axelrod and Jim Gillette, became famous for discovering an enzyme system that could detoxify foreign chemicals—that is, render them nontoxic and therefore harmless and ready to be excreted from the body altogether. Really, it was an enzyme supersystem, composed of more than fifty different kinds of enzymes, each with its own gene. In time, it was given a name—the cytochrome P450 system, CYP450 for short. Two scientists working at the McArdle Laboratory at the University of Wisconsin, Jim and Betty Miller, made the further discovery that CYP450 was principally located in the liver.

Then came the discovery that CYP450 was also involved not just in detoxifying toxins but in metabolizing substances native to all living cells. This meant that the supersystem did double duty: It protected us against foreign xenobiotics from the outside world and from toxic bacteria produced within our intestinal tracts, *and* it decontaminated the metabolic by-products in cells and got them ready for elimination from the body.

The problem is that this sets up a competition for the CYP450 enzymes. What are they going to do—transform particular products associated with normal metabolism or detoxify specific toxins? Both tasks are profoundly important and complex. Trying to do both at once can make an enzyme system—even an enzyme supersystem—end up cheating one or the other, if not both.

The analogy I use when I talk about this to my students is to ask them to think of the CYP450 enzyme supersystem as a room you're dying to get into. A number of different doors offer entry into the room, and each door is another CYP450 enzyme, but you can enter the room through only one of the doors. Some of these enzyme-doors are big, like sliding-door entryways to major build-ings, while others are narrow openings you have to squeeze into, like the folding doors to phone booths you see in old movies. The differences are of course due to each individual's genetic uniqueness.

So let's suppose that a bunch of substances crowd up trying to get through one of the narrow doors inside you, and they're forced to enter one at a time. Some of those substances will no doubt be friendly substances—hormones just doing their job, for example. But some will also be toxins. The result will be a scramble at the entrance, with hostile toxins and benign friendlies vying with one another to get into the room through that single door, competing against one another to get some of that particular CYP450 enzyme. The result will be a buildup of both toxins and nontoxins, with only a small amount of either able to get through the door to be processed by the body and, in the case of the toxins, rendered harmless and flushed away.

Why is buildup bad? As with many things in life, while a small amount of toxins may not do any serious damage, a crowd of them can do a lot of damage indeed. Have you ever found yourself undone by a spacey feeling? You get the jitters or a headache, start sweating, or feel heart palpitations. These are likely to be early signs of toxic-ity that may come from an overload of the CYP450 detoxification system. That doesn't mean you're suffering serious poisoning, but rather that there is an imbalance in a component of your detoxifica-tion process. For the most part, the adage that "dilution is the solution to pollution" will restore the balance; drink a lot of water, and maybe add some soluble fiber to help flush the toxins out of your body as fast as possible. But such symptoms of toxicity just might signal a serious imbalance that needs to be taken very seriously indeed.

As for the friendly substances racing around in our bodies, while they are certainly essential for sustaining life, they too can become toxic if their level rises too high or drops too low. In other words, Mae West was wrong, at least about the benign substances in our bodies: Too much of a good thing turns out *not* to be wonderful, and the same is true for too little of a good thing.

Fortunately, the body has this process, detoxification, for keeping these substances—toxins and the useful substances that can become toxic—at appropriate levels, thereby controlling the chemical balance within the organism that is us. Keep in mind that the body is a seething mass of chemical reactions going on all the time. Catalyzed by enzymes, big molecules are being broken down by other molecules into smaller molecules, and components of cells are being constantly constructed and transformed. Anything that throws a monkey wrench into that process, altering the structure of a molecule or changing the amount of a certain substance, might compromise the body's ability to detoxify what needs to be detoxified and can throw the whole organism off balance. Needless to say, such an alteration is to be avoided.

There are three main culprits throwing monkey wrenches into our detoxification process—medications, substances let loose into our natural environment, and substances within us. The alterations these three culprits can effect can indeed throw the process off balance and thereby adversely affect our health.

USEFUL CANARIES AND SCARY REACTIONS

To understand why the drugs we take for our health can harm us, we need to remind ourselves of the genetic uniqueness with which each of us comes into the world. Where the detoxification process is concerned, the genetic differences affecting CYP450 enzymes mean that each person detoxifies specific substances in specifically individual ways. Some people show a particular sensitivity to specific toxins; such people can be very useful in alerting the rest of us to possible risk from those toxins, serving the role of the canary in the mine shaft.

As recently as the early twentieth century, no coal miner would head down into the pit unless a canary was brought along. Sensitive to gases like carbon monoxide, the canary served as an early-warning system. If it stopped tweeting and grew ill, that meant that gas was present and it was time to get out of the mine—before the gas sickened or killed the humans working there. People who develop symptoms of toxicity long before the rest of us similarly serve as sentinels of danger, alerting us to the risk of exposure to specific xenobiotics.

Let's go back to Alan and Sue and ask again how it is that Sue can drink eight cups of coffee a day and remain cool, calm, and collected while Alan is aflutter on one cup and would be jumping out of his skin on two. There's a specific CYP450 that detoxifies caffeine preferentially; it's the enzyme that "claims" caffeine. Like all enzymes in the body, its structure has been determined by the message coded for it that was locked into the genome at conception—your genome, my genome, the genomes of Alan and Sue.

Remember SNPs—single nucleotide polymorphisms—from Chapter 2? They're the three million–plus infinitesimal variants that can occur in a single letter in the many-lettered genetic code of the DNA alphabet that makes up the gene. The SNP alteration slightly changes the meaning of the sentence that is the information of that gene, and while most SNPs do not radically affect the function of the body, the effect on the function of an enzyme can be significant—depending upon which letter in the alphabet coding for a specific enzyme gets changed. If you change the third letter in the word "deed" from "e" to "a," for example, that's a significant effect. "Deed" and "dead" are very different from each other.

It's pretty clear that a particular SNP within the CYP450 family of caffeine enzymes in Sue's genome is what lets her sail through the day unperturbed by an amount of the stuff that would leave the great bulk of the population pretty well jazzed. Another single SNP in the CYP450 caffeine family in Alan's genome has him shaking like a leaf on what to Sue would seem a thimbleful of coffee. This makes Alan the canary in the mine for exposure to caffeine; his reaction—that is, the way his CYP450 detoxifies caffeine—alerts us all, except Sue of course, to the potential danger of exposure to this substance.

Can the differences really be that profound—that is, Alan shaking like a leaf on what to Sue would be a thimbleful? Emphatically yes. We know now that the genetic difference in drug detoxification between one person and another can be as much as a thousandfold. That is, the amount of a foreign substance that one individual's physiology could detoxify might need to be a thousand times lower to prevent a toxic reaction in another individual.

Such profound differences have also given rise to the new scientific discipline of pharmacogenomics—the study of how people metabolize certain drugs and the recognition that no one drug fits all. Suppose you're taking two different medications at the same time. We know that both will be detoxified by CYP450, but suppose that both require the same particular CYP450 enzyme for detox. Depending on the uniqueness of your particular SNPs for that CYP450 enzyme, your system could end up with that scramble at the door— that is, the two medications vying for the same CYP450. That might well overload the system and produce an adverse drug reaction—and a spacey feeling and jitters may be the least of it.

Adverse drug reactions have become an increasingly common and increasingly scary health-care phenomenon. It's scary enough to contemplate the estimated 6.7 percent of hospitalized patients who suffer a serious adverse drug reaction to medications that are correctly administered by trained medical professions. It is downright frightening to realize that the most common adverse drug reactions in fact occur from the use of over-the-counter nonsteroidal anti-inflammatories (NSAIDs) or analgesics—especially acetaminophen—used by an estimated 36 million Americans every day without benefit of a doctor's care.* The fact is that an individual's unique genetic makeup is so powerful in shaping his or her detoxification process that you really have no idea what these "simple" over-the-counter drugs may be doing to you.

---

* A number of case reports and well-controlled clinical trials evidenced ADRs between prescription/OTC NSAIDs and alcohol, antihypertensive drugs, methotrexate, and lithium, as well as between frequently prescribed narcotics and other central nervous system depressants.

HOW DETOX WORKS

Why do we need a complicated physiological process to detoxify foreign, hostile substances? Can't our bodies just excrete them directly through the digestive process of elimination via our urine and stool? Can't we just breathe them out or sweat them out?

No. The reason—and therefore the problem—is that many of the most toxic substances behave like fats. Because our blood is principally water and because fats don't dissolve in water, these fatlike toxins tend to stick in the body's fatty regions instead of getting washed out and flushed away. They therefore have to be converted into substances that will dissolve in the blood so they can be transported into the urine and stool and get out of the body. The conversion is a chemical modification that makes the fatlike toxins look less like fats and more like water. That is precisely the first step of the detox process; it renders fatlike toxins into soluble nontoxins, and that is the job done by the CYP450 superfamily of detoxification enzymes. The result of it is a product called an intermediate, which, as its name suggests, is a substance created by one chemical modification and about to be used in another.

That "other" is the second step needed to complete the detox process. This second step is the job of another family of enzymes, also principally found in the liver, called conjugases. If you remember your Latin and the verb *coniugo*, to yoke together, you'll know this is all about joining things. The conjugase enzymes take the intermediate from step one, the now-nontoxic substance, and add a chemical tail to it. There's a huge variety of tails that can be added, but the conjugases will pick the one that is right for the specific intermediate, and the result will be a substance that is able to be transported into the blood and from there into the urine and stool more effectively.

This may seem like a lot more detail than you think you need to know, but here's the punch line: The conjugation reactions depend upon the availability of substances provided through your diet. In other words, specific foods and their nutrients determine or certainly influence the effectiveness of your detoxification process. Compromise the detox process, and a toxic load of substances builds up in the body and poisons your metabolism. Have you ever had a hangover from too much alcohol? It was a result of overloading your detoxification process. You might have been able to stave off the morning-after hangover if you had eaten well the night before and drunk plenty of water along with—or, of course, instead of—the excessive alcohol. You might also have been able to prevent the morning-after effects if you had preceded your consumption of alcohol with the consumption of nutrients known to support alcohol detoxification—sesamin from sesame, magnesium, vitamin B1, vitamin C, coenzyme Q10, and N-aceytlcysteine (NAC). But you didn't take either of those preventive measures, and your overburdened detox process is letting you know it with a headache, nausea, thirst, and a disinclination to look at sunlight.

If you are one of those people with a genetic intolerance of alcohol—that is, your genes don't control the metabolism of alcohol effectively—and if you then consume foods or medications competing for the same CYP450 enzymes as alcohol, drinking could cause you real trouble. I don't mean just a searing headache the next morning; I mean serious health problems. The double whammy of genes and what you ingest can put a real strain on your detox process, with really unfortunate results.

Go back to those adverse drug reactions from common, over-the-counter analgesics like acetaminophen—called paracetamol in much of the world. In the United States, acetaminophen is the source of the most common drug-related toxicity and of more ER visits due to poisoning than any other cause. The toxicity can be especially harsh in people who are taking the drug routinely and in recommended dosages—but while consuming alcohol or eating a poor-quality diet. Here's why.

Step two of detoxifying acetaminophen conjugates the intermediate that results from step one, combining it with a substance called glutathione. You will hear a lot more about glutathione in Chapter 9, but what is important here is that both alcohol and a poor-quality diet deplete the amount of glutathione available in the liver. If you're missing the key ingredient for step two of your detox process and your liver is exposed to a powerful toxin derived from acetaminophen, the detoxification of this powerful toxin is going to be inadequate at best, ineffective at worst. And that's what seems to have happened in the case of many of these people heading to the ER with acetaminophen/paracetamol "poisoning"; the people suffering the reactions were the canaries in the mine for this kind of toxic exposure. Their alcohol intake and/or the foods they typically ingested in their poor-quality diet depleted their liver's supply of glutathione and weakened that organ's ability to detox what they assumed was a simple over-the-counter analgesic.

What do I mean by "poor-quality diet"? In the case of glutathione, important nutrients for its manufacture in the body include the sulfur amino acid cysteine, the amino acid glycine, the trace minerals iron and selenium, vitamin C, and the family of B vitamins. As we'll see, you can get all of those nutrients in foods like garlic, onions, eggs, milk protein, and fish or in supplements.

Figure 3 illustrates all of this in some detail, showing how nutrients influence the process.

FIGURE 3: DETOXIFICATION PROCESS*

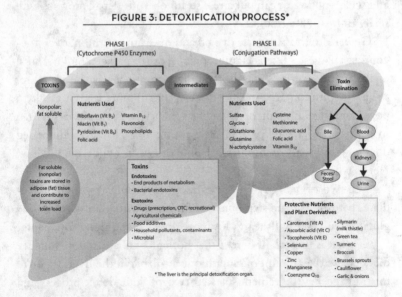

PHASE I
(Cytochrome P450 Enzymes)

PHASE II
(Conjugation Pathways)

TOXINS → Intermediates → Toxin Elimination

Nonpolar: fat soluble

Nutrients Used
Riboflavin (Vit B$_2$)   Vitamin B$_{12}$
Niacin (Vit B$_1$)   Flavonoids
Pyridoxine (Vit B$_6$)   Phospholipids
Folic acid

Nutrients Used
Sulfate   Cysteine
Glycine   Methionine
Glutathione   Glucuronic acid
Glutamine   Folic acid
N-acetylcysteine   Vitamin B$_{12}$

Fat soluble (nonpolar) toxins are stored in adipose (fat) tissue and contribute to increased toxin load

Bile   Blood

Kidneys

Feces/Stool   Urine

Toxins
Endotoxins
· End products of metabolism
· Bacterial endotoxins

Exotoxins
· Drugs (prescription, OTC, recreational)
· Agricultural chemicals
· Food additives
· Household pollutants, contaminants
· Microbial

Protective Nutrients and Plant Derivatives
· Carotenes (Vit A)   · Silymarin (milk thistle)
· Ascorbic acid (Vit C)   · Green tea
· Tocopherols (Vit E)   · Turmeric
· Selenium   · Broccoli
· Copper   · Brussels sprouts
· Zinc   · Cauliflower
· Manganese   · Garlic & onions
· Coenzyme Q$_{10}$

* The liver is the principal detoxification organ.

However you get or fail to get these nutrients, their effect represents an important example of how what we ingest can affect this core physiological process. But it still doesn't adequately explain how and why toxicity is such a common cause of chronic illness. To understand that, we need to go outside.

WHAT RACHEL CARSON TAUGHT ME

Every now and again, someone writes a book that changes the way we think. It reframes the narrative we thought we knew so that we can never again see the world or ourselves in quite the same way. Its impact—culturally, socially, personally—can be enormous. Such a book for me was *Silent Spring* by Rachel Carson, published in 1962 and never out of print. It opened for me, as for millions of readers, a window of understanding into the potentially adverse health effects that low levels of exposure to persistent pesticides—pesticides that don't break down easily into harmless compounds—could have on living organisms.

Carson had earned a graduate degree in zoology and genetics from Johns Hopkins University and in 1937 was working at the Bureau of Fisheries when she concluded that something in the environment was adversely affecting the viability of certain species of fish. Spurred by these observations, she went on for the next twenty-five years to delve deeply into the relationship between pesticide use and living species.

The same year *Silent Spring* was published, its author came to San Diego, California, to deliver a lecture at the local high school on the loss of seabird species due to pesticide accumulation in the birds' fat tissue. I was a senior at that high school, and the lecture changed the course of my life. I decided to study chemistry and environmental sciences and went on to teach both and to make the connection between a healthy population and a healthy environment my lifework. I have always been grateful to Rachel Carson for that.

Carson's work inspired many people and kicked off research all over the world into the kinds of things we do to our natural environment that may prove toxic to living organisms. At first, all we knew was that there was some sort of connection between very low levels of toxic substances—levels far below what traditional toxicologists would define as toxic—and adverse health effects in animals. The first signs of these adverse effects were subtle. They often manifested themselves as changes in an animal's behavior or through an animal showing increased susceptibility to certain diseases. A number of researchers noted that these were the kinds of changes that hinted at alterations in the nervous and immune system functions of the animals.

By the 1980s, a biochemist at the University of Birmingham in England, Dr. Rosemary Waring, researching the relationship between xenobiotic exposure and neurological diseases, had found that animals exposed to low levels of pesticides and other toxic chemicals showed increased incidence of nervous system diseases. Waring later teamed with Dr. Glyn Steventon in the neurology department at the Queen Elizabeth Hospital, also in Birmingham, where for decades the two focused on the effect of long-term exposure to low levels of toxic substances, which can have serious negative influences on human health, often leading to such conditions as Parkinson's and Alzheimer's diseases. Their work demonstrated also that the influence is far greater in those with defective detoxification processes.

The story took another interesting turn in the late 1970s back here in the United States: a group of young men in the Bay Area of northern California presented to their doctors with Parkinson's-like symptoms: tremor, gait disturbance, and postural changes. Parkinson's disease is extremely unusual in younger adults, so this was considered atypical enough to prompt some detailed medical detective work.

One early finding was that the men were all marijuana users. This was at a time when the U.S. government was working with the Mexican government to reduce marijuana trafficking; one of the strategies in their joint effort was to get rid of the stuff at the source by spraying Mexican marijuana fields with the defoliant paraquat. Paraquat, it was learned, degrades under heat—as when a marijuana cigarette is lighted—and is transformed into a powerful neurotoxin called MPTP. Could the exposure to even a low level of MPTP in tainted marijuana have contributed to the Parkinson's-like symptoms? Such a conclusion is in keeping with more recent research showing that such recreational drugs as Ecstasy and even cocaine can contribute to the neurological injuries that lead to Parkinson's and Alzheimer's diseases and possibly even to amyotrophic lateral sclerosis, ALS—Lou Gehrig's disease.

Waring noted the same effect in paint and dye workers, printers, plastics workers, even people working in leather production. Although the level of chemicals they inhaled on the job was below what was traditionally considered toxic, they evidenced a small statistical increase in Parkinson's disease. The level of their exposure, in other words, although low, was enough at least to influence individuals with susceptibility. They were canaries in the mine for these chemicals, as Waring confirmed in evaluating their CYP450 and conjugase activities, which showed one or more detox process inefficiencies.

Some argue that these examples are outliers; they happened only because there was a large exposure to the potential toxin. Yet today, in the era of pharmacogenomics, the truly pertinent question is this: Just how much exposure does it take to present a health risk to a particular individual? In essence, how much exposure constitutes toxicity? That's a difficult question, inviting a far subtler answer than the standard toxicologist's definition of "toxic." For who can say how much exposure *in any single individual* is enough to influence mental state, energy levels, mood, and immune defense? How much is enough to increase the incidence of a disease that takes decades to become serious enough for a diagnosis—a disease like cancer, dementia, heart disease, diabetes, or arthritis? Trying to trace such conditions back to an earlier exposure to low levels of toxins is a little like watching shadow puppets. The exposure may set off movement toward a serious disease, but the effects are not obvious; they take place at the gene and cellular level, unseen and undetected, well before the development of an overt disease.

Yet the twenty-first century is seeing the emergence of just such a scientific discipline—molecular toxicology, the science that Rachel

Carson brought to our attention. Molecular toxicology recognizes that we need to look for different types of toxicity when we are talking about low levels of exposure over the long term. Remember the old saw about the guy looking for his lost keys on the sidewalk under a bright streetlamp? A passerby offers to help and is instructed to look across the street, where it is dark. "If you lost the keys over there," says the passerby, "why are you looking for them over here?"

"Because," answers the guy who lost the keys, "this is the only place where I can see."

If your only definition of a toxic effect is a serious disease that immediately follows exposure to a toxin, then you will never find the keys to understanding the influence of chronic, long-term exposure. You have to look in the shadows—for the molecular toxicity inside the function of cells—to find the keys to the toxicities that lead to chronic illnesses.

THE BPA STORY

It was in the shadows that scientists stumbled upon the story of bisphenol A, a compound common in the environment because it has been used for decades to keep plastics flexible. In fact, it's called a "plasticizer," and you'll find it in water bottles, sports equipment, DVDs, and a range of other commercial products. BPA, as it's known, is a persistent chemical in the environment: it does not break down; rather, it accumulates. Moreover, it concentrates in fats.

BPA was first used in 1957, but even by the 1970s and 1980s, the levels of BPA in the environment remained undetectable by most of the analytical instruments available to measure its presence. The sarcastic maxim, "If you can't measure it, assume it doesn't exist," seemed to be in the ascendant. By the early twenty-first century, however, thanks to significant advances in the technologies for measuring very low levels of chemicals in the environment, BPA was shown to be associated with adverse health effects in certain organisms and in certain environments. Studies were then undertaken to measure the levels of BPA in the urine and fat tissue of humans, and the results showed the presence of levels that had been harmful in other species. The next step was to correlate data on the levels of BPA in children and adults with data on the incidence of certain chronic diseases. The results were shocking.

In 2008, a paper in the prestigious *Journal of the American Medical Association* (*JAMA*) reported on findings from the Peninsula Medical School in Exeter, England, that elevated urinary levels of BPA were associated with the incidence of diabetes in adults. Four years later, a subsequent research paper from Dr. David Melzer's group at the Peninsula College of Medicine and Dentistry, this paper in the journal *Circulation*, reported that elevated urinary levels of BPA in apparently healthy men and women were associated with increased incidence of heart disease. If that weren't enough, Dr. Leonardo Trasande's group at the New York School of Medicine reported that same year in *JAMA* that elevated urinary levels of BPA were strongly associated with obesity in children and adolescents.

Diabetes, heart disease, childhood obesity. Yet what was truly striking about all this varied research was that the level of urinary BPA associated with these health risks was extraordinarily low— so low that it wouldn't even have shown up in the measurements that analysis was capable of taking twenty years previously. In other words, what had not even registered on the radar for nearly five decades of BPA's existence was now demonstrably a potential health threat to humans of all ages.

Why is BPA a threat? It belongs to a large family of chemicals described as endocrine disruptors. The endocrine system is the body's hormonal messaging system, so if it gets disrupted—if messages are altered—the impact on our health can be significant. BPA binds to receptors on cells that the body's natural hormones use to regulate physiological function. In doing so, BPA displaces the natural hormones—basically, knocks them off the receptors and takes their place—and thereby sends different messages to the cells. Moreover, because many of these endocrine-disrupting chemicals are very active, it takes only a very small exposure to create significant changes in health.

This is toxicology on a very basic molecular level, and it is changing the way we think about what is toxic and at what level. You will not be surprised to learn that not everybody is wild about pursuing studies that go this deep. Powerful lobbying forces—namely, the American Chemistry Council, the industry association for chemical manufacturers—worked very hard for many years against a ban on the use of BPA in baby bottles and sippy cups. The ACC relented only when it decided the ban would actually boost consumer confidence in other chemicals. It's a reminder that old perceptions die hard—especially when money is at stake.*

THE "ENEMIES" WITHIN

To the toxins that come from outside our body—the exotoxins that enter us through medications or from substances in the environment—must now be added the endotoxins we produce inside our bodies that disturb the activity of our intestinal bacteria. We know that our enteric microflora perform essential functions that benefit the human organism—functions having to do with energy production, strengthening our immune system, preventing the growth of harmful bacteria, regulating how we store fats, even producing vitamins. So anything we produce that meddles with those functions is going to be potentially harmful.

In a collaborative effort, researchers from my own Functional Medicine Clinical Research Center joined with a remarkable group of investigators at the Catholic University of Leuven in Belgium headed by Professor Nathalie Delzenne and Dr. Patrice Cani to look more closely at this issue. The project explored how alteration of the intestinal bacteria through lifestyle, diet, medications, alcohol, and stress could affect levels of endotoxins in the blood. The project found that since these endotoxins influence the same detoxification

---

* In this regard, I highly recommend the 2007 book by Devra Davis, professor of epidemiology at the University of Pittsburgh, *The Secret History of the War on Cancer*, about the health impact of endocrine-disrupting chemicals and the active efforts of many industrial forces to keep this information suppressed. We'll hear more of Dr. Davis in Chapter 10.

processes as those for the detoxification of exotoxins, the result of increased levels of endotoxins leads to what the group termed a total-load effect. In other words, the researchers concluded that it doesn't matter where the toxins come from. What matters is how big a burden they place on specific participant components in the detoxification process. In a system that is overloaded, toxic substances can slip through the detoxification process, evading certain detox steps and thus adding to the adverse impact on health.

For example, a person with an imbalance in his or her assimilation-elimination process is likely to be more susceptible to the adverse influence of exposure to foreign chemicals and drugs. Yes, on one level, that's simply because the intestinal tract is connected to the liver and what happens in the seat of the assimilation-elimination process, the gut, naturally touches what happens in the seat of the detoxification process, the liver. It is also because the intestinal tract has its own very active detoxification system, located right in the cells of the intestinal lining. That location means that some ingested xenobiotics and potentially toxic by-products derived from intestinal bacteria may start to be detoxified even before they get into the blood.

What do these connections between the assimilation-elimination process and the detoxification process tell us about curing chronic illnesses? They tell us that if we combine the Four R program found in Chapter 4 for intestinal restoration—that is, for managing problems associated with an imbalance in the intestinal microflora—with a detoxification program to manage an imbalance in toxic exposure, we can deal with two major contributors to chronic illness.

DEFINING A DETOX PROGRAM

In the early 1980s, I met a remarkable physician, William Rea, who had been a successful cardiovascular surgeon in Dallas until he became impaired. The impairment was clearly neurological; Dr. Rea's symptoms manifested themselves as a disturbance in his balance and walking ability. He was one of those canaries in the mine shaft, although he didn't yet know it. But he took his impairment very seriously and went hunting for an explanation.

His detective work led him to the hypothesis that his impairment came from a toxic reaction to substances used in the operating room, where he spent most of his working day. In other words, environmental exposures were the cause of his problem. His solution was to make his personal environment as nontoxic as possible—and his symptoms improved dramatically. The experience prompted Rea to establish in 1974 a pioneering environmental medicine clinic to assist patients who suffer from environmental illness. Over the years, he has treated more than thirty thousand patients with varying degrees of such illnesses and has tested and perfected various ways of improving the detoxification process. No wonder in 1988 Dr. Rea was appointed as the first-ever chairman of environmental medicine at the Robens Centre for Public and Environmental Health at the University of Surrey in England.

The Rea program for detoxification follows the principle articulated by Dr. Sidney Baker and reported in Chapter 2: Take away the things that are bad, and replace them with the needed things that are good. This is a wonderful objective, but the devil is in the details. How can we apply it to the individual in need of detox?

Because Dr. Rea often sees the most seriously ill patients, his intervention programs are extremely aggressive; they go beyond what would be required in the case of most chronic illnesses. Patients are tasked rigorously to remove from both home and workplace any and all synthetic materials that might release gases or vapors or contribute residues; that includes all carpeting, paints, and flooring materials. He recommends air and water purification and clothing made only of natural fibers and containing no synthetic materials. He prescribes organic foods only but excludes such common allergy-producing foods as dairy and grain products. No perfumes, colognes, or fragrances. No cell phones; Dr. Rea believes they may cause electromagnetic pollution. In essence, he asks patients to undergo a complete change in lifestyle and environment. If it seems drastic, its results have been dramatic.

Fortunately, for most people with environmentally based chronic illness, the need for change is not nearly so radical. I credit Dr. Jean Monro, a founder of London's Breakspear Hospital, which treats patients ill from environmental exposures, with pointing the way to a kinder, gentler, more temperate detoxification process that can manage mild toxicity problems without requiring a complete change of lifestyle and diet. Dr. Monro is a most remarkable medical doctor; raised in India and medically trained in England, she has a particularly global view of disease and the role that lifestyle and environment play in it.*

I remember meeting one of Dr. Monro's patients, Mia, during a visit to her office several years ago. An advertising executive in her midforties, Mia was a very engaging woman in every way. About a week after returning from a holiday in Spain, she noticed that it was becoming really difficult for her to get out of bed in the morning. Moreover, once she managed to get up and dressed, she unaccountably felt "weak and sore all over," as she put it, and she even thought she experienced a difference in her breathing. When she noticed red patches on her skin, she made an appointment with her doctor.

At first, he thought she might have a form of autoimmune disease like systemic lupus erythematosus—SLE—which is not uncommon in women in their forties and which presents with symptoms like those Mia described. Puzzled, he recommended she see a rheumatologist, and she made an appointment for the following week.

In the meantime, however, a friend at work suggested she see Dr. Monro first. She did so and was curious that Dr. Monro asked about her trip to Spain, questioning her as to whether she had been exposed there to anything unusual. Mia couldn't recall anything that fitted the definition of "unusual" until Dr. Munro asked her whether she had eaten any fried food.

"Oh!" said Mia. "Every day." She had loved the fried seafood at a particular restaurant and had gone there for a meal at least once a day for the entire two weeks of her vacation.

---

* Dr. Monro has been an important contributor to the Functional Medicine Clinical Research Center, adding immeasurably to our understanding of the importance of chronic toxicity as a contributor to illness.

The answer set off bells in Dr. Monro's brain. She knew about the Spanish cooking oil that had been contaminated by an industrial toxin and had been responsible for nearly six hundred deaths in the early 1980s. She put Mia on a strict detoxification diet plan, and within three months, Mia had regained her strength and function—without medication and without hospitalization. She has remained symptom-free ever since.

It sounds simple, yet this outcome and others like it are dramatic evidence of how diet can influence the natural physiological process of detoxification. The evidence was impetus enough for me to want to understand how to develop and apply a diet that would support the body's own detoxification.

One of my first stops along the path to understanding was a visit in 1992 with Dr. Elizabeth Jeffery, a professor at the University of Illinois in the Division of Nutritional Sciences. She and her students have been involved in pioneering work that demonstrates how cruciferous vegetables have a unique ability to promote detoxification. Specifically, these "cross-bearing" plants of the cabbage family—like broccoli, cauliflower, and brussels sprouts (as well as cabbage, of course)—contain specific nutrients called glucosinolates that improve the detoxification function. How? Many of the genes that control the detoxification process are inducible, which means that their function can be turned on and off as a consequence of exposure to specific substances. The glucosinolates in the cruciferous vegetable family are substances that specifically turn on many of the genes that regulate detox. The more of them you consume, therefore, either by eating your vegetables or by taking a food supplement containing the concentrated glucosinolates—such supplements will have names like indole-3 carbinol and sulforaphane—the more powerfully will you activate your detoxification process.

A Rockefeller University professor of biochemistry, Dr. H. Leon Bradlow, has discovered that the same glucosinolates in crucifers that help to detoxify foreign substances also help women safely metabolize and eliminate the estrogen their bodies produce. The basis for that conclusion is Bradlow's finding that the detoxification of estrogen hormones in the body is done by the same CYP450 and conjugase enzymes that are stirred to activity by the glucosinolates in cruciferous vegetables. If you're a woman who may be producing too much estrogen and who, as a consequence, is at risk from your own estrogen for breast cancer, you should know that you can boost your estrogen management with a diet rich in cruciferous vegetables.

Further understanding has come from the work during the 1990s of Dr. Paul Talalay, a physician and the Abel Distinguished Professor of Pharmacology at the Johns Hopkins School of Medicine, who found that the glucosinolate-derived sulforaphane from broccoli and brussels sprouts serves as a protective agent against cancer. How so? Talalay attributes the protective power of sulforaphane to its ability to improve the detoxification of potential cancer-causing substances. The improvement is in the way the sulforaphane talks to genes. Different substances give the genome different messages that turn on the detoxification processes in different and very selective ways. Some food substances affect the CYP450 enzymes; others influence specific conjugation steps. Sulforaphane, says Dr. Talalay, does both; it activates a combination of specific CYP450s and conjugase enzymes that work together to detoxify potential carcinogens. We call phytonutrients like sulforaphane "bifunctional detoxifiers" because they communicate to genes that control both CYP450 and conjugase activities.

Could any of these diet or lifestyle changes work to reduce the amount of BPA that might be stored in our bodies? Over the years, we have actually learned a lot about the specifics of BPA detoxification, and the simple answer to the question is that increasing the dietary intake of soy, kale, cranberry, and green tea as well as of the spices turmeric and rosemary can help eliminate BPA from our bodies. All these foods are known to contain specific substances that increase a particular component of the detoxification process called glucuronidation. In lieu of a detailed explanation, suffice it to say that glucuronidation is a process that makes it easier for intermediates of the metabolic process that relate to BPA detoxification to be transported around the body—and out of it. And that, in turn, is how to eliminate BPA.

Indeed, the scientific explanation of how very specific elements of our diet can influence the detoxification process and help us eliminate toxins is writing a whole new chapter about how what we eat can help us manage chronic illness.

A DETOX DIET?

So if we were looking for the optimal diet plan to support the detoxification process, what would it be? All the signs point to a high intake of vegetables, fruits, beans, and whole grains; moderate consumption of meat, eggs, fish, and dairy products; and low intake of processed foods, fats, and sugars. Such a way of eating is sometimes called an alkaline ash diet. It decreases the production of acid metabolic by-products that may impede the kidneys in their job of eliminating detoxified by-products. Another trick for increasing the elimination of toxins is to consume 1,000 milligrams of potassium citrate in water after each meal; potassium citrate is an alkaline salt, so it too improves the body's acid-alkaline balance.

Here's a list of some other specific foods and beverages that contain phytochemicals known to support the genetic expression that regulates detoxification.

- Green tea, which contains catechins
- Turmeric, which contains curcumin
- Soy, which contains genistein
- Cruciferous vegetables, which contain glucosinolates
- Red grapes and Spanish peanuts, which contain resveratrol (in the skin of the peanuts)
- Watercress and pomegranate, which contain ellagic acid
- Hops, which contain humulones

These foods offer an added benefit: They have a positive influence on the expression of genes that regulate those detoxification processes associated with toxic mineral accumulation. Toxic mineral accumulation is definitely something you do not want.

LEAD, MERCURY, CADMIUM

In 1980, I met a remarkable medical researcher, Dr. Herbert Needleman, at a conference at Harvard University Medical School. Needleman had just published in the *New England Journal of Medicine* an important and highly controversial paper on his work with children in the Boston area; the title of the paper was "Deficits in Psychological and Classroom Performance of Children with Elevated Dentine Lead Levels."

Needleman's study had measured the ability of elementary school children to stay on task—basically, to concentrate. He had then correlated the data with the results of a standard IQ test and with measurements of the level of lead in the children's baby teeth. The results showed a strong correlation between elevated lead levels in the deciduous teeth—baby teeth—and both a lower IQ and lower ability to stay on task. This effect persisted across all socioeconomic backgrounds.

To many people, this conclusion was simply shocking. At the time, lead was everywhere—in gasoline, in the paint that covered the walls of most homes, in batteries, in plumbing, in dozens of common household items. Roadside dust was found to have elevated lead levels, and so was the dirt in school playgrounds.

In a conversation I had with Dr. Needleman twenty-five years after his paper was published, he spoke honestly and feelingly of the extent to which he had underestimated the intensity of the emotional reaction the publication unleashed. He found himself under attack, to put it mildly, by representatives of the industries that use lead in their products. The attacks were not pleasant. The integrity of his research was questioned and his professional bona fides derided. Over time, of course, he was proved right, as the story of what exposure to even low levels of lead can do to brain function in children was confirmed time and again. Today it is recognized that low levels of exposure to mercury and cadmium as well as to lead—from environmental and food sources—can be toxic to the body's nervous, cardiovascular, and immune systems. And they are in us; all three are common environmental contaminants that become more and more concentrated in organisms the higher up the food chain you go.

Against these contaminants, diet is again a factor. Toxic minerals are detoxified not by the CYP450 and conjugase enzyme systems, but rather by a system comprising a family of proteins called metallothioneins. These proteins are genetically programmed to be manufactured within virtually all the cells in the body. Their role is to bind minerals very tightly and to conduct the exit of minerals from the body via elimination in the stool or urine. What stimulates the manufacture of the metallothioneins is pretty much the same set of dietary factors that increase the detoxification of the persistent chemicals that don't break down easily but rather accumulate. We think this shared mode of stimulation is probably due to the fact that both these functions—the genes that control detoxification and those that control the manufacture of metallothionein—sit very close to one another in the genome. It seems likely they would share a mechanism that stimulates their detoxification processes.

What are the foods that put that shared mechanism in motion? Metallothioneins are very high in the sulfur-containing amino acid known as cysteine, which binds minerals very tightly. In fact, this particular kind of binding is called chelation, from a Greek word meaning "clawlike." Metallothioneins containing cysteine almost literally claw lead, mercury, and cadmium out of the body. So proteins with sulfur-rich cysteine—like eggs—as well as sulfur-rich foods like onions, garlic, leeks, and asparagus will spur detoxification. So will foods rich in soluble fiber—like oats, barley, and soy. If you're designing a diet to support detoxification of mineral toxins, these foods are key.

A DETOXIFICATION STORY WITH A HAPPY ENDING

Jennifer was a dental hygienist who suffered serious numbness and tingling in her hands and feet. Her own doctor had ruled out the common causes for her complaints and, unable to find a remedy for her, had referred her to our group to participate in one of our research studies. After similarly ruling out standard diagnoses in their evaluation, our physicians decided to examine the level of mercury in her blood. As a dental professional, could Jennifer have been exposed to enough mercury on the job to create chronic symptoms of toxicity?

Her blood indeed showed a level above the upper limit of acceptable, although not high enough to constitute mercury poisoning. The doctors prescribed a specific, dimercaptosuccinic acid (DMSA), to pull mercury out of her body and release it in the urine, then followed up with a urine test. It showed enough mercury being excreted that it was safe to assume deposits of the mineral were "hidden" in her body.

The doctors put Jennifer on a detoxification program that emphasized the foods high in sulfur including members of the allium family of garlic and onions, eggs, chicken and fish, along with foods that increase the gene expression of the metallothioneins such as grapes with their skins, green tea, zinc, the herb *Andrographis paniculata*, and the phytonutrients curcumin from turmeric and isohumulones from hops, as well as oral capsules of charcoal, which is known to improve the elimination of toxic minerals. They also recommended that she engage in rigorous office hygiene to reduce her exposure to mercury at work.

Progress was slow in the beginning, and there were times that Jennifer felt she would prefer to take a stronger medication approach to her problem. But since she could feel some improvement, she persisted.

First, her fingers, which had seemed to "go to sleep at night," began to feel normal. Within a month, the tingling in her toes and on the soles of her feet had disappeared. Within six months, all of Jennifer's symptoms were gone, and a follow-up blood test indicated that the level of mercury in her blood was now within a low normal range.

Yet there are still people who say there is no such thing as a detoxification diet, and that there is nothing to be done about the signs and symptoms of chronic toxicity. Yes, there are detoxification diets of questionable validity out in the marketplace, but the substance of the process of detoxification and the role of diet in that process are scientifically valid, as is the clinical experience of tens of thousands of patients like Jennifer.

Here's the simple truth of it: an imbalance in the physiological process of detoxification can result in the canary-in-the-mineshaft syndrome, making the individual susceptible to exotoxins and endotoxins that he or she would normally have been able to detoxify and eliminate before they could do harm. Of course, the process intersects with that of assimilation-elimination, which in turn intersects with the core process of defense.

CHAPTER 5 TAKEAWAY

1. Detoxification processes defend the body against exposure to toxins from both the environment and the process of metabolism.
2. Detoxification is genetically controlled and highly individual.
3. The level of toxicity is a result of the total load of exposures to environmental pollutants, dietary contaminants, toxic by-products produced by intestinal bacteria, and substances produced through metabolism.
4. The most common symptoms of toxicity are related to nervous and immune system dysfunction.
5. Children and pregnant women have been found to be particularly susceptible to toxic exposures.
6. Chronic exposure to lead, mercury, and cadmium in the environment has been identified as a significant contributor to toxic symptoms.
7. A program comprising specific steps to reduce exposure to toxins and the use of specific foods and nutrients to eliminate them can improve the detoxification function.

CHAPTER 6

Defense

1. Do you tend to get every cold and flu that goes around?
2. Do you have sore joints that are made worse by modest exercise?
3. Ever get skin rashes of unknown origin?
4. Are you unusually sensitive to the sun?
5. Do your joints swell up?
6. Do you suffer chronic pain in your hands, wrists, ankles, or feet?
7. Is your grip getting weaker?
8. Are you losing muscle?
9. Do you have chronic sinus infections?
10. Are fungal infections like athlete's foot a common occurrence?
11. Do you have frequent bladder or urinary tract infections?
12. Do you have chronic intestinal pain or discomfort?
13. Do you have dental problems associated with periodontal disease?
14. Does it feel to you that your leg or back pain is chronic?
15. Do you take anti-inflammatory medications regularly?
16. Do you frequently take prescribed antibiotics to get over an infection?
17. Have you ever been diagnosed with any of the following

    a Epstein–Barr virus
    b Herpes virus
    c *Candida albicans*

   d Lyme disease (*Borrelia burgdorferi*)
   e A waterborne parasite like *Entamoeba histolytica* or
      cryptosporidium
   f HIV
   g Cytomegalovirus
   h Clostridium

One of the medical doctors on our research team came into my office at the Functional Medicine Clinical Research Center one morning and slapped a newspaper down on my desk. "What do you think of this?" he asked.

"This" was a front-page photograph of two outstretched hands holding sixteen different pills. The caption below the photo identified the person whose hands were pictured as a thirty-eight-year-old mother of three—we'll call her Jane—and it labeled her condition as erythromelalgia, a rare autoimmune disease that periodically causes the ankles and feet or hands and arms to swell, turn red, and become hot to the touch. The condition is so painful that people afflicted with the condition often cannot walk or wear shoes. Jane was unable to stand long enough to prepare meals, couldn't leave the house for any extended period of time, and certainly couldn't wear shoes. The sixteen different pills in the photograph represented the medication regimen she followed to manage her symptoms. The regimen included some very strong painkillers. But Jane was still disabled.

"We can help this woman," my colleague announced emphatically. "Let's see if we can get her into the clinic."

I hesitated. I knew that our research clinic had had no direct experience with this very uncommon autoimmune disease. What made him think we could do something for Jane? "Because," he answered, "our approach has had such tremendous success with other autoimmune diseases like rheumatoid arthritis and lupus. I'm confident it will work here."

By "our approach," he meant the functional medicine approach of a personalized lifestyle program. As he put it to me that day, "At worst it can do no harm, and it has the chance to help her regain some of her lost quality of life."

So began our experience with Jane. She acceded to our request to participate in our clinical research trial, part of a larger study being carried out at the time under the auspices of an independent institutional review board. The trial would evaluate the impact on autoimmune disease of a lifestyle program prescribed on an entirely personalized basis. She would not be asked to change her medication or her traditional treatment regimen; rather, the aim was to assess the influence on her quality of life of a functional medicine treatment program consisting of lifestyle measures personalized for her genetic uniqueness and physiological condition.

Of course, everyone has a lifestyle. Functional medicine understands that lifestyle intersects with the individual's unique genetic legacy to either support good health or contribute to chronic illness—and to influence the outcome of any medical therapy. Prescribing a personalized lifestyle for a patient with a chronic illness will, at the very least, maximize the success of that individual's traditional medical therapy.

Such a program begins, as it did with Jane, by incorporating the diagnostic findings of the patient's traditional-medicine practitioners with a comprehensive patient-centered assessment of her diet, habits and behavior, environment and surroundings, family and personal health histories, and genomic profile. We also carried out a variety of specialized tests to evaluate the functional status of Jane's immune system, endocrine hormonal system, nervous system, and gastrointestinal system.

When the team put all the data together, the findings suggested that some form of foreign exposure was triggering the immune response that underlay Jane's symptoms. The medical literature had no evidence of an environmental trigger for the specific condition of erythromelalgia, but other autoimmune diseases are often triggered by exposure to foreign chemicals, so the next challenge was to determine the specific environmental exposure that might be triggering the response in Jane.

Again, the team started with environmental toxins known to be associated with autoimmune diseases—mercury, certain drugs, specific pesticides, plasticizers, and petrochemical by-products—but came up empty. They finally found a clue in one of the food sensitivity tests administered during the examination phase—namely, an adverse immune reaction to gluten, the common protein in wheat. This seemed slightly odd because Jane showed none of the classic digestive symptoms of gluten sensitivity; that did not necessarily mean, however, that the gluten connection was out of the question. As we saw in Chapter 4, gluten is a family of interrelated proteins found in grains. Each member of the gluten family has its own personality, slightly different from that of the others. So intolerance to different members of the gluten family of proteins can vary from person to person. The team therefore decided that further evaluation was warranted.

More testing confirmed the original finding: Jane's immune system "saw" gluten as a foreigner. That her response was unusual was precisely the point: when Jane's unique immune system confronted what it saw as a foreign protein in her digestive system, it was uniquely activated to respond in its own way, sending a message to the whole body that a foreigner was on board: get ready to do battle.

Yet the team knew that the presence of the foreigner was only part of the answer. It typically takes multiple environmental factors working together to tip a physiological process off balance, so it was essential to explore other factors that might be contributing to Jane's immune imbalance. As we learned in the previous chapter, even small contributors can accumulate into a total load effect that can push the immune system past a certain threshold—the straw that breaks the camel's back—and result in the appearance of an illness. Indeed, the team found that in addition to Jane's unique genetic susceptibility to gluten in her diet, a high intake of other inflammation-stimulating foods—foods containing saturated fats, sugars, and trans fats—an estrogen imbalance, and altered intestinal function all contributed to the aggravation of her erythromelalgia.

The personalized lifestyle medicine program developed for Jane thus focused on diet, eliminating gluten entirely, and recommending specific foods and supplements to rebalance her gastrointestinal function and to boost her estrogen metabolism. The next four months were amazing. Jane's pain and swelling started to subside. Her rheumatologist was able slowly to decrease her multiple medications, eliminating them one by one. Jane had told us she had three wishes for herself—to stand at the kitchen counter long enough to prepare meals for her children, to walk the length of the local shopping mall, and to be able to go outside in the spring and tend her garden. The first two of those wishes came true in those first four months of her personalized lifestyle program. Her kids actually bought her a pair of running shoes and walked *with* her through the mall.

After six months, Jane was taken off virtually all her medication and was reasonably symptom-free. She learned that if she strayed off her program, she could feel the symptoms returning. It was great feedback—sufficient to encourage her continued adherence to her program.

One year after her first visit to the center, Jane returned to present her doctor and nutritionist with a photograph of herself at the end of the hiking trail atop the 4,167-foot Mount Si, near Seattle, Washington. In the photograph, she brandished a sign above her head that thanked both doctor and nutritionist for what she called "the miracle" of her return to health.

If it was a miracle for Jane, it rested on a scientific conclusion derived from our understanding of how the body's physiological process of defense works. The fact remains that because of the immune system's interconnections with the body's other core processes and with the external environment, an imbalance in that system very nearly brought Jane's life to a standstill, adversely affecting her from head to toe. Yet if she is an example of what such an imbalance can do to a life, she also shows us how substantive changes in diet plus a prescribed regimen of supplements can bring the body's process of defense back into balance and cure a disabling chronic illness.

A SIMPLE MATTER OF DEFENSE

True, understanding the immune system is a little like trying to understand particle physics or cosmology: the more you ask about the system, the more it demonstrates its complexity. But science has come a long way in learning how our defense process is influenced by the interactions between our genes and our environment, and that knowledge drives functional medicine's revolutionary approach to the often disabling chronic illnesses that arise from immune system imbalance.

The prevailing view of autoimmune diseases like rheumatoid arthritis, systemic lupus erythematosus (SLE), and multiple sclerosis continues to be that they are inherited genetic conditions that impel the immune system to attack the body. In such a view, some people are simply born with an immune system that sees the rest of the body as a foreigner against which the immune system must mount a defense. What we learned in the genomic revolution, however, doesn't support this characterization.

For one thing, linking specific genes to the entire family of more than eighty different autoimmune diseases just doesn't compute. In fact, we now suspect that the genetics of any specific autoimmune disease can explain only some 30 percent of its origin. The other 70 percent, of course, is in the connection between an individual's genes and his or her environment, diet, and lifestyle.

For another thing, the idea that you're born with a weak or strong constitution and are just stuck with the consequences is genetic determinism all over again. Even without the advances in knowledge in the wake of the genomic revolution, this is pretty obviously not the case. You don't have to be a physician or medical researcher to notice that chronic sinus and intestinal infections can continually alter immune system function. Exposure to drugs, chemicals, and toxic minerals can alter the immune system function. Stress and the hormones that are released during stress can alter immune system function. Activity patterns, exercise, obesity can all alter immune system function. Exposure to sun and other forms of radiation can alter immune system function. And obviously diet and specific nutrients—or their lack—can alter immune system function.

You get my point. Our physiological defense process is in constant communication with how we live, what we eat, and our environment. These factors are continually talking to our immune system, which continually determines whether it is hearing from friend or foe, and which then talks back based on that determination. What we used to think of as immune-related or autoimmune diseases are really functional disorders arising from an altered immune response. And again, what dictates the response is the unique genetic makeup of the individual at its moment of exposure to very specific events or characteristics of the environment.

Remember the celiac disease discussed in Chapter 4? It's a condition in which damage to the small intestine prevents nutrients from being absorbed, and it is associated with a range of digestive symptoms as well as dementia. Celiac is routinely described as an autoimmune disease occurring in genetically predisposed individuals, and it is triggered by gluten, the protein found in wheat, barley, rye, and therefore in many kinds of foods—soups, salads, sauces, cereals, cookies, crackers, and more.

But the relationship between the autoimmune condition and the genetic predisposition works with a certain subtlety, as I've learned from one of the preeminent researchers of the disease, Dr. Alessio Fasano, a pediatric gastroenterologist and director of the Center for Celiac Research at Massachusetts General Hospital and Harvard Medical School. Yes, says Dr. Fasano, there are genes that increase *susceptibility* to celiac, but the individuals carrying those genes in their book of life will not experience the disease unless and until they consume gluten. When they do, the protein, which is well tolerated by most people, can become a toxin; the toxin can trigger a defensive reaction by the immune system, and that reaction produces collateral damage around the body. It's a classic example of the old adage that one man's meat is another man's poison, although in this case it's bread, not meat, that carries the poison—literally.

In the same way, there are autoimmune disorders that result from exposure to specific medications or chemicals in the environment. You probably know someone who cannot tolerate penicillin; you may have a friend who can't go to the theater with you if the show uses a fog machine to create a smoke effect. Each of them has some susceptibility gene that can get defensive in the face of the trigger, and the defense manifests itself as a burning sensation on the skin and a swollen throat if the trigger is penicillin, or as wheezing and teary eyes as the fake fog spreads from the orchestra right up to the balcony.

So the takeaway message vis-à-vis autoimmune diseases is that, with a very, very few exceptions, they are not hardwired in the genes and are thus not inevitable for the person carrying the susceptibility genes. There are indeed important environmental, dietary, and lifestyle triggers that can alter the function of the immune system so that it reacts—even overreacts—and initiates injury to the body itself. But if we alter the environment, diet, and lifestyle behaviors that influence the expression of the genes regulating our immune system processes, we can end, reverse, and avoid the injury.

WHERE IT IS AND HOW IT WORKS

Take a look at the body's defense system, shown here in Figure 4.

As we learned back in Chapter 4, more than half of the body's immune system clusters around the gastrointestinal tract; that is its area of highest concentration. But it also resides in the lymph glands that are distributed throughout the body and are particularly apparent in the armpits, groin, breast, tonsils, and neck. The reason you can say you know you're sick when you have swollen glands in your neck is that the swelling is a result of a spurt of increased activity in the immune system. That spurt indicates that the body is responding to some sort of foreign invasion—or is manifesting a chronic condition.

White cells are the workforce of the immune system, which is divided into two functional units. One unit, the cell-mediated immunity department, is populated by T cells and serves as the immune system's infantry, which is to say that the T cells engage in hand-to-hand combat with foreign invaders. The other unit is the humoral department—the word comes from the old reference to bodily "humors," or fluids; this is the immune system's air force. It launches

FIGURE 4: THE BODY'S DEFENSE PROCESS

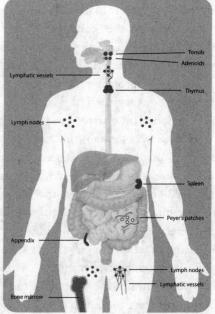

the antibodies that are the system's Patriot missiles. Secreted by specialized cells called B cells within the immune system, the antibodies seek and destroy incoming foreign substances.

It is important to understand that T cells and B cells really do perform two different functions. Our tolerance for things that we may be exposed to across the span of our lives is controlled to a great extent by our B cells, whereas the T cells control our immediate response to a foreigner. Because B cells neutralize toxins by secreting antibodies against them, they have a lot to do with allergic disorders. T cell function, by contrast, defends against viruses, bacteria, and transformed cancer cells.

Armed with these functional units, the system practices what is called immune surveillance, continually patrolling the body looking for enemies to combat. Think of your immune system as a readiness patrol on the lookout at all times for any foreign invaders or attackers.

The patrol has no eyes to see with, but it does have an extraordinarily sensitive sense of touch. Transported by the bloodstream and lymph system around the body, the white blood cells move in and out of tissues and organs. As they do so, they constantly come in contact with other occupants of those tissues and organs. If one of those occupants seems like a foreigner—be it a bacteria, a virus, a transformed human cell, or a foreign chemical or protein—the white blood cells undergo a personality change. They morph from peaceful travelers minding their own business into vigilant warriors ready to do battle.

Once upon a time, it was thought that such constant vigilance and reaction happened only in states of illness. It is now recognized, however, that a low level of immune activity goes on pretty routinely against damaged cells or molecules; this is a good thing, because it keeps those damaged cells or molecules from accumulating in the body and thereby possibly creating disease. It is only when this search-and-destroy function is overly active that we start to see healthy tissues suffering from bystander injury.

But of course, that is always the issue with the defense process (or any physiological process): too much is as bad as too little. The human immune system is a double-edged sword. If it is insufficiently active, we get sick; if it is overly active, we may suffer collateral damage. It must find the resting place that keeps it in balance, that keeps it self-regulating. How do you regulate a double-edged sword? By having the ability to turn it both ways.

Our genes, of course, are the regulators, and that is exactly what they are able to do—modulate the immune system selectively from one edge to the other. The genes assigned to immune system response are on chromosome 6. This chromosome has approximately 2,000 genes out of the total 25,000 in the human code of life; 140 of the 2,000 genes on chromosome 6 constitute what is termed the major histocompatibility complex, the MHC. The MHC genes control the way the white blood cells interact with the various foreign substances or invaders. As they receive, transcribe, and translate the messages they receive from events and factors in the external environment, the MHC genes shift from one sword edge to another. It's not unlike turning the analog dials on a sound system—volume up if the genes sense foreign invaders and need the immune system to be more active, volume down if they sense friends and need to tell the immune system to be less active. They keep turning the dial, shifting the sword, adjusting the system's level of activity in order to find just the right resting place, the immune system's point of perfect balance.

We human beings with reason and willpower have the ability to change, eliminate, or add environmental factors and events sending messages to our gene regulators so that they can turn down a defense process that may be running too hot or turn it up if it has cooled down too far.

And here's something that I find absolutely fascinating and very, very pertinent. Located on the same chromosome 6 are the genes for such autoimmune diseases as rheumatoid arthritis, SLE, celiac disease, ankylosing spondylitis—the "bamboo spine" that typically afflicts young men—and the autoimmune disease known as Hashimoto's thyroiditis, a condition with alternating bouts of hypothyroidism and hyperthyroidism and with symptoms that can affect the entire body. Is it a coincidence that the genes for these diseases are colocalized with the genes that control the function of the immune defense system that triggers these diseases—and that have turned the dial so that one edge of the sword has gone wildly hyperactive? I think not. And neither do many other experts in the fields of autoimmunity and genetics.

The colocation of these genes tells me that in most cases, we are not born with an autoimmune disease. Rather, we are born with genes that sense factors and events in our environment, lifestyle, and diet as either friend or foe and then respond accordingly. If the response is extreme, we call it an immune disease. If the genes that control the immune response sense the exposure as less threatening, then we have intermittent chronic symptoms. Either way, the focus needs to be on the gene-environment intersection.

I can't claim to be the sole or original progenitor of this thinking. When I was working at the Linus Pauling Institute of Science and Medicine in 1982, Pauling recounted an exchange he had had in 1940 with Nobel laureate Karl Landsteiner. Their exchange concerned the function of the immune system and the formation of antibody proteins, the things B cells create to give us long-term immunity. Conceding that he was neither a biologist nor an immunologist, Pauling told Landsteiner that he nevertheless believed that the way immune antibodies work must have something to do with their structure. That night, after the exchange between the two men, Pauling went home and read Dr. Landsteiner's book on the immune system; the next day he sent Landsteiner a sketch of how antibodies might be formed and how they might work as immune agents capable of developing tolerance in us toward substances to which we have never previously been exposed. Pauling's sketch became the classic model from which researchers were eventually able to elucidate the immune defense process in which the antibody binds to a toxin it has perceived, the antigen, forming a complex that initiates the immune response.

Fifty-one years after sketching that model, Dr. Pauling remained convinced that understanding the origin of immune-related diseases was rooted in how the structure of the immune system altered its function when exposed to different environmental factors or events. Now that it has been reported that the third leading cause of premature death in the United States is the burden of autoimmune diseases, it may be time to consider that the eighty different autoimmune diseases may be more similar in origin than we thought, and that the differences derive from a mismatch between an individual's genes and his or her environment.

For most of us, however, the question is a bit more mundane and far simpler: How do we address whatever may be disturbing our core defense process? How do we help the immune system find its resting balance and stay there?

YOUR DEFENSE PROCESS: MODULATING THE IMMUNE SYSTEM FUNCTION

We have long known that a number of specific nutrients play important roles in supporting immune system balance. A deficiency in any of these nutrients can adversely influence the functions of T cells and B cells in the immune system—each in a specific way:

Zinc
Omega-3 fatty acids derived from fish
Vitamin A
B vitamins—especially folic acid
Iron
Copper
Amino acids L-lysine and L-arginine
Vitamins C and E

In addition to these nutrients, a number of plants and plant foods have been recognized as containing active substances that can keep the immune system's thermostat working well. Among these are:

Blueberries
Cranberries
Garlic
Pomegranate
Echinacea purpurea and *Andrographis paniculata*

Let me give you just a few examples of how specific nutrients can influence gene expression to modulate the defense process and keep it in balance. Let me start with one of the most powerful nutrients of all, ascorbic acid or vitamin C.

To begin with, I must confess to some bias on this topic thanks to my association with Dr. Pauling, whose 1970 book, *Vitamin C and the Common Cold*, was an immediate—and continuing—best seller. Simply put, it advanced the idea that vitamin C was needed daily at levels significantly greater than those recommended by the Food and Nutrition Board, the influential food-advisory arm of the Institute of Medicine. The book also argued that in cases of viral infections or illness, the need for vitamin C intake was even higher.

Pauling had refined his thinking on the subject through discussions with Dr. Irwin Stone, the biochemist and chemical engineer credited as the first person to advocate the use of vitamin C as a preservative in food processing. Stone had argued that millions of years ago, when humans lost the ability to make vitamin C in the liver, as most animals do, they began to become increasingly vulnerable to infection and toxins. As the American diet grew more and more top-heavy with animal products and reduced the intake of plant foods, that vulnerability accelerated and expanded. The result? Stone proclaimed the vitamin C intake of most humans in this country simply insufficient for optimal immune function.

How much is sufficient? Dr. Pauling liked to compare humans with goats. The latter, about the same size as humans, produce their own vitamin C, as we humans do not. The vitamin is produced in the goat's liver to the tune of approximately 1,000 milligrams per day per goat under normal circumstances. Under the stress of illness, however, a goat can make as much as 10,000 milligrams per day to meet its increased needs for the nutrient. Dr. Mark Levine, a leading endocrinology researcher, has been exploring the question of recommended daily doses of vitamins for decades.* His research group has found that humans can increase the levels of vitamin C in the blood through daily oral intake up to a point of saturation—in most healthy people, after an intake not exceeding 1,000 milligrams. If the person is ill, however, the turnover of vitamin C is increased, and a bigger oral dose may be required to keep the blood level saturated.

Yet what is the recommended daily allowance that the Food and Nutrition Board suggests? As I write this, the RDA for the average adult nineteen years old or older is 90 milligrams a day for a man and 75 milligrams a day for a woman—more for a pregnant woman, even more for a nursing mother, and much more for a smoker. That's

---

* Dr. Levine is a research endocrinologist at the National Institutes of Health in Bethesda, Maryland, and chief of molecular and clinical nutrition within the Digestive Disease Branch of the NIH.

quite different from the recommendation suggested by Nobel laureate Pauling for optimal immune function and by endocrinology expert Levine to saturate the blood.

The reason for the difference is simple: the RDAs are intended for that elusive average human we've met before; they're based on preventing nutrient deficiency and hedged about with a margin of safety.

It isn't that RDAs are wrong. It's that the Food and Nutrition Board is answering a different question. They're recommending an amount humans need to prevent such nutritional-deficiency diseases as scurvy, beriberi, pellagra, and rickets. For one thing, those are short-latency disorders; that is, it doesn't take that long between the stimulation that sets a disease in motion and the appearance of symptoms. Yet, as Dr. Robert Heaney, one of the nation's foremost nutrition researchers, has pointed out, making a short-term vitamin deficiency disease the marker for establishing daily nutrient intake makes no sense when we know that our most pressing chronic health problems stem from inadequate nutrient intake that dates back years.* For example, although these illnesses remain latent for a long time before becoming evident, we can trace osteoporosis to insufficient vitamin D and calcium, and we know that certain cancers are due to insufficient folic acid intake. Wouldn't greater daily intake make more sense for these long-latency disorders? Shouldn't they be factored into the equation for recommended daily allowance?

There's an even better strategy for determining nutrient intake, and that is a strategy based on the concept of biochemical individuality. My experience over forty years in the field is that vitamin C has a greater impact on immune system function than any other single nutrient. I take 2,000 milligrams per day unless I am sick, in which case I take more.

I well remember a particular lecture about vitamin-deficiency diseases that I attended back when I was a university student in the early 1960s. The lecturer was Casimir Funk, the great Polish

---

* Dr. Robert Heaney is research endocrinologist at the Creighton School of Medicine in Omaha, Nebraska, and recipient of the 2003 E. V. McCollum Award.

biochemist who both "discovered" vitamins, isolating thiamine (vitamin B1) from rice polish in 1912, and named them "vital amines"—vitamins—life-giving chemical compounds in the amine family. Dr. Funk ended the lecture with a stirring peroration about how much there was still to be discovered about the role of vitamins in promoting health. That was in 1963. Now here we are in the twenty-first century, and scientists are learning more every day about how nutrients can influence gene expression and cellular function so that they can be biologically based alternatives to drugs. It's exciting.

Some of this work is taking place at the Jean Mayer Human Nutrition Research Center on Aging at Tufts University outside Boston. One of the extraordinary researchers there is Dr. Simin Meydani. Dr. Meydani is both a nutritionist and a veterinary doctor, as well as the founder of the nutritional immunology laboratory at Tufts. The focus of her pioneering research has been to understand the role of nutrition in the function of the immune system—particularly among the aging. Specifically, her group has delved into the importance of nutritional support in improving the resistance of the elderly to infectious diseases—particularly upper respiratory infections (URIs), which can be a serious medical problem in seniors. Dr. Meydani's group has demonstrated that such nutrients as vitamin E—and a particular form of vitamin E called tocotrienols—as well as omega-3 fatty acids, epigallocatechin gallate (EGCG) from green tea, vitamin D, and mushrooms all play important roles in supporting the immune system's defense against viruses that cause URIs.

I expect that some of these nutrients may be new to you. Tocotrienols, for example, are relatives of vitamin E that are found in high levels in palm oil—and can be obtained as supplements as well. A study of women who took 400 milligrams of tocotrienols daily, following an immunization for tetanus, showed an increased B cell antibody response. Similar results were achieved among older individuals who took tocotrienols along with the other natural forms of vitamin E.

Vitamin D is a nutrient we've known about for a long time, but its story turns out to be far more complex than just preventing rickets, the bone disease that remains a childhood disease in some of the world's poorest countries. In fact, it is now well recognized that vitamin D is not truly a vitamin at all, but rather a pro-hormone. That means it is a kind of precursor of a hormone, with little hormonal effect of its own until it is converted into the hormonal form of vitamin D and amplifies its effect. The conversion takes place through metabolic transformation in the liver and kidney by none other than our old friends from Chapter 5, some members of the CYP450 family of enzymes. The hormonal form of vitamin D that results from the conversion has been identified as a central player in regulating the immune system because of its ability to control the expression of the genes that regulate the system.

As with vitamin C, the RDA for vitamin D—600 international units (IU)—seems low for supporting improved immune function. The medical diagnosis of vitamin D status—that is, figuring out how much you have—happens in a blood test for another hormonal precursor, this one called 25-hydroxyvitamin D3. According to the National Institutes of Health, this value should be greater than 30 nanomoles per liter for proper—that is, healthy—vitamin D status.*

Yet a great many people who consume 600 IU of vitamin D per day are nevertheless below this 30 nmol/L level. At the Functional Medicine Clinical Research Center, the suggested norm was 2,000 IU per day—with a caution. Sometimes, excessive vitamin D intake can lead to elevated calcium levels in the blood, a condition that has been associated with heart disease. So it is important not to jump to the conclusion that if a little bit is good, a lot more is better.

Our institute research team has participated in clinical research on vitamin D with Dr. Michael Holick, one of the world's leaders in vitamin D.† Holick did his doctoral work at the University of Wisconsin under Dr. Hector DeLuca, who discovered vitamin D in

---

* A nanomole is a unit of measurement in chemistry; it is one thousand-millionth of a mole, which in turn is measured in molecules. In other words, we're talking very, very small measures.

† Michael Holick, MD, PhD, is a professor of medicine, physiology, and biophysics at Boston University Medical School.

1968, and the two men collaborated in creating the diagnosis for vitamin D status using 25-hydroxyvitamin D3 in 1973. In Dr. Holick's view, we have reached a point with vitamin D similar to the situation with vitamin C. That is, as a consequence of people spending so much time indoors, not to mention the use of sun-blocking skin creams that decrease the production of vitamin D in the skin, we're no longer getting optimal levels of vitamin D.

According to Holick, there is a substantial difference between the level of vitamin D needed to prevent rickets and the level of vitamin D desirable to promote optimal immune function; the latter goes much higher than the standard guidelines. Holick also points out that the explosion of genetic information now available makes it clear that there are considerable genetic differences among individuals in the way they manufacture and metabolize vitamin D in their bodies—which also means there are considerable differences among individuals in how much vitamin D they need. From my own experience, I would suggest that a person with a known imbalance in his or her defense process should start with a daily supplement of 1,000 IU of vitamin D3. This book's self-assessments for whether or not you might have such an imbalance can be a signal to supplement your defense process, and of course, a health-care provider trained in functional medicine can perform the blood test that DeLuca and Holick devised and interpret it to evaluate your particular need for vitamin D.

Let me give you one final example of a nutritional product that can strengthen your immune system's ability to self-regulate for balance: the mushroom. Right down the road from our Functional Medicine Clinical Research Center in Gig Harbor, Washington, is a world-class mycologist named Paul Stamets. His particular expertise in the field of medicinal mushrooms is without parallel, and he is a passionate advocate of the benefits of mushrooms in supporting the immune system's defensive function.*

What mushrooms bring to the battle is a class of unique substances

---

* Paul Stamets is also the author of the 2005 book *Mycelium Running: How Mushrooms Can Help Save the World*—among other works.

called mucopolysaccharides, which have a specific affinity for sending messages to the T and B cells, which then activate the genes responsible for their function. The National Institutes of Health, to take just one example, has funded clinical studies on the adjunctive effect of specific types of mushrooms in cancer patients and in patients with HIV. For good reason: studies have shown that regular consumption of the common white button mushroom, *Agaricus bisporus*, is associated with reduced incidence of breast cancer. And Dr. Meydani's group at Tufts found that the mucopolysaccharides of white button mushroom concentrate activated natural killer activities as part of cell-mediated T cell action.

"A GOOD DEFENSE IS THE BEST OFFENSE"

So we come full circle back to Jane. Her success was a matter not of luck but of asking the right questions about how her genes were responding to her environment in such a way as to make her body present with the disease erythromelalgia. She worked hard carrying out her personalized functional medicine program; compliance was key in helping her win her battle with her immune system and once again make it her friend.

Now there *are* diseases for which genetic alteration of immune system function is so profound that it is the cause of the disease. They are literally inborn immune diseases; among them are agammaglobulinemia, in which the body does not generate mature B cells; Chediak-Higashi syndrome, afflicting its victims with neuropathy, albinism, and frequent and sometimes fatal infections; congenital IgA deficiency, presenting with a total lack of immunoglobulins; and Wiskott Aldrich syndrome, characterized by skin eruptions and eczema. As a family of congenital immune diseases, however, these represent but a minuscule fraction of the total number of diseases or conditions associated with immune imbalances. For the vast majority of chronic immune problems, the cause is the impact of environmental messages on genetic expression.

The functional medicine approach to these immune system

imbalances focuses on that intersection between genes and environment. Its aim is to modulate the factors of the latter to influence the former so as to return the immune system to its resting place and restore its balance. One reason it can do so is that cells, tissues, and organs—everything within the physiological network—are in constant communication.

CHAPTER 6 TAKEAWAY

1. The immune system controls the defense against both infectious and inflammatory diseases.
2. Various environmental chemicals, some constituents of food such as gluten, certain types of intestinal bacteria, and a number of pharmaceuticals can cause chronic inflammatory diseases.
3. Specific nutrients—for example, vitamins C and D—have been shown to have a strengthening effect on immune defense system function when the nutrients are consumed at levels higher than the recommended dietary allowance.
4. Phytochemicals in certain plant foods and botanical medicines have been shown to reduce chronic inflammatory conditions.
5. A program that integrates changes in lifestyle and diet along with specific nutrient supplementation can be effective in restoring proper immune defense processes.

CHAPTER 7

Cellular Communications

1. Do you suffer from arthritis-like pain or inflammation?
2. Do you have night sweats?
3. Does a change in the weather produce joint pain?
4. Do your joints swell after physical activities?
5. Do you suffer from a feeling of low energy in the morning that takes until noon to overcome?
6. Do the stresses of your life affect your health?
7. Do you feel "wired and tired"?
8. Is your libido low for your age?
9. Are you chronically depressed—and do you feel you shouldn't be?
10. Do you think you're more forgetful than you should be—and does that concern you?
11. Is it difficult to get to sleep? To stay asleep?
12. Do you have chronic infections of the sinuses, tonsils, intestines, skin, or mouth?
13. Do you routinely take anti-inflammatory medications, either over-the-counter or by prescription?
14. Are you on blood pressure medication?
15. Do you take antidepressants?

Say wha'?

Ever been involved in a conversation in which something or other keeps you from communicating? Of course you have. We all have.

The technical process of communication just gets interrupted. There you are, walking along the sidewalk with your friend—let's call him Bill—and he has something to say. That means that his voice vibrates the air in a very specific pattern that you pick up through your receiver—namely, your eardrum and the sensitive parts of your inner ear. That receiver mechanism translates the movement of air Bill stirred up into a signal in your nervous system, and your brain translates the signal into a meaning you instantly apprehend.

Unless a car blaring its radio passes by in the middle of the process and you miss the last half of what Bill is saying. Or unless your brain is suddenly distracted by a guy on Rollerblades barreling toward you along the sidewalk and your attention focuses on that. Bill sees the guy too and raises his voice, increasing the intensity of the signal he's sending to get your attention back on him. And it works.

But just as you're ready to answer Bill, a bus lumbers along in the street beside you, and you have to raise your voice. And as cars honk and riders pour out of the bus and start talking on their cell phones, the ambient noise gets louder, and pretty soon you and Bill are yelling at the top of your lungs just to have a conversation.

In principle, much the same thing happens when one cell of the body wants to communicate with another. It sends a message—not by stirring the air, obviously, but in the form of a chemical substance or an electrical impulse through the nerves. There is a huge range of such messenger chemicals—hormones, neurotransmitters, inflammatory mediators, and more; think of them as different little language structures the cells can choose from to communicate with one another. They all carry the message through the bloodstream to the receptor on the cell for which the message is intended, and the receptor translates the signal just as your brain translated what Bill had to say.

And by the same token, just as your brain cut out when there was too much other noise to hear, cell receptors sometimes don't get the message either. Physiologists call it resistance; the receptor can't hear or isn't listening. Then the messengers must, like Bill, intensify the content of their message—only they do it by sending more of the messenger chemical. The problem is that increasing the number of messenger chemicals may actually increase the resistance to the message—the equivalent of you and Bill yelling at the top of your lungs. Even worse, it can begin to damage other parts of the body.

What happens when two people have to shout to hear one another? The din becomes painful, and people around cover their ears. This result is mirrored, metaphorically, in cellular communications. One of the central realities of chronic illness is a cellular messaging system locked into a shouting match, an alarm state of communication that causes persistent collateral damage to innocent bystander cells.

In this chapter, we'll learn how the cellular communications process works and why tipping the balance into a shouting match underlies virtually every chronic illness. What can redress the balance? Follow along with Figure 5. We'll follow the path from the vegetable garden and the

FIGURE 5: THE HORMONAL COMMUNICATION PROCESS

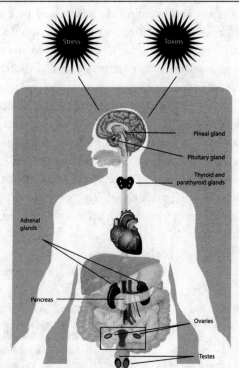

fruit orchard to the very core of your genome, so you can see how some important compounds in fruits and vegetables can influence your cellular communications balance and keep you free of chronic disease.

STRESSED OUT

First of all, it's essential to realize that our cells are communicating with one another all the time. Remember that our bodies are teeming factories of chemical reactions, which are stimulated by the messages of the cellular communications system, going on around the clock, whether we wake or sleep. These messages, signals, alerts, and in many cases alarms are what maintain the dynamic tension between inside and outside our bodies. Cellular communications sustain the interdependence of the core physiological processes and keep the human organism that is us in balance. The word for it is homeostasis, a kind of perfect equilibrium that is sustained precisely through constant messaging and adjusting, signal and response, alterations, rearrangements, corrections, repairs, renewals, and change.

The scientist who really turbocharged our clinical understanding of how the cellular communications process may get out of balance was Dr. Hans Selye, the world-renowned endocrinologist who coined the term "stress" to describe the physiological response of animals to a change in their environment. As we noted back in Chapter 2, the term has since become the most widely used English word in medicine and physiology. It's pretty pervasive in daily speech as well, probably because Selye's book, *The Stress of Life*, published in 1956, became an instant classic and has been reprinted in virtually every major language.[*]

Basically, it's all about the fight-or-flight response; simply put, here's what happens. Under conditions that an individual perceives

---

[*] Selye's work has prompted tens of thousands of other investigations in laboratories around the world, as scientists deepen our understanding of stress and disease. I note particularly Dr. Robert Sapolsky at Stanford University and Dr. Bruce McEwen at Rockefeller University, both of whom have contributed significantly to the incorporation of stress physiology into the functional medicine operating system.

as threatening and therefore stressful, the cellular communication system swings into action in all its locations: in the brain and in the hypothalamus within the brain, in the thyroid gland, in the adrenal glands that reside on your kidneys, and in your sex glands—ovaries in women and testes in men. Once activated, the system begins releasing the chemical messengers adrenaline and noradrenaline, which stimulate further message activity in numerous other cells.

All this responding to stressors is called allostasis, a concept developed by renowned stress researcher Dr. Bruce McEwen.* The term refers to that process by which the human organism makes adjustments and effects change precisely in order to regain the stability of homeostasis. In response to each of these stressor messages, your organism either fights or flees, either combats the stress or runs from it.

Fight-or-flight is a basic response mechanism. It helps us humans escape from danger or do things that seem beyond our normal capability; the classic example is of a mother lifting a car under which one of her children was pinned. And to the extent that our system is resilient enough to let us recover from its effects, it is a very important mechanism.

What Selye learned from his extensive studies on more than 15,000 animals, however, is that continual reliance on the fight-or-flight system to cope with daily life produces a resistance to the message; the body hears the message so much it stops listening. He termed it "adaptation," and he tracked the sequence of events in the clinical process he dubbed the general adaptation syndrome (GAS).

First comes arousal as the communication system is activated and adrenaline and other stress hormones are released. You feel a nervous tension. Your mind races, your muscles tighten, you're on adrenaline overload.

But after repeated instances of arousal in response to stress, the receptors on the stress hormone cells resist the message—they've heard it too often, and you fail to feel the jittery tenseness from

---

* Bruce S. McEwen, PhD, Alfred E. Mirsky Professor, is head of the Harold and Margaret Milliken Hatch Laboratory of Neuroendocrinology at the Rockefeller University.

high adrenaline that the threat may actually warrant. That is called allostatic load—the cumulative effect of too many responses.* It now takes a much higher level of chemical messengers to get the threat message through these now-resistant receptors, but that can be costly. Remember that too much of anything in the body can be toxic, and that is the case here. Higher levels of these messengers producing heavier allostatic load can have damaging effects on a whole bunch of innocent-bystander organs: the brain, heart, and blood vessels, your digestive system, your bones, skin, muscles, and kidneys. And these damaging effects often manifest themselves in the form of chronic illness. These effects are due to the production of stress-related substances in the body that are friends at low levels, but at high levels of exposure for a long time they become toxic to cells. This once again reminds us that we shouldn't put labels on substances in our body, saying some are good and others are bad. Everything produced by the body can be either good or bad. It is all about amounts and balance. Too much of anything, including air and water, can be toxic.

What you feel now is disturbance manifesting itself as chronic sleep problems, mood swings, fatigue, inability to concentrate, worry over impending concerns in your life. The levels of fats and sugar in your blood rise too high, and you're probably in chronic pain.

Finally, you reach a point of exhaustion. The still rising allostatic load has tipped the balance; it now overwhelms your body's ability to produce stress hormones. Your communication system is unable to get back into balance, while the control mechanism that keeps trying for homeostasis is simply depleted. In some people, the result is what used to be called a nervous breakdown; today, we just call it burnout. In the third stage of the general adaptation syndrome, in other words, people just run out of GAS.

Because the body's organs are so closely interconnected through the chemical communication system, however, when the system runs out of GAS, all sorts of other organs feel adverse effects. People

---

* See Bruce McEwen's book, *The End of Stress as We Know It*, for more on allostatic load.

often complain of low thyroid function. Women feel the loss of estrogen; studies of women going through menopause show that those under high allostatic load suffer more night sweats, hot flashes, sleep disturbances, mood swings, and depression than do women with a lower allostatic load.

Men suffer equivalently. Surely you've seen the rash of advertisements for testosterone-replacement medications for men with "low T." It's true enough that men who are going through the climacteric—hormonal changes similar to those experienced by menopausal women—experience worse loss of energy and muscle mass, a greater feeling of weakness, and more severe mood swings as a consequence of high allostatic load. Of course, the testosterone-replacement medications will treat only the symptoms of the general adaptation syndrome, which is precisely what this is, rather than addressing the cause of the syndrome—the imbalance in the core process of cellular communication.

Nor is it solely the feeling that the body really is running out of GAS. Dementia, heart attack and stroke, ulcers and inflammatory bowel disease, osteoporosis from bone loss, muscle loss, high blood pressure, diabetes, and chronic kidney disease are among the end products of the imbalance in cellular communications.

BEYOND THE STRESS RESPONSE

Yet the stress response, GAS, and the allostatic load are only the start of our understanding of how imbalance in cellular communications causes chronic illness. Emergent science has found the origin of many chronic diseases in the way the imbalance alters the body's regulation of inflammation. Some scientists—notably physicians Paul Ridker and Peter Libby of Boston's Brigham and Women's Hospital and Harvard Medical School—have suggested that chronic inflammation associated with the alteration of cellular communication is a hallmark of most chronic diseases.

Ridker and his research group pioneered the identification of a substance produced by the liver that is a messenger of inflammation.

It is called high-sensitivity C-reactive protein, or hs-CRP. The level of hs-CRP in the blood has been found to be a biomarker indicating a shift in the balance of cellular communication toward chronic inflammation. Levels of this blood biomarker above 2 milligrams per 100 milliliters of blood are also associated with an increased risk of heart disease, early stages of arthritis, obesity, and type 2 diabetes. Imbalance in the cellular communications process to inflammation to disease: the links are there.

Peter Libby's group has found that chronic states of inflammation are associated with alteration in a number of substances that control cellular communication. These substances as a group are called cytokines, although they also have such individual names as interleukin 1, interleukin 6, and tumor necrosis factor alpha, and they are created by genes of cells within the immune system. Something in the environment activates these genes in the immune system; the genes control the production of cytokines; the cytokines control the communication of inflammation among organs. Once the cytokines are released into the bloodstream, that triggers a cascading release of other substances that control specific types of inflammation in specific parts of the body.

That's how and why inflammation doesn't stay isolated in one organ even though the symptoms—pain, redness, and swelling—might be seen in just one place in the body. Nevertheless, the inflammation messengers are zipping through the bloodstream, exerting their personality all over the body. Chronic inflammation is thus a systemic issue.*

But even systemic inflammation is a factor in chronic illness only when it is off balance, when something has altered the communication

---

* Not so with acute inflammation. That's usually the result of an injury, and the inflammation stays there. If you get a scrape on your arm, for example, the reddening of the skin as blood and fluids rush to the site remains local, and it eventually subsides as the skin heals. If you get shin splints from too much jogging, that's the only place where you hurt—so long as you stay off the running track. On the other hand, if you resume the exercise before the injury is truly healed, the acute local inflammation can indeed turn chronic and influence function throughout the body.

process that regulates it. Otherwise, the inflammation mechanism is an important part of healing—essential for the maintenance of health. Suppress that process, as many medications do, and you may also be turning off the body's normal repair processes and unbalancing the healthy level of inflammation needed to prevent both infection and chronic illness.

THE NSAIDs ISSUE

A great deal has been written about the most common medications used to influence inflammation—nonsteroidal anti-inflammatory drugs, NSAIDs. They include aspirin, ibuprofen, indomethacin, and ketoprofen among others, and we take them for all sorts of ailments. Have a headache? Pop a pair of aspirins. Muscle pain? Whether it's from tennis elbow or Parkinson's, take ibuprofen. Gout, arthritis, fever, menstrual pain: NSAIDs are nonnarcotic and nonaddictive, and they relieve your pain.

They work by blocking one of the cellular communication processes associated with inflammation; this particular process is one that stirs increased activity of the enzyme in cells called cyclooxygenase, or COX. The resulting enzyme reaction converts one substance into another substance that amplifies the inflammation process, just like the amplifier in your sound system. If the inflammation messenger hs-CRP hits a certain level in your bloodstream, it means that COX activity is working overtime—your natural defense or self-healing mechanism is in high gear. Actually, there are two forms of COX. COX-1 helps maintain healthy function and keeps the inflammation process in balance; COX-2 is turned on selectively anytime an inflammation response is activated.

Most NSAIDs block both. That means even if you are taking the NSAID for a temporary acute ailment, you are nevertheless blocking the good features of COX-1. Do it often enough, and you may be setting yourself up for such predicaments as ulcers, kidney problems, and heart disease. Since more than 100,000 people per year are brought to a hospital emergency room with internal bleeding due to

NSAID overuse, and since more than 10,000 die each year from this cause, we can say with some certainty that way too many of us are taking way too many NSAIDs way too often.

What can we do about this? How can we relieve pain and let the body manage the inflammation process in its own way? To find the answer, we need to dig still deeper into how that process works.

Keep in mind that the process of inflammation is initiated when something somewhere triggers an alarm reaction in the immune system. It is not unlike what happens when exposure to stress activates the release of stress hormones. In the case of stress, however, the hormone messengers are released by the endocrine system; in the case of inflammation, the cellular communication messengers, the cytokines, are released by the immune system.

They then travel in the bloodstream to receptors on the surface of cells. The surface receptors pick up the inflammation signal and transfer the message through the cellular membrane to the inside of the cell. This triggers a process called intercellular signal transduction—basically, converting a signal from outside the cell into a set of responses inside the cell.

It happens like a relay race within the cell. When the surface receptors push the inflammation signal through the cellular membrane, the gun goes off, and runner after runner—substances known as kinases—carries the signal deeper and deeper into the cell, each kinase handing off the message to the next kinase. The kinase-messenger for the anchor leg of the relay—the final leg—is a substance called nuclear factor kappa beta. NF-kB carries the inflammation signal smack-dab into the nucleus of the cell where the genome resides, and it crosses the finish line when it gains access to the coding in your book of life that controls the production of inflammation communication agents. That's when it activates the cell's gene expression, and the message of inflammation is sent out globally throughout the body.

The whole relay-race process of signal transduction is very carefully controlled within the cell because maintaining a balance of inflammation is so important for health. Each kinase-runner in the race is controlled by a specific gene, and each of these genes is unique to the individual. So here it is once again: response to the environment by the cellular communication system is absolutely individualized. That's key because it is in the gene expression part of the process that inflammation is regulated—by turning on or off the release of NF-kB, by letting it go or preventing it from going.

Yet NSAIDs work by blocking the final action of signal transduction—the action of one of the last substances that create inflammation—thus stepping right into the middle of the individual's natural process of controlling inflammation. Whereas the body controls inflammation upstream of gene expression, anti-inflammatory drugs control inflammation at the symptom level downstream of the genetic regulatory process. In a sense, the anti-inflammatory drugs hijack the process by which inflammation messaging is so intricately controlled.

PHYTONUTRIENTS AND THEIR EFFECT

Back in 2002, our functional medicine research group took a look at how the body manages the control of cellular information messaging so that we could perhaps find a way to regulate it at the point of genetic expression rather than downstream in blockading COX. The idea was to maintain the proper balance of inflammation and anti-inflammation control while reducing the risk of the adverse side effects seen with NSAIDs. We felt, to put it very simply, that this was a case where nature knew best and where we should try to find a way to mimic nature's grand design.

We initiated our first screening studies in 2003. The objective was to determine whether certain natural substances could mimic the natural inflammation process. It was what is called a high-risk research project, meaning that we had absolutely no idea if the screening could work at all.

The question for each substance we screened was whether it worked as a traditional NSAID by blocking COX-1 and COX-2, or whether it worked upstream by influencing the way the inflammatory signal influenced gene expression. We started with natural substances that had a history of use by various cultures for anti-inflammatory effects; among these were ginger, frankincense (*Boswellia serrata*), and curcumin from the spice turmeric. The results of the study were revealing—and fascinating. Some of the nearly three hundred natural substances we analyzed did indeed exert their mild anti-inflammatory activity by blocking COX-1 and COX-2; they worked like NSAIDs. Another group, however, did not block COX directly but rather controlled the expression of genes that regulate the production of the inflammatory mediators; they mimicked nature's design.

The surprise of the study—its real revelation—was that the best in class of all the natural substances screened was a family of compounds called isohumulones derived from hops. The anti-inflammatory activity of the hops concentrate containing the isohumulones was significantly higher than that of the natural products that blocked COX-1 and COX-2.

Did this mean we should all just go out and drink as much beer as possible to control any inflammation? Not quite. Instead, the finding spurred further research, and it produced what I believe to have been the most significant discovery of my forty years in scientific research. It came about thanks to the scientific intuition of my colleague Dr. Matthew Tripp, at the time the vice president of research and development at MetaProteomics, at whose lab the research was proceeding. Matt is a cellular biologist who, while working on the control of gene expression decades before, had made discoveries that contributed to the recognition of what was then a major new family of regulatory substances in cells—our friends, the kinases, the runners on the relay race team for signal transduction. More than 300 kinases have now been discovered; they control how chemical messengers outside the cell can speak to the genes inside and regulate gene expression. So that kind of gives you an idea of where Matt Tripp's head is.

On this particular day, Matt walked into my office and set a colored chart down on my desk. He didn't say anything, just stood there to see how I would react. So I leaned over and took a good hard look at the data on the chart. And what I saw there hit me like a ton of bricks: I was looking at a representation of how specific substances in plants—called phytonutrients—selectively influence the way substances outside the cell can communicate with specific regions of the genome. To me, it was like having a private audience with God.

What was so stunning about the data on the chart? First, let's back up for a second to understand what phytonutrients are and do. They are chemical compounds in plants—*phyto* is Greek for plant—that react and interact. They evolved to become the protective capacity of the plant world. After all, a plant cannot run away and hide from sun, pests, mold, or blight, so it must produce substances that defend it from its own hazardous environment—and by the way that also give fruits and vegetables their color, fragrance, and taste.

Many phytonutrients are not well absorbed by cells—that is, they do not pass through the cellular membrane; yet the data showed clearly they could selectively affect cellular function. How? Matthew Tripp's chart suggested that they bind to specific receptors on the cell surface, then translate their message into the cell via the kinase network, which takes specific information in the message to the appropriate specific regions in your genome to be read or expressed by your genes. Since different plants have different phytonutrients, they influence the kinase network in different ways.

It means that different plant foods—as well as the botanical medicines derived from plants—can influence cellular function in different ways based on how they modulate the kinase network. And thus we humans eating those plant foods can reap the benefits of a range of protective capabilities built into the plants through evolution. That was the great discovery of 2005, the most significant scientific discovery in which I have been personally involved. As scientists do, we of course gave a name to this effect—selective kinase response modulation—and called the phytonutrients that produce the effect SKRMs, selective kinase response modulators.

Since then, numerous other researchers have confirmed the SKRM influence of specific phytonutrients in such plant foods as licorice, green tea, red grape skins, cranberries, pomegranate, and blueberries, to take just a few examples. And the many publications from scientists in Matt Tripp's team of PhDs and MDs* have expanded our knowledge and understanding of the potentially important role that these SKRMs play in balancing cellular communication—and in designing a personalized program to address an imbalance in the core process of communication.

THE KINASE NETWORK: COMPLEXITY AND DIVERSITY

That deeper understanding of the kinase network showed how very complex it is—a network of many interacting components. There isn't just a single route a signal travels from the cell surface to the genome; rather, there are numerous intersecting routes. But there is a purpose to that complexity; it answers nature's compelling interest in stability. The more complex a system needs to be to do its job, the greater the diversity of pathways and methods for getting it done, and the less vulnerable it will therefore be to catastrophe. Diversity means stability. This is true inside a cell, and it is mirrored in the environment at large.

Have you ever been in a rain forest? From forest floor to the top of the canopy, it swarms with species diversity—plants, flowers, epiphytes, trees of every sort, and animals ranging from the tiniest insects to the biggest predators, from beetles and butterflies to amphibians and reptiles, from birds of every size and shape and color to mammals of nearly every description. If one organism in the rain forest's ecological system becomes extinct, that's sad, but the rain forest can still survive because it contains so many other organisms that can fill the functional niche left by the extinct organism.

Now go stand in a cornfield. There is no diversity at all; one species of plant stretches as far as the eye can see on the prairie of Iowa or the sandy flatlands of New Jersey. If a pest or disease attacks the

---

* Robert Lerman, MD, PhD; Joseph Lamb, MD; Jacob Kornberg, MD; Veera Konda, PhD; Anu Desai, PhD; Gary Darland, PhD; Brian Carroll, PhD; Deanna Minich, PhD; and Jan Urban, PhD.

corn, the whole ecosystem is in jeopardy, and the entire crop may be doomed. That is why farmers turn to pesticides, herbicides, and other plant drugs. These synthetic killers of pests and disease compensate for the absence of diversity and protect against the instability that is a result of that absence of diversity.

Diversity means stability in human physiology too. The heart rhythm of a trained athlete is much more complex—has far greater diversity of resources—than that of a sedentary couch potato. In fact, the simplest heart rhythms are in people with heart disease. The sicker the heart becomes, the more it loses complexity; the less complexity it has, the more unstable it becomes in the face of any changes in the person's environment; it lacks the diverse resources that might be able to adapt to or defy such changes. As people go from a state of wellness to that of disease, the complexity of their physiological system continues to decline until, in an end-stage disease state, just a few of the critical characteristics that support basic physiology remain. If one of these is jeopardized, the person probably dies; more than one and death is certain.

All of which is simply to emphasize that the complexity of the kinase network, the network that controls communication within the cell, is essential to its ability to fine-tune its translation of the messages coming in from outside and headed for the genome. Families of kinases work together within the cell to regulate that translation. They do it through a rich and highly diverse vocabulary that allows for very precise communication to the genes. Such precision is what provides physiological resilience in the face of changing environmental situations.

We spoke earlier of resilience vis-à-vis recovering from the fight-or-flight response to stress, and how a failure of resilience signaled adaptation to stress and an imbalance in the cellular communication process. Lowered resilience is also associated with diminished organ reserve and an increased biological age, so it is a key factor in our health or lack of health. It is here at the cellular level that resilience is created—in the highly intricate communications along the kinase network. The functional state of that network is therefore essential to human health.

And indeed it has been found that in severe diseases like cancer, the cause may be that a gene for a specific kinase has become damaged or has mutated. That single change to one single kinase in the regulatory network is then capable of changing the physiology of the cell from normal to cancerous.

As I write this, addressing that change has become the breakthrough thrust of cancer research and cancer treatment. The technology is straightforward: A genetic analysis of the genome of the cancer cell can diagnose the presence of a rogue kinase. A specific kinase-inhibiting drug can then be administered, tailored to that rogue kinase in that patient. There are now genomic diagnostic laboratories at virtually every major cancer treatment center in the country, and the newer cancer drugs now being developed are specific inhibitors of mutated kinases that have gone rogue. Meanwhile, research in this area is advancing rapidly at the Van Andel Institute in Grand Rapids, Michigan, at the Broad Institute in Cambridge, Massachusetts, and in many other academic and commercial cancer laboratories. It represents the increasing application of personalized medicine in the treatment of acute diseases.

SKRMs AND HUMAN HEALTH

Once our research group understood how the natural phytonutrients in food substances could influence the kinase network, we began to look at whether specific phytonutrients could influence a specific family of kinases. The answer was that they did not affect any one kinase in their kinase family as strongly as a kinase-inhibiting drug could; rather, the phytonutrients influenced many kinases in the family, and the influence was mild, not dramatic as with the drug. In the language of traditional pharmacology, the bioactive agents in the phytonutrients qualified as low-potency "dirty drugs," meaning they didn't have the level of pinpoint control of a kinase that a good drug could achieve.

We wondered why evolution should have favored the development of such a response to these bioactive agents in food—namely, a response that altered many kinases within a family, and did so mildly. The answer seemed obvious: if the bioactive agents in our food produced a druglike effect, then every meal and snack would jolt our physiology, changing it dramatically and pushing and pulling our cellular functioning up and down like a yo-yo. The fact that the phytonutrients in our food speak to our genes more gently and quietly, unraveling the needed information and parceling it out to the genes at different locations around the regulatory network, provides the stability of cellular function we equate with resilience—and therefore with good health.

It's a different effect from that of vitamins; their absence from our diet can result in nutrient-deficiency diseases. Instead, the effects of phytonutrients are more subtle and more intricate as they control how our genes respond to environmental changes. Remember that these are chemicals the plants produce to defend themselves against the stresses of their hostile environment. We know for a fact that the greater the stress on them, the more phytonutrients plants manufacture. It's one reason why organic fruits and vegetables are considered preferable to nonorganic. Since organic farmers eschew pesticides or herbicides or any other plant medicines, organic plants are forced to defend themselves more vigorously from environmental threats. Hence they produce more phytonutrients. When we humans consume the food of plants, these antistress agents go to work for us, in their converted form as messengers to our genes, to increase our physiological resilience.

So the next question was whether the SKRM effect from particular foods had any clinical value in improving cellular function in humans and diminishing the symptoms of chronic illness. Our first clinical proof-of-concept studies, as they are called, were performed at the Functional Medicine Clinical Research Center.* From 2005 through 2012, a series of human clinical trials evaluated the influence of specific isohumulone phytonutrients derived from hops on such inflammatory disorders as osteoarthritis and degenerative joint disease, two of the most common conditions treated with NSAIDs. (As

---

* The studies were performed under the medical direction of Joseph Lamb, MD; Robert Lerman, PhD; Jack Kornberg, MD; Daniel Lukaczer, ND; Barbara Schiltz, RN, MS; and Lincoln Bouillon, MS, MBA.

is standard with all clinical trials using human participants, an out-side institutional review board examined and approved all protocols of these trials for safety and scientific rigor.)

The studies concluded that the SKRM-capable phytonutrients played a clinically important role in reducing the pain and inflam-mation of osteoarthritis *and* were found to be safe for the digestive tract, kidneys, and blood vessels. In other words, we had shown that nature's intelligence was built into these substances. In the study par-ticipants with osteoarthritis, we observed declines in the biomarkers of inflammation in those taking the SKRM phytonutrients versus those consuming a placebo. But the study made it clear that these phytonutrients are not potent inhibitors of COX like the NSAIDs.

The bottom line? The studies confirmed that there are substances in certain foods that send messages to our genes through the in-fluence of the kinase regulatory network, and that these messages control the production and release of inflammatory mediators. Food really is information for our genes, and its role in modulating the ex-pression of genes associated with inflammation has a clear and certain effect on our physiological resilience and our overall health.

WHAT FOOD PROCESSING DOES TO PHYTONUTRIENTS

That is precisely why food processing can be so harmful to our health, for one of its core purposes is to remove phytonutrients from the products. Why? Phytonutrients often impart a bitter taste; remember, they are a plant's stress fighters, and they "bite." To the food industry, there is therefore a flavor advantage in removing them. Indeed, the phytonutrient index defining the amount of phytonutrients present in the diet makes it clear that the more processed food a person con-sumes, the more his or her phytonutrient index declines.*

By contrast, high phytonutrient indexes are the norm among

---

* Created by Heather Vincent, PhD, and her research group at the University of Florida at Gainesville.

populations in which chronic diseases least frequently occur. In blue zones like our island of Ikaria, Costa Rica, Sardinia, Okinawa, and Loma Linda, California, all places where people live longer, healthier lives, the population consumes many more vegetable products in their diets.

I know what you're thinking: Loma Linda? Right smack in the middle of San Bernardino County? The city with a defense plant that has leached chemicals into the water and westerly winds bringing pollutants from Los Angeles? A place you'd expect would share the disease patterns of all the other populations in the region? *That* Loma Linda?

None other—for the reason that Loma Linda is home to a large population of Seventh-Day Adventists who follow a vegetarian diet rich in nuts and beans *and* are kosher, eschewing certain foods they deem "unclean." They also do not smoke, drink alcohol, or do drugs, and they scrupulously observe their Sabbath day of rest. Even though the Loma Linda Adventists represent diverse genetic backgrounds, these practices are enough to make their city stand out statistically for greater longevity *despite* the polluted air and water. And it demonstrates once again that it isn't our genes that determine our life span and life's health, but rather how we communicate with our genes.

Processed foods have very few phytonutrients. Foods high in sugar and fat, animal foods, and white-flour food products have the very lowest phytonutrient content. Some foods, on the other hand, are particularly high in phytonutrients. As noted, organic fruits and vegetables have a higher phytonutrient index than their nonorganic equivalents. Remember that an organic vegetable or fruit has to work harder to defend itself from the stress of its environment. It therefore manufactures more phytonutrient stress-fighters than do foods coddled by pesticides, herbicides, and fungicides that do the stress-fighting for them. If you really want to send some powerful health messages to influence the kinase network, try organic berries, red grapes, celery, green pepper, capers, dill, watercress, cruciferous vegetables, hops, tomato, rhubarb, garlic, spinach, and adzuki beans.

In situations where the phytonutrient intake from the diet is not sufficient to influence the kinase cellular communication network, it is now possible to provide a nutritional supplement containing concentrated forms of SKRMs. It is not uncommon for this phytonutrient nutritional gap to go unrecognized, but the development of this supplement represents an exciting new chapter in our ability to use specific nutrients to address health issues.

It is also important to observe once again that the need for specific phytonutrients can vary considerably from person to person based upon genetic predisposition. Dr. Kenneth Kornman and his colleagues at the laboratory of Interleukin Genetics in Waltham, Massachusetts, reported in 2007 that people with a specific SNP—a particular variant—of the gene that codes the receptor of the inflammatory mediator interleukin-1 have increased response thanks to a phytonutrient supplement of particular vegetable concentrates. These concentrates contain specific SKRMs that modulate the cellular communication of this particular inflammatory gene SNP. This is a direct application of the newly emergent field known as nutrigenomics, which charts the level of specific nutrients an individual should intake to promote optimal function. It opens a new era of nutrition, one in which nutritional products can be formulated to meet specific genetic needs based on the evaluation of each individual's genome pattern.

THE RIGHT TOOL FOR THE JOB

Until the turn of the millennium there was little interest in how nutrition could influence cellular communications. But since 2000 there has been a virtual explosion of information in this field. As we've learned in this chapter, it is now well known that imbalances in the cellular communications network are associated with virtually every chronic disease. And we also now recognize the impact of diet, lifestyle, and environmental factors on kinase function and thus on influencing balance in the body's cellular communication process. The bottom line is a new and elemental understanding of the role of phytonutrients and their SKRM capabilities in changing gene expression and thus restoring or maintaining balance in core processes.

So is there still a place for pharmaceutical products in the management of chronic disease? The answer is a resounding yes—with the qualification that the health-care consumer must ask the right questions about their use. Remember that these medications have been approved by the Food and Drug Administration specifically for the symptoms of a particular illness or condition. Remember also that they are designed to deliver a specific effect with high potency—most often the effect of blocking a specific, overly active physiological process downstream of the process of genetic expression. Examples include the blocking by statins of an enzyme in the body that controls the manufacture of cholesterol in the liver, the blocking by antacids of the physiological process by which stomach acid is secreted, the blocking by certain blood pressure medications of the activity of hormones that control the elasticity of the blood vessels, the blocking by certain antidepressants of the way the neurotransmitter serotonin is eliminated from the body, and the blocking by NSAIDs of the COX enzyme effects on the production of inflammatory substances. All of these medications do their job very well, but precisely because they are so potent, their effect can range off-target to touch other functions in the body and thereby possibly cause or contribute to adverse drug reactions.

They are also meant to be used on a temporary basis; most receive FDA approval based on clinical studies performed over one or two years of use. If use continues past that point, the body may become accustomed to the medication, and it may require a bigger dose to achieve the same effect as initially achieved with a small dose. This also increases the possibility of an adverse reaction.

This problem is particularly pertinent for sufferers of chronic illness, the medications for which may be used for tens of years even though data on their long-term safety doesn't go beyond the two years of the clinical studies. Potentially adverse effects from using the drugs over the longer time periods are simply a black box; nobody knows what might happen. The concern becomes even more acute against the background of the significant genetic variation in how medication affects us.

The bottom line on all this? Pharmaceutical medications are very effective in managing short-term health problems, but their long-term use in managing chronic illness raises some critical concerns about safety and effectiveness. Phytonutrients can influence the expression of genes in ways that can beneficially affect our physiological resilience and our overall health, although diet and lifestyle changes may have no immediate impact on short-term health problems or acute pain.

It's a trade-off.

And it is why the functional medicine approach to imbalances in the cellular communications process is to begin with a program of lifestyle and nutritional changes that can mediate the way that specific genes are expressed while minimizing the potential for long-term adverse effects. Start early with such a program and reverse the chronic illness or avoid it altogether, but if you can't, save the drugs for later on if and when the condition becomes more severe.

Such a personalized plan is in keeping with what we might call the longest-running human experiment to design safe medical treatments—evolution. Over millions of years, living organisms have selectively survived to arrive at the right fit between the bioactive substances in food and the maintenance of health, creating a relationship between certain anti-stress substances in food and their use as anti-stress substances in humans. The bioactive substances in food just might turn out to be better at modulating chronic illness over the years than drugs, which are good for short-term therapies but have potential adverse long-term effects. Further studies will clarify that point.

For now, we have clarified how cellular messages are created and what their effects are in modulating the function of the body, and we have learned that managing stress through lifestyle, diet, and environment is a primary therapeutic objective for the management of chronic illnesses caused by an imbalance in our cellular communications process. Well might we ask, therefore, how these cellular messages get from one part of the body to another. It is this question that leads us to the fifth core physiological process, which we will discuss in the next chapter: cellular transport.

CHAPTER 7 TAKEAWAY

1. Complex symptoms associated with chronic diseases are caused by altered cellular communication processes.
2. Influenced by stress or allostatic load, environmental toxins, diet, fitness levels, and specific phytochemicals, altered cellular communication can produce inflammatory responses that are part of almost all chronic diseases.
3. Inflammation, which is a function of genetic expression in response to lifestyle, diet, and environment, will vary widely from individual to individual.
4. Food processing removes many of the important regulatory substances that positively influence cellular communication.
5. Altered cellular communication can cause imbalances in the levels of such hormones as estrogen, testosterone, and insulin.
6. A program to improve cellular communication through the evaluation of hs-CRP, insulin, estrogen, testosterone, and other biomarkers can be effective in averting or curing many chronic diseases.

Cellular Transport

1. Do you frequently experience brain fog and find it hard to focus?
2. Is your blood sugar count higher than it should be?
3. Do you frequently suffer from digestive problems if you eat high-protein foods?
4. Do you feel sleepy from time to time, especially after meals?
5. Have you gained weight—especially around the middle?
6. Have your blood triglyceride levels gone up?
7. Do you have high blood pressure?
8. Have you noticed a loss of muscle over the last few years?
9. Is your LDL cholesterol higher than it should be?
10. Do you take a statin drug?
11. Have you been told that you have low albumin or hematocrit levels in your blood?
12. Has your doctor told to cut back on the amount of cholesterol in your diet?
13. Have you been told you that you have reduced kidney function?
14. Is your vision as sharp as it once was?
15. Do you have any concerns about the health of your heart and blood vessels?

The supermarket has a plentiful supply of food, but your cupboards at home are bare. How do you solve this problem if you are hungry? Simple: you go to the store; carry the food home via your trusty means of transport—your car or bike or feet; prepare it; and consume it. Problem solved.

Our cells are hungry too. They need nourishment to keep on doing the jobs they do, and they too rely on a transport system that brings essential nutrition from where it's stored into and through the bloodstream, which is the highway of the transport system, right to the door of the cells, so the cells can take in the nutrition they need to support your body's health functioning.

In fact, all three categories of essential nutrients required by our cells—fats, carbohydrates, and proteins—have their own separate carriers, their own particular transport systems. As you will guess, each of these carriers is also genetically unique to the individual and naturally is influenced by that individual's lifestyle, diet, and environment.

How do these carriers operate? The carrier for fats essentially has to mask its fat "personality" in order to do its job. This is because fats are not soluble and therefore do not dissolve in the blood, which is principally made up of water. These carriers are called lipoproteins; you know them as forms of cholesterol—very-low-density lipoproteins, or VLDL; low-density lipoproteins, or LDL; and high-density lipoproteins, or HDL.

Carbohydrates, by contrast, can be transported into the blood directly as glucose, a soluble carrier. Once the glucose gets to the cell, however, its transport into it is controlled by a complex regulatory system of hormones, of which the most important is insulin.

The carriers for protein, needed by all cells in the body to maintain cellular structure and function, are amino acids and the blood protein albumin, which, like cholesterol, is made in the liver.

Vitamins and minerals have their own carriers as well. Vitamins A, D, E, and K, which are fat-soluble vitamins, are carried by the same lipoproteins that carry fat. Other vitamins, which are water-soluble, are carried by a range of different protein transporters.

These transport carrier systems are all tightly controlled; they need to be if they're going to get the right nutrients, not to mention all those communicating hormones and signaling substances, to the right cells needed for the maintenance of health—and to *all* the cells that need to get the nutrients. Any sort of glitch in any of these carriers anywhere along the route of transport can produce a state of malnourishment in the cells the carrier serves. Such a glitch works like any standard traffic jam on any road or highway: as the line of traffic slows and then comes to a halt, there's too much of a buildup at the end of the line, in the storage tissues. Obviously, that means that not enough of the substance is getting to the cells of the tissues and organs where it is needed.

In an automobile traffic jam, the cars get there eventually—if they don't turn around and go home. In your body, there are damaging consequences when not enough nutrients get to your cells. In due course, the deficiency produces a change in the function of the body for which the cells are responsible. Over time, if not corrected, that alteration constitutes a damaging defect that can lead to conditions of chronic illness. Defects in fat transport have been associated with heart disease and stroke, defects in the carbohydrate transport process with diabetes and dementia, defects in the protein transport process with muscle loss, and defects in the transport of vitamins and minerals with such nutrient-related diseases as osteoporosis and various forms of anemia.

What is particularly notable about glitches in the body's transport process, however, is the extent to which the chronic illnesses they lead to can be prevented and reversed through changes in diet and lifestyle. That's particularly lucky, because some of the standard drugs that treat these illnesses can cause adverse reactions along with their benefits. A case in point is the class of drugs widely used today to combat the heart disease that too often results from an imbalance in the fat transport system.

FAT TRANSPORT AND HEART DISEASE

I'm pretty sure you know what plaque is. It's a deposit of fat clinging to an artery wall and clogging the artery. But did you know that its discovery goes back to the late nineteenth century, when Dr. Rudolf

Virchow in Germany noted the connection between such deposits and heart disease, a health problem that was far less common at that time? Confirmation of the connection came later when the Russian physiologist Nikolai Anitschkow produced this same type of plaque in rabbits by feeding them diets high in fat and cholesterol.

The connection—fat and cholesterol, cholesterol and plaque, plaque and heart disease—was explored further in 1948, when the Framingham Heart Study got under way in Massachusetts. The aim was to evaluate the behavior and habits of people in the town of Framingham—some 5,000 of them at first—to see if there was a relationship between the incidence of heart disease caused by plaque in the arteries and Framinghamers' diet and daily habits. As I write this, the Framingham study is in its third generation. Much has been learned, and among the results the study has yielded is the famous list of cardiac risk factors—among them, the substance fingered as the cause of plaque, elevated levels of cholesterol in the blood.

Actually, only about 10 percent of the cholesterol in blood comes directly from the cholesterol in animal products in the diet; most of the cholesterol in the blood is made in the liver and is not a result of direct consumption of food. It is transported by the lipoproteins from the liver through the bloodstream to the arteries. The Framingham study found that if the cholesterol was carried by low-density or very-low-density lipoproteins—LDL or VLDL—there was an increased incidence of heart disease, but if the cholesterol was carried by the high-density HDL, the incidence was reduced.

Why would one form of cholesterol be a risk for heart disease and another form act as protection from the very same disease? The answer is not in the cholesterol, although we popularly speak of "good" cholesterol and "bad" cholesterol—erroneously and inaccurately. Rather, the answer is all in the transport experience.

The first thing to understand in this regard is that cholesterol is very important to the proper functioning of the body—when it is available in the right form in the right place. It performs three essential functions. First, cholesterol is used by all cells of the body in the construction of the membrane that keeps each cell intact. Second, it serves as the source material from which testosterone, estrogen, and the steroid hormones like cortisol are made. Finally, cholesterol is used to make the bile salts that are necessary in the digestion and assimilation of fats. If there isn't enough cholesterol available, then these important functions can be compromised. The result? Numerous health problems like low libido, poor tolerance of stress, and even altered immunity.

LDL, the so-called bad cholesterol, is transported from the liver on a specific protein carrier whose job is to deliver it to the artery wall, where it can then be used by cells within a range of different tissues. HDL, or good cholesterol, however, is transported by a different protein carrier whose particular task is to pick up the cholesterol from the artery wall and take it back to the liver to be broken down and excreted. The balance between the cholesterol influx into the artery wall and the cholesterol efflux out of the artery wall determines how this cholesterol influences health and disease.

So in this as in just about everything having to do with our health, balance is everything. If the transport tilts too much toward the to-the-artery side, our LDL will be too high and our HDL too low, leading to a definite risk of heart disease. But it's all too easy to surmise that the exact opposite—a tilt to the lowest LDL cholesterol levels—would equate with peak health. It does not. Peak health comes with the proper balance between LDL and HDL levels; both transporters are needed, but in the correct proportional relationship.

LDL cholesterol, for example, is found in neurosteroids that are critical in regulating brain function and mood, so too low a level of LDL is not healthy for the brain. Studies show a correlation of very low cholesterol levels with depression and even with suicidal thoughts and behaviors. So not enough of it is not good for happiness in general and perhaps for survival in particular. Deficiencies of LDL can also mean insufficient protection by the fat-soluble vitamins A, D, E, and K, which means deficiency in needed nutrients, and away the system goes—like a dog chasing its tail in a loop of increasing health risks.

There's another factor that should probably be mentioned here, and that's stress, a major agent of cholesterol imbalance. I saw this up close one day some years ago when a patient who had just had a blood test left our lab, got into her car, and promptly backed right into a tree in the parking lot. She was uninjured but in mild shock when she came back into the laboratory. We took her blood again. She had certainly not consumed any food or drink between blood draws, yet her LDL cholesterol level had shot up nearly 30 percent post-accident.

Studies on competitive athletes confirm this effect of stress on LDL level. I'm told that the elite Formula One drivers at the twenty-four-hour Le Mans auto race experience elevated levels of LDL during the race despite the fact that they do not take in any food. In fact, their LDL levels stay high for some time after the race. It's only when their bodies have had a chance to adjust to the absence of competition and danger and the accompanying stresses that the cholesterol levels of these typically very fit athletes come back into balance.

What happens in these cases? There is now evidence that stress hormones mobilize cholesterol from the body and bring it into the blood to elevate LDL cholesterol. The cholesterol is in a sense an alarm chemical; when your physiology is under stress, your LDL cholesterol spikes in the blood as a signal of that stress.

STATINS

But now fast-forward from the Framingham study to the early 1970s, and travel across the globe to the research laboratory of microbiologist Akira Endo at the Sankyo Company in Japan. Endo, who had grown up on a farm, had been fascinated as a boy by Alexander Fleming's discovery of penicillin from mold. His desire was to follow in his idol's footsteps, and at Sankyo, he was being tasked to do pretty much that; his job was to find substances of industrial value in fungi. At the time of this story, Endo was looking at specific enzymes made by fungi that could be used to process fruit juice, but his interests were much broader than that. And indeed, in screening the effects of various types of fungi, Endo came across one species, *Penicillium citrinum*, which produced something that prevented animals from making cholesterol. From this unlikely discovery, the family of statin drugs was born.

At the Merck Research Laboratories, Dr. Alfred Alberts picked up on Endo's discovery to develop the first FDA-approved statin drug for the treatment of high levels of cholesterol in the blood, lovastatin (Mevacor). From that, the most widely prescribed drug in the world, the statin Lipitor, was developed by Dr. Roger Newton, a colleague and good friend of mine, and his atherosclerosis research team at what was then Warner-Lambert/Parke-Davis.

As is well known, statins block the manufacture of cholesterol in the liver. That obviously means less LDL is being delivered to the artery wall. Often, there is an accompanying decrease in the amount of HDL picking up cholesterol from the artery wall as well, but the impact of the reduced rate of delivery *to* the artery wall is greater than the effect of the lowered rate of removal *from* it—a slight tip in the balance. This means that blood cholesterol levels go down, and so does the risk of heart disease.

But hold on. A reduction in blood cholesterol is associated with a lower incidence of heart disease: Does that necessarily mean that cholesterol causes heart disease? No. Not necessarily. Association does not prove causality.

And now the story of statins and cholesterol gets quite interesting. Yes, medical studies confirm that people who have had a heart attack can prevent a second by taking statin drugs. And yes, studies find that men with elevated LDL blood cholesterol levels may prevent a first heart attack by taking statins; the benefit is small but definable and occurs only in men. In women, who suffer a different type of heart disease from men, there is no general first-heart-attack pre-vention benefit in taking statins. In fact, there is some evidence that postmenopausal women taking statins have a greater risk of type 2 diabetes from taking the drug.

What these varied responses to statins tell us is that the activity of statins seems to be more than just a matter of inhibiting choles-terol synthesis; rather, the statins serve as agents that block inflam-mation at the artery wall. And since such inflammation normally causes damage to the LDL carrier of cholesterol, literally oxidizing it, what statins effectively end up doing by blocking the inflammation is preventing injury to the artery wall.* This is a finding that takes us back to the future, for Rudolf Virchow, the discoverer of plaque, first proposed in 1879 that atherosclerosis was due to an injury—his word exactly—to the artery wall. Now here we are in the early twenty-first century finding that Virchow's model is in fact correct. The inflammation triggers an immune response that leaves the fatty deposit behind. That fatty deposit in turn triggers more immune responses, and more plaque builds up, degrading the artery wall further. So the injury to the artery is caused by inflammation—in part, anyway—and statins seem to be uniquely able to prevent the type of inflammation that causes that arterial injury.

Statins may also produce adverse side effects, however; one in particular is that in blocking the production of coenzyme Q10, statin use can lead to muscle pain, often serious.

Some time ago, I was introduced to the high-powered senior executive of a major insurance company—let's call him Doug. He was a very fit, healthy-looking guy, a man of disciplined habits—nonsmoker, exercised regularly, healthy diet—but a definite type A personality. Whatever he did, he went above and beyond what was required and what was expected. That was probably why his cardiologist, noting that Doug's LDL cholesterol level was a "little too high" at 110 milligrams per deciliter, put him on a statin drug; the doctor wanted Doug's cholesterol count to be under 100. The statin worked: Doug's LDL went down to 85. At his next cardiology appointment, however, the doctor announced that the new LDL standard for optimal health was to get the level below 60, and he increased the dose of the statin.

When Doug and I met, some months thereafter, he told me how little energy he had; he felt his memory had become spongy and he was losing his male vigor. Doug wondered if all of it—and especially

---

* By the way, the health tip from this is to cook animal products, the only foods containing cholesterol, at low temperatures; this will mitigate the oxidation process.

the erectile dysfunction—could have anything to do with the statin he was taking. Perhaps not the statin itself, I suggested, but rather the dose; it could well be causing an imbalance in his transporters, resulting in a cellular cholesterol deficiency.

That was indeed the case. Doug asked his cardiologist to adjust the statin dose, and his adverse symptoms resolved—without raising his cardiovascular risk excessively. He and his physician together had worked out the right balance—neither too much LDL *nor* too much statin drug.

So while statin drugs may indeed be highly beneficial for people with serious or advanced heart disease, they may also incite some adverse effects and may block some beneficial effects. Isn't it therefore worth asking whether or not there may be other paths to preventing LDL oxidation and arterial injury?

The answer is yes, there are. Let's start by going back to the future again—this time all the way back to the Tang dynasty in ninth-century China. Prevailing medical lore at that time held that red yeast rice, as it was known—actually, rice on which a specific red-colored mold had grown—could "purify" the blood. In our time, controlled studies in humans on the impact of red yeast rice on blood cholesterol levels have confirmed this effect. Trials at the Center for Human Nutrition at the UCLA Medical School* found that eating red yeast rice indeed lowers LDL cholesterol; these findings complement other studies that have found that red yeast rice also reduces oxidized LDL. The reason is simple: The red mold that grows on the rice contains the very same type of substances that statins are composed of.

As it turns out, red yeast rice is only the beginning of the dietary pathways to lowering LDL cholesterol levels in the blood. A class of phytonutrients called phytosterols in particular is now known to lower LDL levels. Phytosterols are found in many plant foods—soy being a prime example, but also nuts, berries, and vegetable oils.

---

* Directed by David Heber, MD, PhD, director of the Center for Human Nutrition at the UCLA Medical School—and an old friend and colleague of mine.

Well-known cholesterol researcher Daniel Steinberg, who tracked how lifestyle behaviors can increase oxidized LDL, also shows us how the increased intake of particular phytonutrients can prevent the formation of oxidized LDL. In particular, foods rich in flavonoids and polyphenols—nuts and berries again but also garlic and onions, grapes, cocoa, black rice, and citrus—seem able to match statins in their power to prevent inflammation. And other classes of phytonutrients found in such vegetables and herbs as virgin olive oil, flaxseed, garlic, psyllium fiber, green tea, and curcumin from turmeric also both lower LDL cholesterol levels and reduce oxidized LDL. So once again, we see the potential of fruits and vegetables to prevent or fight the process that leads to atherosclerosis—that is, hardened arteries and cardiovascular failure.

It is also recognized that vitamin B3, niacin, when administered in doses of 2 to 3 grams a day, lowers LDL and raises HDL. Be aware that there is controversy over the clinical benefit of niacin in high doses; it can produce flushing of the skin that may be extreme in some people. At those levels of dosage, however, the individual is using the vitamin as a drug to achieve druglike effects, not as a nutritional substance. At appropriate doses, niacin is an effective nutritional therapy that can alter the pattern of cholesterol transporters from LDL to HDL.

One of the most widely studied effects of a nutritional substance on transport of fats and cholesterol in the blood is that of fish oil. Elevated levels of very-low-density lipoprotein—VLDL—found in people with high blood levels of a form of fat called triglycerides, are reduced through frequent consumption of such cold-water fish as salmon, herring, and sardines, or through a nutritional supplement of 3 grams of omega-3 fish oil daily. Omega-3 fatty acids, as I'm sure you know, are the essential fatty acids that are vital to human metabolism.

There is an interesting addendum to this, as we have now learned that vitamins D and A can also reduce the levels of oxidized LDL and improve control of cholesterol transport. What emerges from this added knowledge is that the use of a combination of omega-3 fatty acids from fish with balanced levels of vitamins D and A is proving to be a highly effective and significant way to support the healthy transport of cholesterol.

Is there a single natural source of all three of these nutrients—omega-3 fatty acids, vitamin D, and vitamin A? There is: cod liver oil. Decades ago I met Dale Alexander, the health activist affectionately known during the 1960s and 1970s as the "cod father" for his advocacy of cod liver oil as the solution to a range of health problems, including arthritis and joint pain. Alexander was resoundingly criticized by the medical community at the time because there was no scientific explanation for the connection between fish oil and inflammation. Forty years later, there is such an explanation. We now know that the omega-3 oils eicosapentaenoic acid (EPA) and docasahexaenoic acid (DHA), which exist in high levels in cod liver oil, do in fact reduce the inflammatory signaling process and therefore have an anti-inflammatory effect. It is also now known that the vitamins A and D in cod liver oil are beneficial to the gene expression controlling the health of the heart and of blood vessels; the vitamins also help prevent the oxidation of LDL. So Dale Alexander was not really wrong, just possibly a little overzealous. For with cod liver oil as with many things, a little is good, but a whole lot is not so good; vitamins A and D in particular can produce adverse effects if consumed at too high a dose.

What we have found at the Functional Medicine Clinical Research Center is that 2 to 3 grams of a clean source of cod liver oil is a safe and effective daily dose. By "clean" I mean that you want to be sure the oil you use is not from cod caught in the Atlantic Ocean; livers of Atlantic cod have been found to be contaminated with pesticides and dioxins. The source of the cod liver oil should be identified on the label, so look for oil from the livers of cod caught in the Alaskan waters of the Pacific Ocean. They're not only cleaner; they also have a uniquely beneficial balance of EPA and DHA with vitamins A and D—no doubt a result of the particular food sources available to these fish.

But it isn't only particular foods that can help us keep the right cholesterol balance. As we are forever hearing from our parents, our children, First Lady Michelle Obama, various celebrity fitness gurus, and of course our doctors, exercise is all-important.

And in fact, the science is crystal clear that all those preaching the benefits of exercise are right. Regular aerobic activity causes a change in the transport of fats in the blood; specifically, it increases the level of HDL cholesterol in the blood and decreases LDL and VLDL. It also reduces stress. At one time, people who had survived heart attacks were advised by their doctors not to exercise. Times have changed. Today, a cardiologist who failed to start his or her patient on a cardiac rehabilitation program would be considered negligent at best and might be sued for malpractice at worst. Meanwhile, the field of aerobics, started by the U.S. Air Force's Dr. Ken Cooper as a test of fitness, has become a recognized form of therapy, and sports medicine has become a valid medical discipline, as we have learned how exercise turns on the genes that regulate rehabilitation of the cardiovascular system.

But there's another important reason why exercise is so important. The bloodstream is not the only highway along which fat carriers can travel. There's another transport system for fats—namely, the lymphatic system, the network that connects the glands of the body and across which lymphatic fluid transports hormones and other substances.

FATS, HEART DISEASE, AND LYMPHATIC TRANSPORT

I learned a lot about the lymphatic system from prominent cardiovascular surgeon Gerald Lemole, who, among other accomplishments, performed the first coronary bypass operation in Turkey in 1982. Lemole has some very clear ideas about the role of defective lymphatic transport in cardiovascular disease, ideas based on thirty years of observations as a cardiovascular specialist. Here's what Lemole says about heart disease.

First, it is poorly correlated with blood cholesterol levels. Yes, there is a connection, but it is not as tight or as mutual as is generally believed. By itself, in other words, cholesterol is not the cause of heart disease. Second, cardiovascular disease occurs primarily in the arteries of the unmuscled regions of the body, places where the lymphatic system plays an important physiological role in the transport of lipoproteins and cholesterol, including oxidized LDL. Third, people who get cardiovascular disease often have damaged lymphatic systems as well. And finally, a sedentary lifestyle absolutely increases an individual's risk of cardiovascular disease.

The key point that connects these factors, according to Lemole, is that the lymphatic system does not have a pump; the heart is the pump for the circulatory system, but the lymphatic system has none. The only way that things get moved through the lymphatic system is by the body's own mechanical motion. A body at rest is a body with lymphostasis; that is, the lymphatic fluid necessary to transport lipoproteins is moving slowly, if at all, through the system. Defective lymphatic flow or lymphatic flow slowed to inactivity can be a causative factor in cardiovascular disease.

That means that it is only your own physical activity and, secondarily, manipulations like massage, yoga, acupressure, Reiki, or shiatsu that keep things flowing through the lymphatic system. There is no substitute for these physical or manipulative activities. No pill, powder, or potion can accomplish what physical activity does to keep fats and cholesterol moving through the lymphatic system, getting them to where they need to get to, and ensuring that they get cleared out of the body as well.

I have seen the results of exercise and manipulative therapy in a great many people with high LDL and low HDL cholesterol levels and who have the biomarkers of early cardiovascular disease. Many start off with just a daily walk and a massage focused on lymphatic transport, then work up to more activity and more sustained activity, combined with a personalized dietary program. There is simply no better way to lower cardiovascular disease risk while improving functional health and a sense of well-being.

TRANSPORTING CARBOHYDRATE

The body is made up primarily of water, protein, fat, minerals in bone, and a small amount of carbohydrate, mostly in the form of the sugar known as glucose. This small amount of carbohydrate in our bodies is nevertheless critical, for glucose is the principal source of energy for the body's cells.

Since it is a sugar, glucose dissolves in water, so unlike fat, it can be transported directly across the gastrointestinal barrier and into the bloodstream after it has been ingested. No transport chaperone is needed. This means that when we eat a candy bar, all the sugar it contains is in our blood within about fifteen minutes. Since the total amount of glucose in our blood in general is approximately 5 grams, and since the amount of glucose in a single half-ounce candy bar can be 15 grams—even as much as 20 grams—the math is pretty clear: Eating the candy bar will take about a quarter of an hour to multiply the level of sugar in the blood by at least three. This would produce a condition of elevated blood sugar on a par with diabetes.

It doesn't happen, thank heavens, because the normally functioning body transports the glucose out of the bloodstream into the tissues very, very fast. The transport operates through a tightly regulated process controlled to a great extent by the hormone insulin. Insulin—as well as its opposite number, glucagon, which raises blood sugar—is secreted by specialized cells in the pancreas, the gland adjacent to the liver on the right side of your abdomen. After you eat a meal or snack containing carbohydrate, these specialized cells, called the islets of Langerhans, secrete insulin into the bloodstream, where it is transported to all the cells of the body. Its job is to instruct the cells to let the glucose in through specialized doors called glucose transporters. That's how the glucose gets out of the blood—and how you avoid getting diabetes from eating just a single candy bar. It all works wonderfully well as long as this complicated system of transport and cellular communication is operating as it should.

All too often, however, there is a glitch in the transport system, and this obviously causes a communication problem between insulin and the cell. If the cell's communication apparatus doesn't understand the transport message from insulin—if it resists the insulin message—then the pancreas puts out more insulin in an ongoing attempt to get the glucose out of the blood and into the cell. (Remember how cellular communication will "talk louder"—that is, send more of the messenger chemical to get the message across?) This insulin resistance represents the early stage of the chronic illness that is on the rise worldwide in epidemic proportions—type 2 diabetes.

Originally known as adult-onset diabetes to differentiate it from the juvenile form of the disease, it has been renamed "type 2" because so many adolescents and children are now being diagnosed with the adult form. Type 1 diabetes is due to an autoimmune response that destroys the islets of Langerhans cells so that the pancreas simply *cannot* secrete insulin, while type 2 diabetes stems from an imbalance in glucose transport due to a mismatch of the individual's genes with his or her diet, lifestyle, and environment. There is no cure as yet for type 1 diabetes; for type 2, which constitutes nearly 80 percent of the global incidence of this disease, the cure is clearly in diet and lifestyle behavior to correct the transport imbalance.

We have learned so much in recent years about this physiological imbalance that it even has a name—metabolic syndrome.

INSULIN RESISTANCE AND METABOLIC SYNDROME

In 1976, I was a speaker at a medical conference on diabetes in Seattle, Washington. My talk was about the years-long transition that takes people from a state of balanced glucose transport through insulin resistance to the defect in glucose transport that today we diagnose as type 2 diabetes. After my presentation, a prominent diabetes specialist raised his hand and commented that there was "no such thing" as the transition I had described. "Either you have diabetes or you don't," he said emphatically.

His contention was a common one among medical practitioners, yet much work refuting the contention had already been done by the time he delivered it. In 1949, Dr. Harold Himsworth, dean of the University College Hospital and Medical School in London, published a seminal paper in *The Lancet* about a form of diabetes that, he said, was caused by lack of proper glucose transport; the transport defect, according to Himsworth, was due to a defective action of insulin, not to the inability of the pancreas to secrete insulin.

In 1968, Drs. John Farquhar and Gerald Reaven at Stanford University Medicine School published work on insulin resistance that defined it as part of a syndrome between proper glucose transport and type 2 diabetes. Twenty years later, in a famous lecture, Reaven, one of the nation's most prominent endocrinologists, elaborated on this syndrome. He articulated the cluster of conditions that constitutes the functional imbalance in physiology and that derives from a dysfunctional intersection between a person's genes and lifestyle— what we today call metabolic syndrome. Emphasizing that metabolic syndrome is not a disease, Reaven ticked off the biomarkers that characterize it: a high level of triglycerides in the blood, low HDL levels, elevated blood pressure, high levels of blood glucose, and what is called central obesity—meaning an apple-shaped body that is significantly overweight or obese. All of these characteristics, Reaven contended, derive from the common cause of insulin resistance and an imbalance in glucose transport that impairs glucose tolerance.[*]

Today, physicians use this cluster of conditions as diagnostic criteria to test whether a patient may be on the way to type 2 diabetes and, potentially, heart disease, dementia, gout, fatty liver disease, and other ailments. The more of these diagnostic criteria an individual has and the more the individual's values deviate from normal, the closer she or he is to type 2 diabetes.

If you know you have some or all of these conditions, or if your

---

[*] Specifically:

Fasting triglycerides in the blood: greater than 150 mg/dL

Reduced HDL cholesterol: less than 40 mg/dL in males, less than 50 mg/dL in females

Elevated blood pressure (BP): systolic BP greater than 130 or diastolic BP greater than 85 mm Hg, or treatment of previously diagnosed hypertension

Raised blood glucose (FPG): greater than 100 mg/dL after fasting

Central obesity with a waist-to-hip ratio greater than 0.90 in males and greater than 0.85 in females, or with a body mass index (BMI) greater than 30

Urinary albumin to creatinine excretion ratio greater than 30 mg/g doctor has spoken to you about metabolic syndrome, don't think that you are alone. By 2011, a study reported in the journal *Diabetes Care* concluded that more than a quarter of the adult population in the United States has metabolic syndrome; in some specific genetic groups marked by racial or ethnic distinctions, the prevalence is above 50 percent, as was the case among the Pima Indians.

And as we saw with the Pima, the condition took root at the intersection between genes and environmental factors. For the Pima, it was the radical change in diet and activity patterns that over time interrupted their transport and cellular communications processes and led to insulin resistance. Yet, as we know, there are numerous genetic variations in the regulatory network that controls insulin signaling and glucose transport, and these can be highly individualistic. So the idea that everyone with metabolic syndrome has the same disorder and should get the same therapy makes no sense whatsoever. The constellation of conditions that we conveniently describe as metabolic syndrome can be as individual as fingerprints.

A DIFFERENT WAY TO MANAGE METABOLIC SYNDROME

Metabolic syndrome and type 2 diabetes have been a twin focus at the Functional Medicine Clinical Research Center for some time—with important results from clinical trials involving patients with one or the other.

One trial consisted of a diet plan we might describe as "modified Mediterranean" along with a program of daily walking. It is termed "modified" because the amount of refined carbohydrate is limited. The Mediterranean-style diet, as you probably know, has been shown in a number of studies to improve insulin sensitivity and to ameliorate the adverse symptoms of metabolic syndrome and type 2 diabetes. It is a low-glycemic-load diet, which means that its foods don't spike the level of sugar in the blood after eating. This lessens the demand on the pancreas to secrete insulin, and it lowers the need to immediately transport glucose into the tissues.

Participants in our clinical trial were given no calorie limits; rather, they were encouraged to eat as much as they wanted of foods on the approved low–glycemic-load list while avoiding everything on a list of such high-glycemic-load contributors as sugary foods, white flour foods, convenience and snack foods, and sweetened beverages. In our view, the taste of sweetness, whether through sugar or through artificial sweeteners, sets up an entirely different response to foods and alters the glycemic response.

The control group followed this modified Mediterranean eating plan exclusively. But a second study group added to it a medical food containing specific phytonutrients. This food had been developed by our research team to improve glucose transport by stabilizing insulin signaling; the clinical trial was its first test.

Both groups also followed the daily walking program, which was simplicity itself: a minimum of twenty minutes daily at a walking pace, not a stroll. Regular walking, as the research makes clear, can improve insulin sensitivity in sedentary people.

The most visible result after the twelve-week trial was weight loss; participants on average lost about a pound of body fat per week. Test results were equally positive: in all participants, 70 percent of the markers for insulin resistance and metabolic syndrome simply disappeared.

The most remarkable outcome, however, was the effect of the medical food, loaded with the specific phytonutrients, taken by the special study group. Their results trumped even the positive results of the control group. In fact, the difference between the two groups was so significant that it was evident the moment we put the data onto a spreadsheet and looked at the comparison participant by participant. The phytonutrient-supplemented study group experienced better than a 30 percent improvement in reduced LDL, increased HDL, and reduced triglycerides. In other words, our study demonstrated that the excellent results the Mediterranean diet can achieve in terms of managing insulin resistance can be even further improved if the diet is supplemented with specific phytonutrients that support the glucose transport process.* We believe this was the first clinical trial showing that patients with insulin resistance and metabolic syndrome get an even better health outcome if their Mediterranean-style diet is supplemented with specific phytonutrients than from the diet alone.

PHYTONUTRIENTS AND GLUCOSE TRANSPORT

What *were* the phytonutrients in the medical food that supplemented the Mediterranean diet? They came from all over the world and were selected after extensive screening of more than 200 plant and spice extracts that medical anthropology tells us are used by indigenous cultures to manage the disease we call diabetes. The screening was carried out by Dr. John Babish, a onetime Cornell University research pharmacologist and the lead scientist for the trials, in a series of experiments to evaluate how each extract might influence glucose transport. Babish's tests confirmed that the highest beneficial activity came from those substances that worked as selective kinase response modulators—SKRMs—in influencing the insulin signaling network. They were highly active when tested in diabetic animals, and they proved equally active in humans in our clinical trials.

The most active SKRM phytonutrients in supporting insulin sensitivity and balanced glucose transport? Here are the top five: soy-derived phytosterols, lignans, and isoflavones; hops-derived reduced isohumulones; and anthocyanins derived from the bark of the *Acacia nilotica* tree. This tree, found in equatorial Africa, has been used medicinally for centuries—mostly in a tea made from the bark and given to people with the symptoms of diabetes. Both on its home ground and in our lab, this extract proved powerful, and the combination of these top five phytonutrients, formulated

---

* A larger follow-up study, also for twelve weeks, confirmed the results. Participants with metabolic syndrome were tested in trials at the University of Connecticut, the University of Florida College of Medicine, and the University of California, Irvine, School of Medicine. The results again demonstrated the superiority of the program supplemented with the phytonutrient-enriched medical food.

into a medical food, clearly improved insulin signaling and glucose transport in the trial participants.

LESSONS LEARNED: ON A PERSONAL NOTE

For me, these results had particular resonance. As a scientist engaged for nearly fifty years in basic and clinical research, I was struck by the extraordinary consistency of the data in the trials—from cell biology screening experiments to animal testing in different diabetic models to human clinical trials. The lesson it brought home to me was the extent to which and the power with which the bioactive compounds manufactured in the plant kingdom's own laboratory can influence human physiology and health in very specific ways, simply through their influence on cellular communications and transport.

The results of the trials also, in my view, open the door wider to an expanded role for medical foods in the safe and effective management of chronic illness. Defined as foods specially formulated and intended for the dietary management of a disease the nutritional needs of which cannot be met by normal diet alone, medical foods are regulated under the FDA's 1988 Orphan Drug Act amendments and are subject to the general food and safety labeling requirements of the Federal Food, Drug, and Cosmetic Act. They are also one of the key tools that functional medicine practitioners use in implementing medical nutrition therapy.

Finally, the trials confirm yet again the significance of the need to individualize any therapeutic program in order to optimize the unique genetic potential of each patient or participant. There is no such thing as one perfect diet for everyone any more than there is one perfect drug for everyone. General considerations may guide us in constructing an overall plan, but the overall approach must always be fine-tuned for the individual. It means that health practitioners need to be very careful not to set rules for everyone to follow, but rather should offer guidelines and objectives that can then be personalized for the individual. More on this in Chapter 11.

CHAPTER 8 TAKEAWAY

1. Defects in cellular transport of nutrients, hormones, or other cellular messenger substances can contribute to many chronic diseases—among them, heart disease and type 2 diabetes. The latter may result from poor glucose transport caused by resistance to insulin signaling.

2. Statins reduce cholesterol in cells but may also diminish such other important cellular substances as CoQ10 and neurosteroids.

3. Omega-3 fatty acids are important cellular building materials for ensuring proper brain, eye, heart, and kidney function. Cod liver oil is an excellent source of omega-3 fatty acids and has the added value of containing vitamins A and D.

4. Lymphatic system function, essential for the efficient transport of fats and fat-soluble vitamins, is improved through physical activity and manipulative therapies.

5. A personalized therapeutic lifestyle program containing supplemental phytonutrients has been shown to improve insulin sensitivity.

CHAPTER 9

Energy

1. Do you routinely feel a fatigue you can't explain or justify?
2. Are eight hours of sleep not enough for you?
3. Do you get muscle pain after even moderate exercise or activity?
4. Ever feel brain fog? Feel it often?
5. Do you have trouble walking comfortably up a flight of stairs? Are you excessively winded when doing so?
6. Do you lack ambition? Is your energy level low?
7. Ever find that you just can't tolerate disturbances around you that you used to be able to ignore or dismiss or manage?
8. Do you worry about undertaking an activity that incorporates exercise because you know you won't feel good afterward?
9. Are you ever bone-weary? Often?
10. Do you feel you just don't have the energy to cope with the issues of daily living?
11. Do you frequently get headaches for no known reason?
12. Have your senses of smell and taste gotten worse?
13. Are you forgetting things you shouldn't be forgetting?
14. Do you feel older than your age?
15. Does a regular old cold wipe you out for a prolonged period of time?

John just turned sixty. It has brought him up short; he finds himself thinking about his life and his health in ways he never has before.

One reason may have been his birthday celebration. Not the main one—that was at home with his wife, plus the kids and their spouses showing up via Skype with their good wishes. No, the birthday party that really got to him was the morning golf game and lunch at the club with The Guys, the group of eight good friends who have been golfing and lunching together since they were all in their thirties. Back then, the conversation had been about work and sports and politics. Lately, and especially at the birthday celebration, talk focused mostly on how they felt they were "getting on," their aches and pains, the discomforts and growing list of limitations that every-one knows are just part of the aging process.

Not that any of The Guys are sick. All are blessedly free of the serious diseases that many of them watched their parents suffer through, and some of their contemporaries as well—arthritis, heart problems, diabetes, cancer. It's just that most of them feel that they simply don't have the energy they once used to count on. Like John, they're tired but can't seem to get a really good night's sleep. Once, they woke up every morning feeling rested, refreshed, ready to go go go. Not anymore. "It's just part of getting old," said one of them, resigned. The others nodded.

Well, Philip didn't nod, and neither did Larry. But then, those guys always looked and acted younger than the other six—more vital, with much more energy, and with a kind of zest John doesn't think he can manage anymore. His only explanation is that it's the luck of the genetic draw. He said as much to Philip as they were packing up their clubs and heading out—something about how Philip had been "dealt a better hand when they were passing out the energy genes."

Phil chuckled, then slapped John on the back. "Don't you believe it, Birthday Boy. I created this energy. You could even say I work at it. I'm aging, all right. But it's healthy aging."

John thought about that all the way home. Healthy aging sounded a lot better than his own lackluster progression toward more aches and pains, more limitations, and way less energy for life.

We all know what energy is. It's the strength and vitality that are just there—available to power us through our daily activities of work and play. It's mental as well as physical, and it's typically something we feel we can recharge with physical rest or through some mental or even emotional agitation.

"Bioenergetics" is the scientific term for the constellation of cellular processes that keeps our physiological energy flowing; it's the way the energy to power a living organism is harnessed, made available, used, transformed to support our physiological processes. It's how our personal energy works.

Energy is produced inside us in the mitochondrion of the cell. Check it out in Figure 6. As we learned in Chapter 2, the mitochondrion is an organelle in the cell; that is, it serves a specific purpose in the cell just as organs serve specific purposes in the body. The mitochondrion's specific purpose is to convert the fat, protein, and carbohydrate from the food we eat into energy. It does this through

FIGURE 6: CELL MITOCHONDRION AND ENERGY PROCESS

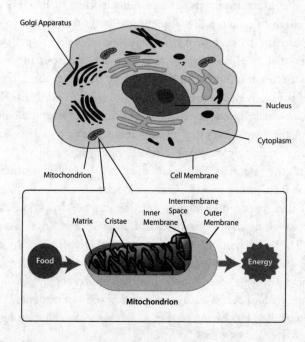

the highly sophisticated, highly complicated process known as metabolism. As we age, this mitochondrial bioenergetics—the transformative process that creates energy in the mitochondria—diminishes, which is why six of The Guys, including John, feel they have a lot less energy and grow more tired more quickly than they used to. The question is why our bioenergetics diminishes.

Let's start with how the energy gets produced. Again, that process takes place in the mitochondria and is called metabolism—specifically, aerobic metabolism. Simply put, the food matter you have ingested is burned—that is, combined with oxygen. This particular act of burning isn't like throwing a log on the fire, however. On the contrary. The combustion process in the mitochondria is controlled very carefully so that the energy from the food does not wholly burn away like the heat from a wood fire in your fireplace. Instead, the process of mitochondrial bioenergetics captures the energy liberated during metabolism and stores it in the form of three specific chemical compounds—adenosine triphosphate, or ATP; nicotinamide dinucleotide, NADH; and flavin adenine dinucleotide, or FADH. These storage chemicals then allow the energy to be transferred to other sites within the tissue where the energy powers up the cells to do the work that cells do—contracting muscles, transporting signals, keeping the brain moving, repairing tissue, and everything else that supports the body's core physiological processes. ATP, NADH, and FADH are our cells' energy fuels. In essence, everything we do depends on the production and management of these cellular energy fuels that in turn rely on proper mitochondrial function.

If that's the case, what's the secret to ensuring proper mitochondrial function? Remember back in Chapter 2 when we talked about how some of the genetic information in our mitochondria comes exclusively from our mother—our maternal DNA? That means that our mitochondrial bioenergetics is to some extent inherited, but only just. In reality, mitochondrial function is regulated by thousands of genes, the vast majority of which are influenced in their expression by our lifestyle, environment, and diet. That also means that most of our energy as we age is controlled by the interaction of our genes with environmental and lifestyle factors. Our surroundings, what we eat, how and how much we exercise: all these factors influence our energy level because all send messages to the genes that regulate our mitochondrial function. So the secret to ensuring mitochondrial function is, once again, what happens at that intersection between environment and our genes.

Yes, the core physiological process of mitochondrial bioenergetics diminishes as we grow older, but by adjusting our environment, lifestyle behaviors, and diet, we clearly have a shot at making our bioenergetics more efficient, thereby retarding that diminution or keeping it at bay a lot longer. What should we know, therefore, especially as we age, about the particular factors that can influence the genetic expression regulating our mitochondrial function? That's what this chapter is all about.

MITOCHONDRIA AND BIOLOGICAL AGING

Our physiological ability to metabolize food with oxygen in the mitochondria gives us an energy advantage over organisms that do not use oxygen for their energy production. Organisms that can't use oxygen can't really squeeze all the energy out of the food as we can, breaking it down completely into carbon dioxide and water, urea, and inorganic salts. In a competition for energy in the world, those that use oxygen more efficiently win.

The problem is that the use of oxygen is a double-edged sword. One edge gives us the energy advantage; the other edge is corrosive. Just as oxygen can rust iron, so too can it "rust," or oxidize, cells. The resulting damage accelerates biological aging and therefore advances the progression of many chronic illnesses—heart disease, diabetes, kidney disease, arthritis, dementia and such other degenerative neurological diseases as Parkinson's disease, and loss of muscle.

In the 1950s, a medical scientist at the University of Nebraska College of Medicine, Denham Harman, proposed an interesting and at the time controversial theory on aging. He likened the corrosive effects of oxygen in the mitochondria to a kind of chemical reaction called free radical chemistry. Free radicals are highly reactive—indeed, explosive; in fact, the phrase originally was coined for fireworks. Harman called oxygen's damaging effect on mitochondria "free radical pathology," characterizing it as an explosive increase in corrosive activity over time.

The analogy is what happens if you leave a stick of butter out on the kitchen counter. For the first few days, the butter looks and smells like butter. Then all of a sudden it has turned into a glob of goo that smells and tastes rancid. Rancidity is the result of free radical chemistry; once all the antioxidants in the butter have been used up defusing harmful oxygen, the next corrosive reactions meet no defensive action; the butter just goes off and becomes rank. Dr. Harman suggested that aging and the diseases of age were to some degree a form of biological rancidity related to free radical pathology.

I remember sharing the lecture stage with Denham Harman at a medical conference in Germany in 1983, when we both wondered how long it might take the scientific establishment to recognize his hypothesis as an important contribution to the science of disease. Now we know: After more than fifty years of research by thousands of investigators, the first decade of the twenty-first century finally saw the medical community accept the theory, while the pharmaceutical industry has embraced it, developing several successful drugs that treat diseases associated with free radical pathology.

Not that the mitochondria don't have their own protections against the corrosive effects of oxygen. Over tens of millions of years of evolution, the mitochondria have developed numerous protections so they can keep on converting food to energy—even if they must constantly defend themselves against the damaging effects of oxygen as they do so.

Some of these antioxidants, as the protections are called, are vitamins—vitamins C and E, for example. Others are enzymes produced within the mitochondrial cell specifically to defuse damaging forms of oxygen before they can cause injury; among these are superoxide dismutase (SOD), catalase, and glutathione peroxidase.

Glutathione is the most important of these protectors. You may remember that in Chapter 5, it played a key role as a conjugase in the detoxification process against toxins. Here in Chapter 9, it also provides protection against mitochondrial injury from oxygen. To carry out these important and varied roles, glutathione is made up of three amino acids: glutamic acid, cysteine, and glycine. Cysteine is a sulfur-containing amino acid, and we need a sufficient supply of it to produce glutathione. We get our cysteine supply from high-quality protein. So an individual on a low-protein diet or consuming protein that does not contain enough sulfur-containing amino acids is probably compromising his or her ability to produce enough glutathione to meet the body's needs. Poor-quality diet in general, as well as heavy alcohol use and exposure to chemicals, can overload the glutathione protection system and render the mitochondria susceptible to damage from oxidation.

But glutathione is not the only defense against mitochondrial injury. An entire antioxidant team works cooperatively to defuse corrosive forms of oxygen. We've already noted vitamins C and E—the latter best consumed in its natural form containing not just the collection of tocopherols that typically constitute this vitamin, but also super antioxidants called tocotrienols. (The best sources of both are brown rice, whole grains, and soy.) Also on the antioxidant team are such members of the B-complex vitamin family as thiamine (vitamin B1), riboflavin (vitamin B2), and niacin (vitamin B3). Mitochondrial defense also depends on minerals like selenium and magnesium to activate specific antioxidant enzymes in the mitochondria—among them superoxide dismutase (SOD), catalase, glutathione reductase, and glutathione oxidase.

But the big news is the ongoing research into the many phytonutrients that also selectively activate the antioxidant enzyme system by turning on the expression of genes that control its activity. Phytonutrients from berries, green tea, grape and peanut skins, and such fragrant spices as rosemary, thyme, basil, and turmeric have all been found to regulate genetic expression in ways that control oxidation damage to the mitochondria.

So does exercise. And with exercise, it's all relative. A well-trained athlete has more than twice the metabolic capacity in her muscle mitochondria as a sedentary person. One reason is that exercise actually stimulates the production of more mitochondria in the cells. It's called mitochondrial biogenesis, and it literally multiplies the number of mitochondria.

What we have now learned is that some forms of exercise are more effective in stimulating mitochondrial biogenesis than others—specifically, cross-training between aerobic cardiovascular conditioning and anaerobic strength conditioning. Practically speaking, that means that the most highly recommended form of exercise is to alternate moderate-intensity aerobic exercise—jogging, bicycling, swimming, stair-climbing, rowing, dancing—with such anaerobic activities as weight training, isometrics, heavy calisthenics, or any resistance exercise done at high intensity for shorter periods of time. The objective is to build oxygen-using capacity by conditioning the lungs and heart while at the same time stimulating mitochondrial biogenesis by creating oxygen debt in the muscles—that is, by stressing the mitochondria and sending a message to the genes to increase the number of mitochondria in response.

It is fascinating to compare the microscope images of the muscle tissue of people who do this kind of cross-training regularly with images of people who are engaged only in aerobics or people who are sedentary. You can actually see that the people on the cross-training program have the most mitochondria in each cell; the aerobic-trained folks have slightly fewer mitochondria; and the sedentary group have far fewer than either of the other two. Clearly, exercise speaks to the genes; the louder it speaks, the more cellular bioenergetics is increased.

What we also understand is that exercise should be regularly performed, part of the normal routine of life. John thought about that as he drove away from the club after his birthday golf outing and his chat with Philip. He hadn't played a round of golf in some time, and he was feeling it in his arms and across his back. Both Philip and Larry, he knew, were gym rats; they belonged to health clubs and attended regularly, and Philip, he also knew, did yoga, which The Guys used to kid him about. John himself had never bothered with a regular exercise routine; his travel-heavy job as head of sales made it difficult, and his own fitness made it unnecessary, or so he thought. He could put in a week of sixteen-hour days on the road, going to meetings, hosting rich lunches and richer dinners for clients, sleeping five hours a night in a different time zone each night, and barely feel it. He'd still come home on the weekend and think nothing of playing a full eighteen holes. Now, after nine holes, his muscles ached.

The reason is simple. John's unconditioned body had exceeded the capacity of his mitochondria to provide the energy needed to fuel his body's activity, so every swing of the club after that point started producing waste called lactic acid. It happens in your body as well. When the buildup of lactic acid hits a certain level in the tissues, that stimulates the nerves to send a pain message to your brain. And while any form of vigorous activity will signal the genome to increase mitochondrial function, a once-in-a-while golf game is nowhere near enough to extend the point at which the tissues start accumulating lactic acid—and keep that threshold out there. It is only through regular conditioning, particularly the cross-training kind, that you can do more and more activity before your body gets to the point where it starts producing lactic acid and you feel pain. Such conditioning builds the increased capacity, and the regularity of an exercise routine sustains it.

Sustained exercise is not only great for muscular stamina and endurance; it also affects pain conditions throughout the body. Did you know that a common form of headache is associated with mitochondrial insufficiency? Like a muscle accumulating too much lactic acid, the mitochondrial reserve in the neurons of the brain can also exceed its capacity. The same regular cross-training routine that conditions muscles can also condition the neurons of the brain. It means exercise is a pain antidote from head to toe.

GOOD OXIDANTS

So if oxidants can be damaging, does that mean that the absence of oxidants is good? As you will have guessed by this point in this book, the answer is no. Our physiology is never all or nothing; too little of something is as upsetting to the balance as too much. And it is the balance that counts. It is that often complex, sometimes very delicate equilibrium within and among all the processes that keeps us ticking over and in health.

In fact, of course, the body uses oxidants for a number of important functions, one of which is immunity. One of the ways a white blood cell "kills" a foreign invading cell is through the release of a caustic form of oxygen known as hypochlorite. You probably have some in the house; it's bleaching agent. Hypochlorite is produced by the T cells; when the cells come into contact with a foreign invading organism, they send out the hypochlorite literally to bleach the invader to death. Too much bleach, however, can cause collateral damage to the adjacent healthy cells and injure their energy-producing mitochondria.

The bottom line? We need enough oxidation to produce energy and defend ourselves from invaders and the harm they can do, but not so much that the defensive action injures the mitochondria and other components of the cell.

And the best way to maintain the balance of our energy process, maintain efficiency in our bioenergetics, and keep biological aging at bay is with a substantially plant-based diet rich in phytonutrients—a glass of fresh-squeezed vegetable juice daily would help—and a regular program of cross-training exercise.

But what happens when the process goes out of balance and our bioenergetics is affected? Let's turn to that next.

CAUSTIC OXIDATION

It is in the mitochondria that the greatest number of caustic forms of oxygen are produced, and they are produced, paradoxically, by a lack of oxygen. I think of it as the dialectic of mitochondria—thesis and antithesis together, each mitochondrion creating the seeds of its own destruction. We see this condition in high-altitude climbers—you've heard of the Death Zone on Mount Everest?—or among extreme athletes who push themselves beyond their aerobic limit for prolonged periods, or in people who are deprived of oxygen because of an injury or problem with circulation of the blood carrying oxygen, or even in people with severe anemia. When the tissues are starved for oxygen—it's called hypoxia—the mitochondria begin producing caustic oxygen substances that injure the tissue or organ that is the site of the deprivation. Most of the time, the caustic oxygen substances are trapped and decontaminated by the antioxidant protection systems in the cell, but when the production of toxins exceeds the ability of the system to manage them, injury results, and the consequence is a diminution of bioenergetics.

It's why even a regular exercise program should not push too hard. While regular conditioning extends the pain threshold, extensive exercise to the point of exhaustion can increase the risk of mitochondrial injury. In a number of extreme adventure racing and ultra-marathon events, post-event blood tests have shown that some individuals are indeed damaging themselves. Even worse, we've seen some who go beyond their aerobic limit for so long that their bodies shut down and they collapse on the event course.

We've also learned, through the extraordinary work of Dr. Bruce Ames, professor emeritus in biochemistry at the University of California at Berkeley, that the process of caustic oxidation can deface and eventually damage the book of life itself. That's tough to do because the DNA in our genome is locked in a vault that is far more secure than Fort Knox. Still, excessive exposure to caustic forms of oxygen produced in the cell can breach that security and damage the DNA—and with it the clarity of the genetic message in the genome.

The consequences for our health range from adverse to catastrophic, depending on where the injury to the DNA occurs and how well it can be recognized and repaired by the cell. But cancer, arthritis, heart disease, and degeneration of the nervous system and brain can all be triggered by such injury. The brain is particularly vulnerable because, oddly, it has a very poor antioxidant defense system.

I learned of the connection between caustic oxidants and such diseases of the brain as Alzheimer's, Parkinson's, and Lou Gehrig's disease back in 1990, when I first met Drs. Wayne Matson, of the

Massachusetts Institute of Technology, and Flint Beal, at the time a research neurologist at Harvard Medical School and the Brigham and Women's Hospital in Boston. They had spent the late 1980s exploring whether Denham Harman's theory of free radical pathology could in some way explain the injury to the brain that characterizes so many neurodegenerative diseases. Specifically, Matson and Beal wanted to know what caused the production of the caustic oxidation substances. They found that the brain cells themselves produce caustic forms of oxygen. They do so when they receive a message of alarm from their environment—maybe a toxic chemical, a stress reaction, or an inflammatory message from the immune system. Any and all of these can trigger mitochondrial dysfunction in the brain cells.

To the extent that substances in the diet contribute to the inflammatory response, this alarm reaction can be transferred to specific cells in the brain and, potentially, to such genetic susceptibility factors as the ApoE4 gene. This is the gene identified over the past two decades as occurring in people showing a much higher incidence of both Alzheimer's and heart disease than the population at large. Further exploration of the ApoE4 gene revealed that this gene made the people who carried it more susceptible to the production of caustic oxidation and to its effects and more sensitive to the adverse effects of saturated fats in their diet.

This was actually good news for carriers of the ApoE4 genetic marker. It told them that the gene does not doom them to Alzheimer's or heart disease; rather, it's a signal to them to personalize their lifestyle, environment, and diet to mitigate their susceptibility to both. Clearly, people who carry the ApoE4 genetic marker should, for starters, minimize their intake of saturated fat and maximize their intake of protective antioxidants and phytonutrients.

Ongoing research confirms these conclusions, as we find that the risk of neurodegenerative disease is greater in people with insulin resistance and type 2 diabetes, two other conditions influenced by the same dietary issues. Remember the work directed by Dr. Suzanne Craft about a type 3 diabetes—diabetes of the brain? Craft's "discovery" of this was based on conclusive evidence that as type 2 diabetics age, their risk of dementia increases. The correlation between diet and disease is too potent to ignore.

Too potent by far: additional research has found that people who do not smoke, whose diet is plant-based, who consume minimal sugar and saturated fat, and who exercise regularly show a greater than 50 percent reduction in the incidence of Alzheimer's disease versus those who follow none of those habits. I don't know about you, but my guess is that if the pharmaceutical industry came up with a drug that cut in half the incidence of Alzheimer's disease, we would all want it—no matter the price. Yet here it is: At the rather low cost of making some changes in diet and lifestyle, we can protect the body and brain against injury to the mitochondria and against the effects that the release of caustic forms of oxygen have on brain health and function. That's a big reward at a cheap price.

CHRONIC FATIGUE SYNDROME AND MITOCHONDRIAL ENERGY

The southwestern United States seems an odd place to find chronic fatigue syndrome, yet that's exactly where the first cases of the syndrome were discovered and reported in the 1980s. The physician credited with analyzing the condition as a syndrome is Paul Cheney, both an MD and a PhD, who at the time was working as an internist in Incline Village, Nevada.

Cheney described the syndrome as characterized by bone-weary fatigue, muscle weakness, swollen glands, brain fog, intolerance of exercise that was previously well tolerated, and the desire to sleep through the day. At first there was just a small cluster of patients, but reports on the syndrome grew rapidly until it had become a recognized global health problem. Originally given a number of different names—one was myalgic encephalitis, meaning sore muscles associated with an inflammation of the brain—it was eventually universally known as chronic fatigue syndrome, or CFS.

Medical investigators around the world searched for the cause of the syndrome. Most leaned toward the theory that it originated in a chronic viral infection, but the world's foremost virologists were unable to find a specific virus that could be the source. Over time, it became clear that the condition had multiple causes that worked together to alter the function of the immune system.

I first met Paul Cheney through my good friend Scott Rigden, a talented family doctor in Scottsdale, Arizona, and in the late 1980s, our research group at the center joined with both physicians in trying to identify biomarkers of the syndrome that would help define its cause with more precision. By 1990, our data suggested that CFS was an issue of reduced mitochondrial bioenergetics as a consequence of something "poisoning" the mitochondria. We initiated a small clinical research study in a group of thirty CFS patients and found exceptionally high incidence of biomarkers signaling caustic forms of oxygen as a result of mitochondrial dysfunction. In particular, the biomarkers measured serum lipid peroxides, providing a measurement of rancidity in the blood, and damage to DNA from caustic oxygen substances called 8-hydroxydeoxyguanosine, or 8-OHdG.

The thirty patients were then put on a twelve-week program aimed at improving their mitochondrial bioenergetics and reducing the effects of the caustic forms of oxygen. The program required them to consume a low-allergy diet enriched with rice protein and to supplement with high levels of nutrients necessary to support mitochondrial function—zinc, coenzyme Q10, lipoic acid, and vitamin E, for example. At the end of the twelve weeks, the biomarkers of mitochondrial dysfunction had improved markedly; so had the patients' CFS symptoms.

The published results of our study evoked a response from Dr. Martin Pall, a biochemistry professor at Washington State University. He introduced himself as a former CFS patient. Because Dr. Pall felt the initial symptoms of fatigue and brain fog following a flight back to the United States from Europe, he originally attributed his illness to jet lag. But as the symptoms worsened, and as his once sharp memory began to fade, he realized that he needed to take a leave of absence from his academic position and focus on getting well. Pall's way of doing that was to use all his remaining energy—and all his biochemistry training and experience—to understand his condition and find a solution for it.

It took two years of full-time work. Pall culled all the research he could find, including our work and that of others looking at dysfunctional mitochondrial bioenergetics, and leveraged it with his understanding of mitochondrial function.

A key source was the work done at the Center for Molecular Medicine at Emory University School of Medicine in Atlanta—specifically, research exploring how to manage children born with genetic imperfections in their mitochondrial function. The center's researchers had found that the nutritionally related substances N-acetyl carnitine, coenzyme Q10, lipoic acid, and N-acetylcysteine could mitigate the symptoms of mitochondrial dysfunction in these children.

Putting it all together, Pall developed the working hypothesis that the mitochondria of CFS patients are injured by activation of the immune system. He then came up with a treatment plan consisting of high doses of the nutritional substances that support mitochondria in their job of producing ATP and fueling metabolism. Pall himself became the first test patient for his plan, and a year later, he was well.

His plan has since been taken up by numerous other physicians in treating their own CFS patients. But it was Paul Cheney himself who gave the approach its name; he calls it mitochondrial resuscitation.

Martin Pall's hypothesis that activation of the immune system injures the mitochondria in CFS patients throws into sharp relief the kind of adverse influence stress can have on mitochondrial health and our bioenergetics. It is one of the loudest signals our lifestyle and environment can give to the genes regulating our mitochondrial function. Simply put, if there is too much stress for too long a time, the stress hormone adrenaline can cause the mitochondria to commit suicide.

I suppose that's one reason I find it so interesting that in blue zones like Ikaria, where people live longer and healthier lives, one of the characteristics that define their lifestyle is the sense of community, and another is the preservation of downtime. The sense of community means that even the most do-it-yourself loner knows that help is available if needed and that others are looking out for him. The preservation of downtime means that everyone is expected to spend a prescribed amount of time restoring his or her body, mind, and soul; it's considered an integral and essential part of life, and again, everyone knows it and counts on it. Both of these certain expectations, which seem a far cry from lives spent in isolated, 24/7 interaction with the Internet, are associated with a reduced allostatic load and decreased levels of stress hormones. The mitochondria in blue zoners don't have to self-destruct; they're not damaged by lifestyle behavior or poisoned by caustic oxidants. The result? Blue zoners preserve their cellular energy reserves and show a lower biological age than the rest of us. They live longer, healthier lives.

SPECIAL NUTRIENTS FOR MITOCHONDRIAL PROTECTION

Regular exercise and a healthy, plant-based diet can keep our mitochondrial function healthy and efficient. But when damage occurs, something more may be needed. The role of phytonutrients not just as protectors of mitochondrial function but as treatment mechanisms for mitochondrial damage is an emerging science, and it has prompted important discoveries in the way these plant-derived compounds can influence health.

A good framework for understanding this influence is the concept of hormesis, a term revived precisely in this context around the turn of the millennium by Dr. Edward Calabrese, a professor at the School of Public Health at the University of Massachusetts. The term refers to an unexpectedly large biological effect from a very low level of exposure to a particular treatment. Instead of the effect of the treatment increasing as the dosage is increased, hormetic substances realize a bigger impact at a lower dose.

When it comes to mitochondrial protection, we've learned that specific phytonutrients at very low levels of exposure can influence genetic expression at precisely the right control points for regulating the complex process of mitochondrial function.* What this means is that even a small amount of the right phytonutrient taken at the right time can influence health much more than would have been expected from the amount consumed and absorbed.

It's a little bit like acupuncture—that is, a small influence at just the right point on the body can effect significant change. At issue here, however, are metabolic control points—the specific regulation points in our complex network of genes where a small influence can promote a substantive shift in genetic expression. One example is the positive clinical effect on health outcome in CFS patients with very low doses of specific types of omega-3 fatty acids and phospholipids derived from marine sources. Dr. Garth Nicolson, director of the Institute for Molecular Medicine, administered as little as 3 grams per day of these substances to his CFS patients. Given that the body contains more than 15,000 grams of fat, it would be logical to expect that 3 grams of specific fats would soon be diluted by all the other fats in the body. In this case, however, as Nicolson concluded, the influence is hormetic: although the dosage was minimal, the impact of the specific substances regulated the genes that control signal transduction in the cell, which in turn influenced genetic expression affecting the patients' symptoms.

Which phytonutrients are known to have hormetic influences on mitochondrial function? Resveratrol from grape skins and peanuts, epigallocatechin gallate (EGCG) from green tea, curcumin from turmeric, isohumulones from hops, quercetin from buckwheat, watercress, and dill all work—optimally, when found in whole, minimally processed foods and supplements.

---

* From the work of Dr. Mark Mattson and his research team at the Laboratory for Neurosciences at the National Institute on Aging. The work examined the hormesis mechanism with phytonutrients shown to have a positive effect on mitochondrial function.

CALORIE RESTRICTION

Here's another of the characteristics associated with blue zoners: not only is their food minimally processed and plant-based, it's also relatively lower in calories. Despite all the lovely fresh fruit, wine, and olive oil of Ikaria, for example, by comparison with most developed-economy cultures, Ikarians live on a calorie-restricted diet.

This is not a particularly revolutionary concept, and the impact of partial calorie restriction on mitochondrial bioenergetics has been the focus of considerable research for some time. That calorie restriction could be a way to preserve health and extend the life span was first observed in a laboratory setting by Professor Clive McCay at Cornell University in the 1950s, when he and his students recorded an increase in life expectancy of nearly 35 percent in rats fed a diet of 25 percent fewer calories than the control group. Similar results have been found in many other species of animals from flatworms to monkeys: calorie restriction results in a lower incidence of disease and a longer life.

The research with monkeys has been particularly important—especially the twenty-year study carried out at the University of Wisconsin that is the longest controlled study of calorie restriction in a primate model thus far. The animals in both the control group and the calorie-restricted group were all about the same age at the start of the study; by the end of it, the results were obvious—and remarkable. The control monkeys looked like geriatric cases. They were stooped over; their fur's texture was poor and its color faded; and they had limited mobility. The control group also suffered many more deaths than the calorie-restricted group of monkeys, which not only looked and acted much younger than the control group but also recorded far healthier blood biomarkers. The conclusion was again evident; calorie restriction was shown to improve health and life expectancy over the long term.

The question is why. The answer in large part seems to be found in the difference in the number and type of genes that are expressed in the calorie-restricted group of animals versus those that are eating ad lib. The genetic expression of the calorie-restricted group effected low stress response and increased maintenance of mitochondrial function over time.

From this evidence, we conclude that too many calories over too long a time results in a kind of mitochondrial burnout—particularly if the calories come from such fast-acting energy sources as sugars, processed flour products, concentrated fats and oils, and excessive animal protein.

An added point of interest to the calorie restriction effect is the recent finding that many of the phytonutrients that have hormetic effects on mitochondrial function mimic the influence on genetic expression that is seen with calorie restriction. This means that a diet centered on plant foods along with a modest calorie reduction, which often accompanies the switch to a plant-based diet, can produce a double-whammy impact on the genes that regulate mitochondrial bioenergetics, supporting mitochondrial function while also reducing the potential for adverse effects of the caustic effects of oxidation.

Denham Harman was right back in the 1950s when he predicted that the next century would teach us much more about the effect of diet on free radical pathology and its influence on health, disease, and aging. We're learning new lessons every day.

Yet so much of what we're learning is not being applied. I am reminded of the senior residence where my mother lives—a community of about a hundred retired seniors with an average age in the eighties. Many of the residents have one or more of three main health problems—type 2 diabetes, dementia, and macular degeneration with impending blindness. The same is true in other senior residence facilities across the nation and the world. But the tragic circumstance of these facilities is not that the residents are old and need assistance in their daily lives. No, the real tragedy is in the kitchen.

It is as if the foods being served are intentionally designed to increase the production of caustic oxygen substances and send residents' mitochondria on a path to suicide. Meals consist of high-glycemic-load foods, are filled with sugars and saturated fats, and are virtually devoid of any fresh food at all except a salad of store-sourced lettuce covered in a dressing with sufficient fat and sugar to rob it of any positive nutritional value. I find this criminal as well as tragic.

Yes, meals are important for more reasons than food. These are the times of day when residents get together, socialize, engage in conversation. And certainly, the food that is served should support residents' comfort and, to be sure, their enjoyment. But those aims can be achieved with just a little creative menu planning; such planning should be based on a commitment to the importance of nutrition in preventing the diseases of aging that result from mitochondrial catastrophe.

I've seen other places too—enlightened senior living facilities where low-glycemic-load menus are offered, sugars are minimized, and nutrient-rich foods are plentiful. In such facilities, I see fewer people who are losing their memory, walking with a walker or motorized scooter, or losing their eyesight.

But I am not surprised to hear my mother's co-residents complaining of fatigue, low energy, forgetfulness, and weakness—all symptomatic of mitochondrial impairment, all serious issues that rob quality of life from people *and* propel them to the use of expensive medical services. It's a real-world example of what the loss of mitochondrial bioenergetics means in the reality of people's lives. And in a world where we are all living longer, it's an object lesson in how not to ensure healthy aging.

Okay, I've said my piece.

JOHN AND THE GUYS

By the time he got home, John had remembered that both Philip and Larry had had one beer each in contrast to the two or three drinks the rest of them downed during lunch. He also seemed to recall that the two younger-looking, more vital-seeming guys had said no to the dessert even though both of them had eaten only a salad for their main course. There was a pattern here, a method to the madness Philip and Larry seemed to represent, and John began to wonder whether doing as they did might help him regain the energy he lost.

I know the rest of this story because John called Philip and asked for a referral to his doctor, a functional medicine practitioner who told me what happened. John made some changes in his life; they amounted to his taking charge of his own bioenergetics and health.

No, he did not join the health club—not his thing. But he set himself a regular program of walking and stuck to it. His wife soon joined him, and lately, they've both taken up cycling as well. They also changed their diet; John described it as "switching places," meaning that meat became a side dish—and a less and less frequent occurrence—and vegetables became the center of the meal. Sweets and processed food pretty much went away and, to John's surprise, were not missed.

It did not take long for John to become an energy gainer instead of an energy loser. In addition, his body has taken on a new shape and form, one consistent with the genetic expression of his vitality genes and not his aging genes. To me, the change in John is a classic example of Linus Pauling's axiom that if you get the structure right, the function will follow.

The truth is that structure can tell you a lot about function, which is why we'll turn to structure next.

CHAPTER 9 TAKEAWAY

1. Our energy is produced by the mitochondria in cells; it is in the mitochondria that carbohydrate, protein, and fat are metabolized, producing cellular energy.
2. This energy-producing process is dependent upon proper intake of vitamins, minerals, omega-3 fatty acids, and phytonutrients.
3. Altered mitochondrial function can result in cellular damage associated with accelerated biological aging and chronic disease.
4. Specific antioxidants such as vitamin E, selenium, vitamin C, coenzyme Q10, lipoic acid, and N-acetylcysteine can protect against mitochondrial damage.
5. Cross-training exercise that alternates aerobic and anaerobic conditioning helps to strengthen mitochondrial function and improve cellular energy production.

6. Chronic fatigue syndrome is related to altered mitochondrial function.
7. Insulin resistance and its related condition, type 2 diabetes, can reduce the mitochondrial function in the brain and contribute to dementia.
8. A mitochondrial resuscitation program can improve cellular energy production.

CHAPTER 10

Structure

1. Do you feel you're getting shorter over time?
2. Have any back problems?
3. Do you ever get a sore neck? Frequently? Often?
4. Are you a cell phone user? Sometimes? Exclusively?
5. Have you been told that you have elevated hemoglobin A1c?
6. Do charbroiled foods show up frequently in your diet?
7. Any memory problems?
8. Do you have a weight problem even though you watch your calories like a hawk?
9. Is your waist-to-hip ratio greater than 1?
10. Do you eat a lot of foods and drinks stored in plastic containers?
11. Are you one of those people who are "cold all the time"?
12. Have you been told you have reduced bone mass?
13. Are you menopausal?
14. Do you pretty much avoid dairy products?
15. Do you eat proportionally way more animal protein than vegetables?

In 1951, the proceedings of the august National Academy of Sciences featured seven studies by the same two authors, chemists Linus Pauling and Robert Corey, reporting on their research on protein structure and its relationship to protein function. That same year, Pauling delivered a lecture entitled "Molecular Medicine," the term he had first coined two years earlier and one that crystallized the practical application of the seven collaborative papers in the proceedings. Practically speaking, Pauling stated that if we understand the structure of human biology at the molecular level, we can understand how and why it functions as it does. As he is reputed to have put it, "Get the structure right, and the function will follow."

We think of physiological structure as our skeleton, muscles, connective tissue, and organs—see Figure 7—and we assume the structure to be immutable and permanent. Not so. For one thing, everything in our body is replaced on a regular basis—our red blood cells every three months, the mucosa of our digestive tract every few days, our bones every few years. At the molecular level, the level of the smallest building blocks of those structural elements, the

FIGURE 7: HOW STRUCTURE AND FUNCTION ARE CONNECTED

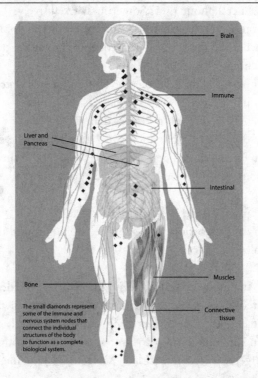

Brain

Immune

Liver and Pancreas

Intestinal

Muscles

Bone

Connective tissue

The small diamonds represent some of the immune and nervous system nodes that connect the individual structures of the body to function as a complete biological system.

proteins that make up our organs and connective tissue, the calcium compound—called hydroxyapatite—that is the bone mineral of our skeleton, plus the lipids of our fat stores, the amino acids of our muscles, and the nucleic acids of our DNA are all being broken down and remade every day. In other words, structure is always changing.

That is significant because structure affects function. When we know what each building block is, why it is where it is, and how it connects to the other building blocks and levels of structure in the body, we can also know *how* the building blocks affect function. And if we follow Pauling's insight about the relationship between structure and function—that is, that our structure at every level can change—we come to understand how function can therefore change as a result.

It is really only now, in the wake of the genomic revolution, that the health implications of that relationship are being fully recognized in medicine. If creating and maintaining structure are ongoing processes from which function emerges, then we can see chronic illnesses as originating precisely in a structural problem in the body manifesting itself as functional symptoms. We can try to correct the functional symptoms, but if the underlying structural problem is not resolved, the condition will continue; in fact, it will progress.

What the genomic revolution has taught us is that we can speak to and affect our structure. Our genes carry information pertinent to the creation of our structure at every level—molecular, cellular, at the level of tissue and organ structure, at the level of the whole organism. As in a hologram, each level of structure is reflected within the others, and each is seen inside the others. But factors of our environment, lifestyle, and diet can reach into all the dimensions of this hologram to influence the way genetic messages are expressed. Environment, lifestyle, and diet can all place epigenetic marks on the genes, turning the volume up or down on specific genes, as we put it in Chapter 2. This means that our structure at every level and therefore our function can change as a result.

This chapter is about how that physiological process works to affect our health.

SPEAKING TO OUR STRUCTURE . . . BUT MAYBE NOT ON A CELL PHONE

It's almost a cliché to talk about the body's structure in terms of architecture, but it is not entirely inappropriate to do so. Like a building—say, a city skyscraper—the human body is engineered for stability; both skyscraper and human are able to withstand the power of nature and the force of gravity over time and remain upright.

But now endow the skyscraper with the ability to move. Will the engineering for stability that went into it when it was stationary still be adequate for the building in motion? Probably not; keeping the structural components aligned is much more complicated in a moving building than in a stationary one. Some reengineering is needed.

Now add another engineering challenge: The skyscraper must not only maintain its stability while it is in motion; at the same time, it must keep all its functions operating—communications, repair, energy production, and mechanical work. That is a formidable engineering challenge requiring a lot of complex interactions. Yet it is exactly what the human body is expected to do.

But this complexity in the body's structural architecture creates its own challenges. Life happens, as they say, and some of its events just may, for example, distort the alignment of the bones, muscles, or nerves. You've probably had a sore neck at some point in your life, or you pulled out your back, or you got tennis elbow even if you never played tennis. These are signals that something structural is out of line.

And when the structural alignment is altered, then, by definition, the function is altered as well. Pain is one such alteration, but so is the appearance of inflammation, or a swelling in the body, or a change you can't see in one or more of the core physiological processes like defense or transport.

These associations between the body's structural alignment and changes in function have been observed since the dawn of medicine in the Ayurvedic and Chinese traditions. Over the course of some two thousand years, the practitioners of these traditions perfected various forms of manipulation—among them therapeutic massage, chiropractic, osteopathy, yoga and other forms of exercise movement, and acupuncture. The driving thrust in all these practices is to create or regain the proper alignment of bones, muscles, and nerves so that the structure can effectively manage the stress and strain of a body in motion.

Here in the West, in at least some sections of the medical establishment, there's a lingering controversy over the efficacy of manipulative therapy, probably because until recently, we had no direct knowledge of a mechanism by which such therapies could alter cellular function and thereby directly affect health or disease. But as with so many of the shibboleths we grew up with, the findings of the genomic revolution have started to change that. Witness the work of academic neurologist Helene Langevin and her colleagues at the University of Vermont College of Medicine, which is offering a new view of the physiological effect of these kinds of physical medicine. Under very carefully controlled conditions, Langevin's group has been measuring the effect on cellular function of inserting an acupuncture needle into the skin. Just below the skin is a whole extracellular matrix—sort of like the glue of our connective tissue—full of nerves constituting a signaling system to the brain and other parts of the body. Pass a feather or even your fingernail lightly along your inner arm and you'll sense this intuitively as you feel a tingling, almost ticklish sensation that is quite pleasant. What is not so intuitive, however, is what Langevin and her group have found out—that this signal going through the skin and the extracellular matrix just below it is also activating specific signal transduction pathways and thereby influencing gene expression. It is regulating cell behavior and therefore cellular function.

If we extrapolate out from the influence of acupuncture on cellular function, we can find implications for various forms of physical medicine—including exercise. It too is a kind of targeted manipulation of the body, and such manipulation, we now know, sends mechanical signals that are translated through the nerves in the extracellular matrix. These signals are received by receptors on the surface of cells within both the nervous and the musculoskeletal systems that then alter the cells' expression of function. What an amazing connection this represents between our genes, our physical environment, and our health.

I can report on just such a connection in my own case, although I too had long been skeptical about physical medicine, even after hearing from patient after patient about how a specific manipulation therapy had solved a long-term health problem that had resisted all other treatments. I simply assumed the "solutions" were the result of a placebo effect.

Then my back, which I injured during my college basketball days and which periodically "goes out" if I move in a certain direction, became a serious issue. I travel thousands of miles a year, and as if airplanes aren't uncomfortable enough, sitting in one for eight or ten or fourteen hours with a bad back can be sheer misery. I finally accepted a referral to a nearby chiropractic physician whose manipulation of my back relieved the pain and discomfort in minutes. I now keep a list of chiropractic and osteopathic physicians around the world so I can keep on keeping on while on the road. I can say without any ambiguity that the effect of these treatments is no placebo; it's real.

There's another interesting example of speaking to our structure, but with a less happy practical application. The idea that there are structures within the body that create and transmit an electromagnetic field was first articulated by Dr. Robert Becker in his 1985 book, *The Body Electric*. After all, as Becker pointed out in the book, brain electroencephalograms—EEGs—and the electrocardial or EKG patterns of the heart are reflections of the body's electromagnetism.

At the cellular level, we also know that when mitochondria convert food to energy, their doing so creates a small electromagnetic field. Controlled studies have demonstrated that when mitochondria are exposed to a high magnetic field, they change their function.

In essence, we are electric beings. Our body's structure operates like an antenna and a transmitter, picking up and sending out certain frequencies of low-energy radiation. What this means is that our structure and the function derived from it influence the electromagnetic environment around us, and the electromagnetic environment around us can influence our physiology.

So we come to the issue of electromagnetic pollution, the term used by Dr. Devra Davis, founder and president of the Environmental Health Trust,* and to the potential health effects from exposure to certain forms of nonionizing radiation. We all know of the health dangers from exposure to the ionizing kind of radiation—namely ultraviolet and X-ray forms of radiation; nonionizing radiation includes certain frequencies of background radiation in the microwave portion of the electromagnetic spectrum, the region of the spectrum used for cell phone communications.

It's an emerging area of study, controversial, and potentially profoundly significant, given that estimates as of 2013 are that there are almost as many cell-phone subscriptions as there are people in the world.† That probably means, among other conclusions, that warnings or even cautions about possible health effects don't have much chance of being heard. That's too bad, because it's an issue that ought to be raised, aired, and examined carefully.

Dr. Davis is not the only expert to contend that the structure of our bodies creates a susceptibility to adverse health effects from these nonionizing forms of electromagnetic radiation, and that the adverse effects primarily influence the nervous and immune systems. The influence is subtle but may be profound with long-term exposure. The World Health Organization has also issued a caution; its International Agency for Research on Cancer asserts that radiofrequency radiation, which cell phones emit, may possibly be carcinogenic to humans.‡

These warnings have not been scientifically proved—yet. But

---

* Also, as noted in Chapter 5, professor of epidemiology at the University of Pittsburgh.

† See http://www.itu.int/en/ITU-D/Statistics/Documents/facts/ICTFacts Figures2013-e.pdf.

‡ http://www.iarc.fr/en/media-centre/pr/2011/pdfs/pr208_E.pdf.

until we know for sure, it probably makes sense to use a headset with your cell phone and to avoid, as much as possible, putting the phone directly against your ear where it is close to the brain.

PROTEIN STRUCTURE AND FUNCTION AND OUR HEALTH

The core message of the seven papers Pauling and Corey published in 1951 was that alteration in the structure of a protein can then modify the function of the protein and therefore of the individual. Much of the work that led to this conclusion was the landmark research on sickle-cell anemia Pauling carried out in the late 1940s in collaboration with biochemist Harvey Itano. The two men showed that the sickle-cell disease resulted from a genetic alteration in one part of the hemoglobin protein molecule. Simply put, the sickle-cell form of hemoglobin has a different shape from that of normal hemoglobin, and the difference makes the sickle-cell form of the protein molecule less flexible. As a consequence, the sickled form distorts the shape of the red blood cell, which then slices through the bloodstream—like a sickle through a wheat field—and in so doing, damages the body. That damage can produce grave symptoms in numerous organs—the kidneys, heart, liver—and in other tissues, all due to the alteration in the shape of one molecule.

That is why Pauling termed it a molecular disease, thus distinguishing it from an infectious disease in which a foreign invader causes a reaction that results in a disease process. You can kill the foreigner with an antibiotic, but you cannot kill a protein produced in the body, even if it has a different structure from other proteins. From a medical point of view, managing a molecular disease deriving from the altered structure of molecules requires a far different strategy from the pharmacology approach that can zap foreign organisms.

Many chronic diseases are the result of an alteration in the shape of specific proteins, and not all such alterations by any means are a result of a genetic characteristic as in sickle-cell anemia. Rather, these diseases result from alterations that occur in the protein cells after they are produced in the body. These changes are called post-translational modifications, and they derive from factors or events in the individual's lifestyle, diet, and environment.

One of the best-known and best-understood examples of this is the altered form of the hemoglobin protein called A1c, or glycohemoglobin, used clinically as a measurement of diabetes. Typically, only a very small amount of the sugar called glucose combines in the blood with hemoglobin, so the level of glucose attached to the hemoglobin protein will be minimal—usually less than 5 percent. But when diabetes is present, with high blood sugar levels, the combination of glucose with the hemoglobin protein produces the altered form of the protein, glycohemoglobin. Levels of A1c above 6 percent are therefore biomarkers of the disease. Just above 6 percent, for example, is considered a signal of early-stage type 2 diabetes, and 8 percent or higher is an indication of poorly controlled diabetes.

Moreover, because the red blood cell where the hemoglobin resides has a four-month lifetime, the level of hemoglobin A1c provides a running record of the average blood sugar level over time. Since a single blood sugar measurement can provide varying results depending on when the person last ate, what he or she ate, and a host of other things going on in the person's life that might influence insulin action, the A1c test provides information about the diabetic's long-term control of blood sugar levels. It has become a key tool not just for diagnosing diabetes but for managing it as well.

COOK UP SOME CRUSTY PROTEINS

Hemoglobin is by no means the only protein connecting with sugar in the blood. This process—the sugar reaction of proteins—is called glycation, and it produces what I call "crusty" proteins. What's crusty about these proteins? Actually, the combination of protein with sugar is precisely similar to what happens when crust forms on the bread you're baking. You put it in the oven as a blob of dough with no distinguishing feature of appearance or taste. But as it bakes, the top layer, where the temperature is hottest, cooks into a crust that looks and tastes quite different from the inner part of the bread. Food chemists call the formation of the crust a Maillard reaction, the chemical reaction that takes place under heat between the glucose from the starch in the flour and the amino acid from the protein in the flour. This is exactly what happens in the blood, without heat, when blood sugar reacts with the hemoglobin protein to form the hemoglobin A1c, which also qualifies as a crusty protein.

In fact, glycation forms a whole bunch of crusty proteins. They are called advanced glycation end-products—AGEs. Each is a protein structure that is basically foreign to the body, and therefore each can stimulate an immune inflammatory response. And indeed, there are receptors on the surface of our immune cells known as receptors for advanced glycation end-products, or—you guessed it—RAGEs.

But here is where the important health story emerges. The more crusty-protein AGEs in the blood and tissues, the greater the risk for various AGE-related chronic diseases sparked by immune system responses. Put it this way: the more AGEs there are, the more the cells become enRAGEd. That is how the story of altered cellular communication associated with insulin resistance and diabetes gets tied together with altered protein structure to increase the risk for heart disease and arthritis. What look like independent diseases are really caused by the same alteration in the core physiological processes.

There's more. We're learning that the glycation products of protein can also be formed in our food and therefore ingested in our diets—with consequences. If you cook foods at high temperatures, advanced glycation end-products turn into glycotoxins. At the Icahn School of Medicine at New York's Mount Sinai Hospital, Dr. Helen Vlassara, professor of geriatrics and palliative medicine, has been evaluating the effects of these glycotoxins in both animals and humans. It's not pretty. The crusting found in charbroiled meats, for example, produces glycotoxins that initiate an immune inflammatory response in the same way that AGEs produced in the body do—with similar adverse effect on health.

Vlassara's work has shown rather convincingly that as our diets have become more processed through heat treatment, our intake of glycotoxins has also increased, and that this increased intake has contributed to the rising incidence of such chronic illnesses as type 2 diabetes, kidney disease, and dementia. In animal studies, the progression of these illnesses goes up when the test animals ingest glycotoxins, which cause an increased inflammatory response. In humans, the evaluations note higher blood levels of glycotoxins in people known to have these diseases. The lesson seems to be to reduce the consumption of charred meats and to lower the cooking temperature in general. Reduced cooking temperatures result in reduced production of glycotoxins.

So the bottom line is that as the structure of proteins is altered, there is an alteration in their physiological effect—an alteration in the way they function—whether the altered structure is produced in the body or ingested.

The extreme example is the case of bovine spongiform encephalopathy, or BSE, first identified in England in 1986. In a way, it all came about thanks to an accident of history. Cattle have traditionally been raised on vegetable foods, and for English cattle, soybean meal was the food supplement of choice for most cattle farmers. But in the early 1980s, the cost of soybean meal began to rise, and since little soy was grown on English farms and no price controls could be put in place, cattlemen turned to an alternative food supplement—namely, the remains of dead and diseased animals, both cows and sheep.

Within a few years after this supplement was introduced, a number of cattle began to show signs of a strange illness. They became unable to stand on all fours, grew aggressive, and seemed demented. After a while, the cattle died. Postmortems showed a spongy degeneration in the brain and spinal cord of the animals; veterinarians gave the disease a name that captured that degeneration—bovine spongiform encephalopathy—but everyone called it mad cow disease. This neurodegenerative disease has a long incubation period, anywhere from about two and a half to eight years; it affects adult cattle between four and five years of age, and it is fatal. But the authorities didn't wait:

after more than 180,000 cattle were found affected, 4.4 million were slaughtered in an all-out eradication program.

The eradication program came too late in one sense, for in time it became clear that the disease had been transmitted to human beings. Those who had eaten products from the animals fed on any of the supplement contaminated with the brain, spinal cord, or digestive tract of the dead animals were affected. The human variant of BSE was given its own name—variant Creutzfeldt–Jakob disease (vCJD or nvCJD). By October 2009, it had killed 166 people in the United Kingdom and 44 elsewhere.

The story then turns to the laboratory of Dr. Stanley Prusiner, a neuroscience researcher at the University of California at San Francisco School of Medicine who was studying CJD. Prusiner's research team found that the infective agent that caused both BSE and CJD was not a virus, as had been proposed, but rather a normal protein that had changed its structure. Prusiner called these altered proteins prions—a combination, sort of, of the words "protein" and "infection." His finding proved to be a classic example of Pauling's structure-function model of disease in action. As Prusiner demonstrated, the prions were natural proteins that had undergone a post-translational modification of their shape; the modification rendered the prion protein stable to cooking temperatures up to 600 degrees Fahrenheit and made it infective. Ironically, the shape of the infective prion protein was what is known as a beta-pleated sheet, a structure that was first defined by Pauling and Corey in their 1951 publications.

This story has an element of intrigue not totally absent from the world of science. Dr. Carleton Gajdusek was a Nobel laureate in Physiology or Medicine in 1976 for his discovery of the origin of kuru, another incurable neurodegenerative disease, similar to CJD, that afflicted the South Fore people of New Guinea in the 1950s. Gajdusek traced the origin of the disease to the tribe's ritual eating of the brains of elders who had died. Once this form of cannibalism was stopped, the disease did not recur.

Gajdusek had long been convinced that kuru was caused by a

slow-reacting virus, but he was never able to isolate or identify it. Nevertheless, when BSE and CJD emerged in the 1980s, he was sure these were other forms of kuru, caused by the same infective virus.

Stanley Prusiner's work of course showed something quite different—that it was not a virus but a structurally modified protein that caused all of these neurodegenerative conditions; in fact, Prusiner added scrapie, affecting sheep and goats, to the list.

The battle was on—a fight between those claiming that an infectious virus was the cause, and those supporting Prusiner's finding that the cause was a structurally modified protein that could be transferred through ingestion. In 1997, the debate was ended when Stanley Prusiner won the Nobel Prize in Physiology or Medicine for his discovery of prions and their role in causing neurodegenerative diseases.

There are many lessons to be learned from this story. One is that the world of science is not free from hubris or an unwillingness to change an opinion in the face of new information. Another is that, for the most part, and even if it takes a while, the truth ultimately wins out. Perhaps the most important lesson is that structure influences function, and that structural information that defines our health and disease can be transmitted through the foods we eat.

Nature is highly selective about the information incorporated into a specific structure. The atoms in a molecule of food are arranged as they are because they constitute a particular piece of coherent information that imparts specific intelligence to the body. When this structure is changed, the information inherent in the structure is changed, and the impact on genetic expression patterns and the way the body therefore functions is also changed.

In chemistry and biology, we talk about "native structure," by which we mean the structure that was present in the plant or animal in its normal state. Did you know that native structure may include handedness—that is, that molecules can be either right-handed or left-handed? Sugars like glucose, for instance, are left-handed, and amino acids are right-handed. If you try to feed someone a right-handed sugar or a left-handed amino acid, that individual will have trouble metabolizing the wrong-handed substance. In fact, the individual is likely to get sick. Yet many synthetically produced substances are an equal mixture of the right- and left-handed versions of a natural substance, only one hand of which is truly natural. A pharmaceutical drug prepared with both right- and left-handed versions can create an adverse effect from the "off-hand" version.

Among other things, this suggests that exceptional care should be taken in messing around with structure—because it is tantamount to messing around with the way the body functions. At the very personal level, the lesson to take away from this bit of science is that the closer to nature the stuff you consume, the more aligned it will be with the functioning of your body—and the better for you. The very rhythm of life is really orchestrated through the structure of substances we ingest. Food is indeed information.

OBESITY IS A STRUCTURAL PROBLEM

Surely one of the dominant health issues of our time is, in structural terms, the adverse health effects associated with an increased waist-to-hip ratio. It's obesity—technically, central obesity, where the fat stores of the body are concentrated around the waist as intra-abdominal fat. It is by now well known that this type of excess fat accumulation is associated with increased incidence of such chronic illnesses as type 2 diabetes, heart disease, stroke, dementia, kidney disease, and both breast and prostate cancers. In fact, the risk of these illnesses is higher from these central fat deposits than from fat residing elsewhere in the body; clearly, this is because the central fat is in direct communication through the bloodstream with the intestinal tract and the liver. Once again, structure—something being where it is in the body—determines function.

To understand how this works—that is, how central deposits of fat so specifically pose a greater risk of chronic diseases than other types of fat—we need to know something about the "personality" of fat deposits. First of all, the cells that make up fat tissue—known as adipose tissue—are called adipocytes. For many years, medicine paid little attention to adipocytes because their only known role was to store extra calories in the form of fat. This all changed starting in the 1990s when further research demonstrated that adipocytes can manufacture and secrete into the bloodstream a family of messenger substances called adipokines. Members of the adipokine family—adiponectin, resistin, and leptin—send messages from the adipose tissue where fat is stored to the rest of the body.

Now here is where the story gets interesting. Adipocytes send two types of adipokine messages; one is friendly, the other angry. Angry messages spur the adipocytes to release particular kinds of substances. Specifically, these are substances that cause what medical students have for generations recited as the hallmarks of inflammation—*rubor, calor, dolor* in the Latin of medical school mnemonics: redness, swelling, and pain. That's what you can get when your adipocytes have been exposed to something they find hostile. By contrast, when the adipocyte is in an environment where its needs are met, its genes express a friendly adipocyte message. Here's how it works:

Suppose you eat a meal that is too high in fat and way too high in sugar. Your gastrointestinal immune system gets alarmed and sends out an alarm message to your white blood cells. They travel through the bloodstream to the adipose tissue where fat is stored, and there they express their anger to the adipocyte. The adipocyte in turn activates its genes to express the angry adipokines, which then race around the body influencing the heart, arteries, liver, brain, kidneys, and pancreas—where, of course, insulin is produced. The adipocytes are basically saying, "I'm fed up and I am not going to take it anymore, and I am sending out adipokines to let everybody know just how angry I am."

And since the original alarm message that ignites this expression of angry fat is received in the immune system of the gastrointestinal tract, most angry fat is found in the nearby central regions of the body. It's the area that gets the first and biggest "hit" from the angry adipokines. For this reason, the greatest risk of chronic illnesses associated with fat accumulation comes from the abdominal fat we see as an out-of-balance waist-to-hip ratio.

But if increased body fat shows risk of chronic illness, it isn't in and of itself a cause of chronic illness; what causes the illness is how angry the fat is. That is why there are plenty of people with significant amounts of excess fat and no chronic illnesses, whereas many leaner folks may suffer type 2 diabetes, heart disease, or any of the other conditions associated with obesity. It is not being fat that causes disease; it's the structure of the fat and its resulting function.

THE CALORIE FALLACY

We have long been told that people become obese because they take in too many calories and don't get enough exercise. This is a very simple expression of the first law of thermodynamics, which states that energy is conserved. So however much energy we take in, measured as calories, that's how much we must use up in activity or we will conserve the unused difference—that is, store it—as fat.

It all sounds so reasonable. But this is neither a complete explanation of nor any kind of answer to the growing global epidemic of obesity. People are not engines that burn fuel; rather, we are complex physiological beings that regulate energy flow and utilization in very sensitive, intricate ways. We saw in Chapter 9, for example, how subtle are the processes of bioenergetics that keep our energy flowing and control its use.

Have you ever noticed that people who carry extra stored calories as fat are often the hungriest people around? And that they often behave as if they have no energy? Why would this be the case when it seems they have more than enough stored energy to meet their needs? I call it "switched metabolism." It is as if the bodies of these people don't recognize how much stored energy they have in their adipose tissue; therefore their bodies demand more quick energy to meet their needs. This turns on the hunger mechanism, which in turn results in more calories stored as fat, and around and around the obesity spiral the person winds.

What causes this? What switches the metabolism? Breakthrough research has finally provided an answer to this question—and it's all about an individual's structure and function. So dismiss, please, the notion that an individual inherits obesity genes. Although we do find that obesity runs in families, no gene that causes it has ever been found; I predict none will ever be found. Rather, what we've learned is that there are many hundreds of genes that regulate the physiological processes that control bioenergetics and its connection to appetite, fat storage, and metabolism.

First, we know that hormones can influence where and how fat is deposited. Higher levels of the estrogen hormone and of the stress hormone cortisol direct fat deposits to the abdominal area. That means that allostatic load, discussed back in Chapter 7, is connected to obesity.

Second, we know that toxic chemicals can poison mitochondria and direct calories to be stored in adipose tissue for a rainy—that is, food-starved—day that never comes. That sounds like our processes of detoxification and defense may be connected to obesity, and in fact, there has been and continues to be a prodigious amount of research in this area.

The story starts in 2005 with a series of papers, now numbering more than a hundred, by two professors working together but some six thousand miles apart. Dr. David Jacobs, professor of public health at the University of Minnesota, and Dr. Duk-Hee Lee, professor of preventive medicine at South Korea's Kyungpook National University School of Medicine, set out to explore the relationship between the level of persistent organic pollutants in the body and obesity and type 2 diabetes. We actually encountered these persistent organic pollutants, POPs, back in Chapter 5 in our discussion of bisphenol-A, BPA, the persistent chemical that simply resists breakdown by any known process. Since such POPs are at large in the environment, they often enter our bodies. Jacobs and Lee wanted to know if there was a statistical correlation between POPs, obesity, and the chronic illness type 2 diabetes.

To find out, they consulted the National Health and Nutrition Examination Survey (NHANES), a comprehensive set of surveys initiated in the early 1960s by the Centers for Disease Control. Aimed at nothing less than assessing the health and nutritional status of adults and children in the United States, the survey is unique in combining interviews with physical examinations. In 1999, NHANES became an ongoing program that examines a nationally representative sample of some 5,000 people in fifteen counties across the country each year. Demographic, socioeconomic, dietary, and health-related measures are tracked along with medical, dental, and physiological measurements. The compiled data offer a comprehensive picture of the nation's health and nutrition and represent a treasure trove of information scientists and the public can access.

On first analyzing the NHANES data, Jacobs and Lee were amazed to find that, contrary to common belief, there was not a strong correlation between obesity and type 2 diabetes—unless the individual also showed a slightly elevated blood level of the enzyme gamma-glutamyl transpeptidase, GGTP. It is a biomarker that has historically signaled liver injury due to alcohol or drug toxicity. For a modest elevation of GGTP level to indicate a relationship between obesity and diabetes in people with neither an alcohol nor a drug problem was unusual in the extreme.

It prompted Jacobs and Lee to search for a connection among the three factors. It was a bit mystifying. They knew that a major function of GGTP in the body is to produce glutathione. Glutathione, as we saw in Chapter 9, protects the mitochondria against injury from caustic forms of oxygen and, as we saw in Chapter 5, is a key component in the detoxification of chemicals. Jacobs and Lee wondered if perhaps the slight increase in GGTP could be a result of exposure to chemicals that the body was trying to detoxify by increasing the production of glutathione.

To check this hypothesis, they examined the level of a number of POPs in the blood of obese people, dividing them into those who had type 2 diabetes and those who did not. The stunning results of this analysis constituted a seismic event in the field of chronic illness research. The results showed a much higher level of POPs and of GGTP levels in the obese people with type 2 diabetes than in those who were obese but did not have diabetes. This suggested that the

POPs had something to do with the origin of diabetes, but it also raised the question as to whether accumulation of POPs might also have some causal relationship with the obesity epidemic.

The two extended their studies to other countries—notably Korea, where obesity and diabetes are rapidly rising—and found the same correlations. The two men now believed they had unlocked a major new understanding of the role of the environment on structure and therefore on function.

Research groups around the world have doubled down on the analyses by Jacobs and Lee and have confirmed their hypothesis. The connection between POPs and obesity is official—official enough to have been given a name: obesogen, a substance that can create obesity.

Let me recap this, because it is essential—not just for understanding our own bodies, but also in providing a clue to the obesity epidemic in which our country and, increasingly, the rest of the developed and developing worlds are now mired.

Obesity is not solely a matter of excess calories. It is a consequence of too many of the wrong type of calories in the presence of an accumulation of environmental POPs. Add it up:

- Bad information from the food we eat creates angry fat.
- POPs poison our mitochondria, reducing their ability to process food into energy, increasing their production of caustic forms of oxygen, and directing unprocessed food calories into storage in fat cells.
- This leads to a change in our structure resulting in a change in the way our physiology functions.

Perhaps a more apt image is that of a vicious circle: We eat foods that cause angry fat, enabling POPs to accumulate in our fat tissue, making it angrier, reducing the bioenergetic capability of our mitochondria, leading to further fat storage—and spinning the circle into chronic illnesses like type 2 diabetes, now on track to become a global pandemic.

BISPHENOL-A AND THE STRUCTURE-FUNCTION RELATIONSHIP

BPA reenters the story in a major way at this point. We explained back in Chapter 5 how this synthetic compound, the plasticizer used globally in bottles and other containers for all kinds of liquids, dislodges naturally occurring hormones from their receptors and sends its own messages to cells regulating physiological function. It is important to note that the levels of BPA in the environment are very low, so low in fact that it was assumed for years that BPA could not possibly have any impact on human physiology.

That assumption was woefully wrong. In 2012, a landmark paper published in *JAMA* reported on research by pediatrics investigators at the New York University School of Medicine. A cross-sectional study of children and adolescents had revealed that levels of BPA in the urine of the study subjects were associated to a significant extent with obesity. In the same year, a study in China reported the same association between BPA levels in children and obesity. Obviously, these studies support the Jacobs and Lee finding of the relationship of POPs to obesity. They make it clear that BPA is an obesogen and a risk factor for such chronic illnesses as diabetes and heart disease, among others.

To me, this raises the question that Rachel Carson posed in *Silent Spring*—namely, how low a level of a substance known to influence human health will produce no effect? What the BPA story tells us is that the answer to this question depends upon the nature of the effect you are looking at. The hormetic effects on structure and function that occur from very low levels of exposure may produce outcomes that are not obvious and that take years to develop.

The studies on BPA in children tell us that obesogens like BPA put epigenetic marks in our book of life and alter the way that genes are expressed. What is even more troubling is to find that some of these epigenetic marks are placed on our genome in germ cells, the cells that can reproduce sexually—that is, eggs in women and sperm in men—and can thus be passed on to subsequent generations. This opens the real possibility that the exposure to a low level of a specific obesogen can alter the genomic expression patterns of the next generation such that the structure and therefore function of that generation's physiology are altered.

The implications are far-reaching. There are obesogens in our environment, and their association with chronic diseases associated with obesity is now much more than a theory. I believe we are looking at a revolutionary new reality about factors that contribute to changing physiological structure and function in people around the world whose societies are undergoing profound change. Have you ever looked at photographs of people from a century ago? Is it possible that the differences in body structure we see between then and now are simply a matter of changing fashions? Surely not. The change is more fundamental.

One of the most fascinating perspectives on this is in the 1939 book *Nutrition and Physical Degeneration* by Weston Price, a dentist living in Baltimore at the turn of the last century. Weston and his wife traveled extensively throughout the world over a period of some thirty years. This was at a time—the first quarter of the twentieth century—when many of the peoples they visited in their travels were just undergoing the transition from their indigenous lifestyles and diets to those of an increasingly industrialized society. Price photographed the same families several different times over the thirty years, and he documented changes in the appearance and health of the children, noting particularly the significant alterations that occurred once white flour and sugar had been incorporated into their diets and in the wake of lifestyle habits made "easier" through advancing technologies. Price has been called the Charles Darwin of nutrition for his detailed recording of these observed changes that so tellingly embody how change in structure results in change in function, and his book, considered a classic, is still available.

Whatever Price's particular observations and whatever his conjectures and conclusions, the question his book raises is an important one. When we consider that in today's children eyesight is declining, dental appliances are increasingly needed to correct tooth alignment, obesity is on the rise, and allergies, asthma, and eczema are all spiraling upward, it's worth pondering whether or not such "developments" aren't the results of epigenetic changes caused by factors of environment, diet, and lifestyle. And it's worth considering what we can do about it.

BROWN FAT, BEIGE FAT, AND OBESOGENS

Obesogens interact with all sorts of different cells in our body in all sorts of different ways, but one of the most important interactions is with the heat-producing cells known as brown fat. There are two types of fat cells—white and brown. White adipocytes store fat; brown adipocytes create heat energy. The brown color comes from the fact that the mitochondria in these cells contain so much iron; it's found in the cytochromes, compounds inside the mitochondrial membrane that are involved in the energy and detoxification processes. (White adipocytes, by contrast, have a different function, storing fat, and therefore a different structure comprising far fewer iron-containing cytochromes.) Thanks to the heat energy that brown fat cells produce, the body can maintain a constant internal temperature even when the external temperature is very low.

Not surprisingly, hibernating animals like bears have high levels of brown fat cells, giving them enough conserved heat energy to get through their dormant period. Infants also have fairly high levels of brown fat. Until recently it was thought that those infant brown fat cells were lost in adulthood, but advanced diagnostic techniques have now identified active brown fat around the neck, shoulders, and upper back of adults.

Obesogens poison brown fat activity, with all sorts of consequences having to do with the production and conservation of heat energy. One consequence is simply that an individual will become increasingly sensitive to cold. Another is obesity: poisoned brown adipocytes may no longer be able to convert a calorie of food into heat, so that calorie will likely be stored as fat in white adipocytes. A sedentary lifestyle is another cause of decreased brown adipocyte activity—it makes them lazy so that they do not convert food to heat very well. It's yet another good reason, if one were needed, for regular exercise. Certain ingredients in food also diminish brown adipocyte activity. One of the most powerful in doing so, and therefore one of the worst offenders when it comes to obesity, is high-fructose corn sweeteners found in many processed foods and beverages.

But just as there are foods that make brown adipocytes lazy, there are also many that wake them up, increase their activity, and therefore help prevent or reverse obesity. Among these are cayenne peppers and other members of the capsicum family of vegetables, apples and peanuts with their skins, grapes, berries, green tea, cinnamon, virgin olive oil, isohumulones from hops, omega-3 fatty oils from fish, and calcium-rich foods like low-fat yogurt.

One of the most exciting new discoveries in this field is the 2008 discovery of beige fat by a professor of cell biology at Harvard, Dr. Bruce Spiegelman.* Spiegelman found the beige adipocytes, as he termed them, embedded in white fat, and he determined that they could be coaxed into becoming heat-producing, active adipocytes through exercise and changes in diet. In other words, activating beige adipocytes can turn angry fat into healthy fat. As you might expect, that in turn has positive effects on insulin sensitivity and lowers the risk of type 2 diabetes and other chronic illnesses.

What does it mean? Simply this: that a couch potato scarfing down supersized portions of junk food who transforms himself into a regular exerciser consuming unprocessed foods rich in phytonutrients will achieve something beyond a sharp reduction in body weight; he can actually create a new, lower set point—that is, the weight at which his body feels natural, and the weight at which it tends to remain.

Such a transformation represents a change in structure and a resulting change in function with long-term positive effects on health. Contrast this with the fad-diet approaches that produce the yo-yo effect—a counterfeit weight loss from which the dieter almost always rebounds, often back to an even higher weight.

---

* Stanley J. Korsmeyer Professor of Cell Biology and Medicine at Harvard Medical School.

THE CONNECTION OF THE SKELETON TO BROWN FAT

And so our story of structure circles back to the skeleton—the first thing that typically comes to mind when we talk about the body's structure. After all, it is the skeleton that keeps our structure upright against the force of gravity and allows us to be mobile and active. That's how I thought of the skeleton when I first began my training years ago; in those days, we had a "real" skeleton hanging in the classroom, and to me, it was a scaffold onto which the body and its parts got attached. I was so wrong.

The human skeleton is the quintessence of getting the structure right and letting the function follow. Of course, the skeleton is bone, but bone consists of the marrow within the mineralized portions of bone, some cortical or compact portions, and some trabecular or meshlike, spongy portions. All are active components that replace themselves throughout our lifetime.

The marrow is where the red and white blood cells in our body are born. Without a healthy bone marrow, we would suffer serious forms of anemia and immune deficiencies. The cortical and trabecular bone, composed of the structural protein called hydroxyapatite, a form of calcium, provides the strength of the skeleton. It also produces signaling substances that talk to other organs in the body, and the other organs in the body produce substances that talk back to the bone. It's a reminder that the skeleton is a part of one of seven core physiological processes, all interconnected, all controlled by genes communicating with one another and with the external environment.

So you will not be surprised to learn that beige adipocytes produce signaling substances that talk to the skeleton in such a way as to improve bone health. For openers, this means that any alteration in the structure and function of fat cells can have an effect on the structure and function of bone. But that's only for openers. Listen in on a conversation, and you'll see what I mean.

The conversation starts when healthy beige adipocytes release a signal called bone morphogenic protein, or BMP, to the bone cells.

In response, the bone cells produce signaling substances called osteo-calcin and osteoprotegerin that influence insulin activity and blood sugar levels. From brown fat to bone to the insulin-secreting pan-creas to the control of blood sugar, the progression is clear: A healthy skeletal structure results in healthy function that can reduce the risk of many chronic diseases.

Another potent example of this is what happens when the skeletal structure is unhealthy—as in the chronic disease known as osteoporo-sis, characterized by bone loss that increases the incidence of fracture in the wrist, hip, and spine. It is a condition seen all too often in post-menopausal women whose ovaries no longer produce the hormone estrogen, which protects the skeleton, but it is seen in men as well.

Medical thinking about osteoporosis saw it not only as the con-sequence of estrogen loss, but also as stemming from not enough calcium and vitamin D in the diet and not enough weight-bearing exercise by the individual. This is in part true, but there is more to the story. We have now learned that ill health in the bone is influ-enced by inflammatory signals from other parts of the body—just like angry fat and arthritis. Indeed, there is a strong connection between osteoporosis, rheumatoid arthritis, and heart disease. If you have one of these chronic illnesses, you are likely to have the others—for the simple reason that they all share common disturbances of the core physiological processes. It is why functional medicine focuses less on the diagnosis of these individual diseases and more on manag-ing the core physiological imbalances and interconnections that have brought them about.

In fact, our research group at the Functional Medicine Clin-ical Research Center in 2009 joined with Dr. Michael Holick, a research endocrinologist at Boston University School of Medicine, in a clinical intervention trial that put a group of postmenopausal women on a fourteen-week Mediterranean-style, low-glycemic-load diet enhanced with selective phytonutrient supplements. The results showed two things: first, significant improvement in the biomark-ers associated with healthy bone versus women of the same age on a standard diet with no phytonutrient supplement; second, lowered inflammation and improved cardiovascular risk factors in the women on the plan. Interconnections indeed.

Have you heard of denosumab—the brand name is Prolia—a fairly recent drug for the treatment of osteoporosis? It works by blocking the inflammatory signal in bone, thereby preventing bone loss. Clearly, it is based on the understanding that bone inflammation is connected to inflammation in other parts of the body, so it is not surprising that the developer of denosumab is exploring this same drug for the treatment of rheumatoid arthritis and other chronic diseases associated with inflammation.

What we are witnessing in medicine are the practical applications of Pauling's revolutionary thinking about structure and its relationship to function derived from his molecular medicine model. As researchers and practitioners increasingly see the ways in which genetic expression is influenced by specific factors of environment, lifestyle, and diet, these applications will continue to expand—and health will improve.

Deborah and Bruce, as I'll call them, are a charming and engaging couple in their early seventies who were referred to our medical and nutritional professionals because they wondered if a change in diet might offer some solution to Bruce's increasing frailty and immobility. A review of Bruce's history, physical evaluation, biomarkers, and functional assessment led to the collective conclusion that he was suffering from sarcopenia, the medical term for loss of muscle mass, which seemed to be due to an underlying chronic inflammatory condition. Bruce showed no signs, however, of a traditional autoimmune disease like arthritis; rather, metabolic factors were contributing to the inflammation. We also gave Bruce a bone density test and found results in the range of an osteoporotic female.

No wonder he felt frail and found it difficult to move. The loss of muscle mass with age is a major contributor to disability and injuries and certainly compromises an individual's strength. Because it happens over time and in increments, it is often not recognized, and of course it is typically thought to be "just a part of aging." This acceptance of loss of muscle mass as inevitable is a principal reason that we see increasing numbers of older adults holding on to a walker or a cane as they try to get around, or using a motorized device. But the truth is that sarcopenia is now recognized as resulting from a number of factors—chronic inflammation, insulin resistance, lack of weight-bearing exercise, and nutritional imbalances.

In Bruce's case, a personalized program was designed that would improve his insulin sensitivity, reduce his inflammation potential, and increase his anabolic hormone activity to rebuild lost muscle. The program included daily strength and conditioning exercises; a diet focused on higher protein content, a lower glycemic load, and of course specific phytonutrients; a prescription for low-dose testosterone replacement therapy; and a nutritional supplement program to close the gap of Bruce's nutritional needs.

We like to give a personalized lifestyle plan at least twelve weeks to work. Everybody is different, of course, but in my view, it takes at least that amount of time to substantially change the structure-function relationship in a person with chronic health problems. Moreover, progress may be slow to start, and not seeing the improvement you hope for in the first days or weeks can be frustrating. If you expect the payoff to take three months, that can often encourage people to stick it out.

That's what happened with Bruce. There was little visible progress in the first few weeks; indeed, it wasn't until week nine that the improvements really accelerated. Yet even when the signs were minimal, Bruce told us he found the experience far more profound than he had ever expected. He felt "empowered," he said, for the first time in his life to take control of his own health, and he was glad to wait the full twelve weeks to know he could be successful at it.

Successful he certainly was. He left his walker behind and became fully mobile without assistance. Our follow-up studies showed increased muscle mass without a significant spike in body weight; in other words, he had replaced fat with muscle. His bone density was showing improvement, as were the biomarkers of inflammation. Most important, he felt "more vital."

There was another benefit as well. Deborah also lost weight

during the twelve weeks, and in her regular checkup, her own doctor commented on a number of improved indicators. In fact, her bone density test had so improved that he said there was no need to prescribe a bone loss drug. "Whatever you're doing," he told her, "keep it up."

The Deborah-Bruce twofer tells us something else about health and well-being—namely, that the structure of our social relationships can also determine how our lives function. Pauling's structure-function model plays out at every level. That is perhaps reflected in the two Nobel Prizes in his own life—one for how structure at the molecular level affects our health, the other, the Peace prize for his global effort to stop atmospheric nuclear weapon testing, at the interplanetary level. In both spheres, what we do to structure can influence how we function.

It is time to put this to work on the personal level. Yours.

CHAPTER 10 TAKEAWAY

1. The structure of the body is related to its function, and nutrition and physical activity play key roles in determining both.

2. Proper structural alignment is important for maintaining good health.

3. Exposure to electromagnetic radiation can result in changes in immune and nervous system function.

4. Elevated blood sugar levels result in the production of glycoproteins that can contribute to many chronic diseases. A low-glycemic-load diet comprising minimally processed foods prevents this problem.

5. Obesity is caused by more than just too many calories; it is also a result of consuming foods that increase inflammation in the body.

6. Exposure to toxins in food and water contributes to obesity.

7. Bone loss can result from such factors as poor nutrition, lack of weight-bearing exercise, digestive problems, inflammation, and insulin resistance.

PART THREE

PERSONALIZING YOUR HEALTH-MANAGEMENT PLAN

The preceding chapters have demonstrated the need for a new way of thinking about medical care and a new role for individuals in managing their health. The chapters that follow set forth the practical basics of this new approach, empowering you to create a personal health-management plan.

A baseline program is the starting point, while a series of eight self-assessment questionnaires help readers address individual process imbalances and restore balance as needed.

CHAPTER 11

A New Approach to Your Health

What do we mean by health? The World Health Organization offered an answer to this question back in 1946. "Health," said the coordinating health authority for the United Nations, "is a state of complete physical, mental and social well-being, and not merely the absence of disease or infirmity." That's a great definition, and it is a lofty goal—one we all hope to achieve. The question is how.

Hippocrates, the legendary physician of classical Greece known as the father of medicine, formulated an answer that has come down to us in its Latin form as *vis medicatrix naturae*, the healing power of nature—the idea that if organisms are provided the right environment, diet, and lifestyle support, they can heal themselves. In our day, the idea has been recast through the lens of the genomic revolution as our ability to shape the way our environment influences the expression of our genes, which in turn shapes our individual health and disease patterns.

Everything laid out in the previous chapters of this book—the discoveries of the genomic revolution and the wisdom captured by looking at chronic illness from a systems biology perspective—comes down to putting that idea to work. Its practical application is the functional medicine model that is our era's revolution in health care. Patient-centered, the model requires that the individual participate fully in managing his or her health. The idea is simple: by creating a personalized health-management program that sets out changes in diet, lifestyle, and environment, we can directly affect how our genes are expressed and thus the patterns of our health.

That's what you're about to do. With the help and support of your chosen health practitioner, you're about to design and execute your own personalized plan to address any health problems you have and to live in a way that optimizes your genetic potential. This chapter gets you started. It prompts you to look at your own health and start putting together the tools to manage it in a whole new way.

Not just new—different as well. In the previous chapters of this book, you have absorbed concepts of medical thinking that diverge markedly from what you've known up to now, and you're about to start applying health interventions and therapies that are likely considerably different from what you're used to. It makes sense, therefore, to review the key tenets of this new thinking before you undertake the new interventions. Basically, they come down to these five.

1. *Our health is not predetermined by our genes.* No single gene controls the presence or absence of a chronic disease. Our pattern of health and illness is determined by how families of genes are expressed, and that expression can be influenced and indeed altered by a range of lifestyle, diet, and environmental factors—exercise, stress, pollutants, radiation, specific foods, phytonutrients, and more—that send signals to the cells of our body.

2. *Chronic illness is a result of an imbalance in one or more of the core physiological processes.* Such an imbalance derives from the interaction between our genome and our lifestyle, diet, and environment. The imbalance alters function. Over time, that altered function is evidenced in specific signs and symptoms that we collectively label a disease. Changes to lifestyle, diet, and environment can bring our core physiological processes back into balance.

3. *The absence of illness does not necessarily equate to the presence of wellness.* A diagnosis of chronic illness comes after a period of declining function. If your ability to function has not yet begun to

decline or has only just begun to decline, now is the best time to execute a personalized lifestyle intervention, for now is when it will have the greatest positive impact on your health.

4. *Each person's physiological response to lifestyle, dietary, and environmental factors is unique to his or her genetic makeup.* Every individual's genetic makeup is unique, and each of us therefore experiences unique responses to lifestyle, diet, and environment. A lifestyle, diet, and environment that are optimal for one individual might be poison for another.

5. *Drugs effective for the management of acute disease may be inappropriate for the long-term management of chronic illness.* Most pharmaceutical drugs are designed for potency in blocking a specific step in the complex physiological network associated with the target condition of ill health. Over time, however, their potency may have a collateral effect off-target, with potential adverse impact. Since most chronic illness needs to be managed for the long term, the safest use of drugs will be as late as possible in the progression of the symptoms of illness and in the lowest dose possible to maintain healthy function.

This is the background against which the functional medicine approach of personalized lifestyle health care has been designed. It focuses on treating the cause of a chronic illness—that is, imbalances in the core physiological processes—not the symptoms and signs that are the effects of the cause.

But the approach is not without precedent. Similar underlying tenets form the foundation of traditional Chinese medicine and of India's Ayurvedic practices. Indeed, long before anything was known about cellular biology, genetics, or pathology, Eastern medical practitioners, through observation, embraced concepts very similar to those we apply today in functional medicine. One of the most gratifying aspects of my role as someone carrying the message of functional medicine around the world is to witness a growing movement to integrate Western and Eastern medical thinking and to consolidate the best practices of both. It is exciting to see how the new ideas born of the genomic revolution are reframing old observations and creating a new medicine in which the individual can take the best of knowledge and experience from many perspectives.

Here again is how we put it all together in our functional medicine operating model.

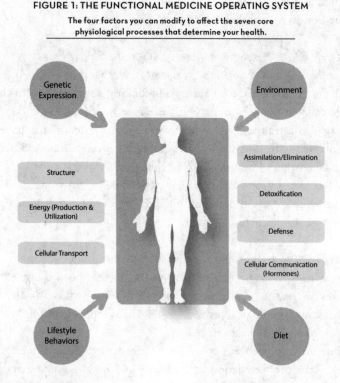

FIGURE 1: THE FUNCTIONAL MEDICINE OPERATING SYSTEM

The four factors you can modify to affect the seven core physiological processes that determine your health.

THE TOOLS OF PERSONALIZED HEALTH MANAGEMENT

What are the capabilities available to you to put the new medicine into effect? We've talked about them throughout this book—lifestyle, diet, environment. They're the tools of health management, and we all own them. Everyone has a lifestyle—a set of behaviors and habits that mark how we live. Everyone has a diet or way of eating. And everyone lives in an environment; more precisely, everyone lives in a range of environments, from big categories such as which hemisphere you live in, whether in a hot or cold climate, whether in a developed or developing nation, city or country, mountain or shore, etc., to the more tightly defined environments of your home, workplace, amenities, and the like. That all three of these factors—lifestyle, diet, environment—play significant roles in determining how our genes are expressed and how our health is shaped over time may seem obvious. But it is not. It is as revolutionary a concept in medical thinking as the idea that bacterial infection causes disease was at the turn of the last century—and will have just as great an impact on medical treatment.

So the decisions you make concerning changes to these three parts of your life can be significant, which is why it's important to make those decisions within a framework of criteria about what your decisions can and cannot affect.

DIET

Let's start with diet because food is the one thing we all think, probably rightly, that we can most definitely control. Moreover, food is a cornerstone of the personalized program; in few other areas is it as clear as it is in this area—literally, as we've noted before—that one man's meat is another man's poison: that the foods that bring health to one individual can be a health disaster for another. Food also has a particularly critical role among the three factors of our plan—environment, diet, lifestyle—because we have to eat. It's a survival essential.

And we know—because we hear it, read it, have it shouted at us on TV—that we should eat a varied diet and in moderate portions. What has become true for many of us in twenty-first-century America is that too many of us are malnourished—not from eating too little, but rather from eating too much of too little. It is called overconsumptive undernutrition, and it is not a deficiency of calories but a surfeit of empty calories, the kind—as you have learned—that send messages of alarm and danger to our genes. This is the malnutrition characterized by obesity, diabetes, heart disease, osteoporosis, dementia, and other chronic illnesses associated with inflammation, which can of course alter all seven core physiological processes.

So the proper diet for you will first and foremost provide adequate amounts of all the essential nutrients that meet your needs based on your genes, as evidenced in the process imbalances you've identified. It will also be satisfying to your taste, will be a pleasure and comfort to eat, and will adhere to the following shoulds and shouldn'ts.

Your Diet Should...	Your Diet Should Not...
have a low glycemic load	raise blood sugar or insulin rapidly after eating
contain a proper balance of omega-3 oils	contain trans fats or partially hydrogenated vegetable oils
provide high levels of phytonutrients aimed at supporting your own healthy genetic expression	contain allergy- or inflammation-inducing foods or ingredients
contain higher levels of specific nutrients necessary to support individual needs	contain empty-calorie snack foods
contain components that help support a healthy balance of enteric microflora	contain overly processed low-fiber foods

In general, of course, we are talking about what is generally known as the Mediterranean diet as the baseline of healthy eating. This is a way of eating that incorporates all the shoulds and shouldn'ts that will guide your personalized plan. It contains a variety of lean proteins from both animal and vegetable products. It is low in sugars and in such processed foods as white flour products. It contains adequate amounts of whole fruits, vegetables, legumes, rice, and spices to meet phytonutrient needs, and it has enough foods containing omega-3 oils to provide a balance of fats.

Study after study has confirmed the efficacy of this way of eating as a baseline for good health. One of the most interesting studies, aimed at evaluating the long-term health impact of a Mediterranean diet, is the Healthy Aging Longitudinal in Europe study, HALE, which reviewed all-cause mortality in 1,507 apparently healthy seventy- to ninety-year-old men and women in eleven western European countries over a ten-year period. The results, published in 2004, showed conclusively that study participants had a death rate 50 percent lower than that of people who did not follow this way of eating or practice similar healthy-lifestyle habits.

A brief aside here: The lack of press coverage about this study makes you wonder about priorities. If a pill had been developed that could reduce death from all causes by half in a population of seventy- to ninety-year-olds, it likely would have been a top headline for weeks, with every senior citizen on earth lining up to get the prescription. The prescription here is a way of eating, and it seems to elicit only indifference from the world's media.

In any event, HALE joins a long list of scientific evidence that the Mediterranean way of eating makes the perfect baseline for positive health outcomes. Only one more ingredient needs to be added, and that is the personalization that should inform your own health-management plan. Use the Mediterranean-diet baseline to meet the should and shouldn't criteria for a general diet plan, then add or subtract the specific foods to meet your own nutritional requirements or avoid adverse immune response, and that will be your optimal plan.

LIFESTYLE

Obviously, this is a huge area. It embraces the personal habits we often label "recreational"; the level and content of your exercise activity; and the allostatic load of stress you may be carrying that is affecting your physiology and function.

Of the first of these, there is really no need to add to what is by now well known: smoking kills; alcohol and drug abuse mess up your life very badly—and then kill. So such habits are to be avoided.

Exercise is so extremely important to all aspects of health that, as with diet, it's a good idea to start with a baseline of general criteria onto which you can add the specifics that personalize your exercise to your needs. Here are the shoulds and shouldn'ts of exercise activity:

Your Exercise Program Should...	Your Exercise Program Shouldn't...
incorporate activities that build endurance, strength, and flexibility	exceed your physical capabilities
bring your pulse and respiration into your aerobic training zone, calculated as 180 minus your age in years	produce serious muscle pain or joint strain
have minimal impact on joints and muscles	total *less* than 120 minutes per week
be something you do routinely 5 to 6 days a week	be only a "weekend warrior" activity of excessive physical demand without proper conditioning

If there is a rock-bottom minimum of 120 minutes of exercise a week, the standard should be five to six sessions of at least 20 minutes per session five or six times a week. The excuse of not enough time is unwarranted. We find time every day to eat, drink, and breathe; exercise is as important to improving our core physiological processes as are those activities, and even with the "additional" time required to dress and undress, shower, warm up, cool down, etc., an exercise session amounts to no more than 4 percent of a day. If we compare the benefits it realizes—the positive messages it sends to your genes—that makes exercise the safest, most rewarding investment an individual can make.

You can enrich the investment further by adding to the baseline criteria more time or effort in any one of the end-goals—endurance, strength, or flexibility—that addresses your particular needs as evidenced in the process imbalances you've identified. More time spent in exercise never hurt anyone, but take care that the additional time does not exceed your capabilities at the time or add too much pressure or strain on muscles or joints.

The important third leg of the lifestyle component of your

personalized health-management plan is dealing with your allostatic load. Clearly, no one can avoid stress altogether. We all occasionally feel the weight of the world on our shoulders, or encounter a back-breaking task, or feel we are going crazy from pressure of one sort or another. The metaphors are telling; allostatic load manifests itself as weight upon our physiology and ability to function.

What we now know is that it isn't the stressor itself but rather our response to it that can amplify our cellular communication process to alarm status—and thereby affect other processes as well. We also know ways to deal with such responses on our part—through various techniques of relaxation and mindfulness that have been put forth over the years to alter the cellular communications process and dampen the alarm. The best advice I've heard on the subject came from one of the most formidable proponents of these ideas, Dr. Robert S. Eliot, the cardiologist and author of the best-selling 1985 book about type A personalities, *Is It Worth Dying For?* Eliot and I lectured together some years ago, and at dinner after-ward, he crystallized his theory as follows: "There are two rules in life," he said. "The first one is easy to understand; it says not to worry about the small stuff. The second one is more complicated; it says everything is the small stuff if it is going to kill us."

I've incorporated that into my own process for keeping my al-lostatic load at bay, and I share it with you here in six steps.

1. Recognize that your allostatic load is affecting your health.
2. Identify the individual contributors to the load.
3. Differentiate those contributors that you have some control over versus those that you do not.
4. Focus on the contributors you can control; act to reduce their load.
5. Don't sweat the small stuff, and anything that isn't going to kill us is the small stuff.
6. Do sweat the big stuff, which is anything that adversely affects your health over the long term.

ENVIRONMENT

How can an individual control his or her environment when environment is the one thing we share with all the communities on the planet? Back in 1968, in an essay in the journal *Science* entitled "The Tragedy of the Commons," ecologist Garrett Hardin of the University of California at Santa Barbara gave voice to that frustration. Air, water, and land, Hardin wrote, are considered "commons" and therefore can be exploited for individual good at the expense of the many. There is no technical solution to this, Hardin went on; rather, it requires a new way of thinking about personal responsibility—an understanding of our individual decisions and actions in the context of the influence they will have on the whole.

Yet once we have that first level of awareness about our personal impact on the environment and how it influences the commons, how is the individual to act? In the wake of the genomic revolution, we have guidelines for that—criteria for managing the environmental messages received by our genes.

- To eat organic foods as much as possible
- To avoid excessive sun exposure
- To drink purified water in metal or glass containers
- To use a headset with our cell phones
- To avoid processed foods and personal care products with synthetic ingredients
- To wash our hands before eating
- To avoid environments that support bad health habits
- To design our own environments to be safe places to live

Everyone can plant a garden. From the window box or shelf of herbs in a small apartment to the urban farming that is increasingly prevalent on building rooftops, every individual can find ways to take some control over his or her environment. It is always possible to send healthy messages to your genes rather than unhealthy ones. It is a matter of making the healthy choice, and in doing so, you also make a healthy contribution to our common environment.

SUPPLEMENTS AND PHARMACEUTICALS

Another key component of your personalized health-management program is the use of such nutritional supplements as nutraceuticals and medical foods,* over-the-counter therapies, and, where appropriate, prescription medications. All are tools that can influence your core processes and your health, and all belong in your health toolbox.

In the functional medicine revolution, dietary supplements, nutraceuticals, or medical foods are the therapies of choice to top up, as needed, an identified nutrient insufficiency in an individual's personalized health-management plan, as we'll discuss in more detail in the next chapter.

Where prescription pharmaceutical drugs are concerned, it's essential, as most physicians will agree, that such therapies work in tandem with a patient's lifestyle, diet, and environment and that they are prescribed to fit that context. One of the most stunning examples of what can happen if a physician is not aware of context is the understanding gained in recent years of the role of grapefruit juice. It has to be one of the more common household staples—a good-for-you fruit juice that families consume routinely. Yet we now know that this juice's unique array of phytonutrients can profoundly affect the metabolism of some widely prescribed drugs. It increases the blood levels in women taking certain birth control pills and alters the effect of those pills. A flavonoid it contains, naringenin, reduces the metabolism of cyclosporine, a drug prescribed after kidney transplant surgery to prevent transplant rejection, and keeps it in the blood longer. These findings remind us again how diet can affect pharmaceuticals and why the control of lifestyle, diet, and environment is so important in any program designed to treat chronic illness.

If you're taking prescription medications at the time you initiate your personalized health-management plan, the likelihood is that your medication doses will in time be reduced or even eliminated as the imbalances in your core physiological processes are rectified.

---

* Medical foods are available by physician recommendation.

But be sure your prescribing health-care practitioner is aware of all your factors of lifestyle, diet, and environment that may affect or be affected by the drugs.

THE TWELVE-WEEK TIME FRAME

Finally, why do we need to give a personalized health-management plan twelve weeks? Years of experience and many clinical studies make it pretty clear that this is the *average* time it takes to make a real change to your cellular biology and patterns of genetic expression. Yes, some people notice the benefits of personalized changes to lifestyle, diet, and environment right away; for others—remember Bruce?—progress is slow in coming.

Keep in mind that changing your lifestyle, diet, and environment is not like taking a drug to cure a specific symptom. The action of a pill or injection is to block or alter the function of one step in a complex physiological network. It can do this reasonably quickly in most cases, immediately in many cases. A program of change, however, is aimed at transforming a pattern of genetic expression and the nature of the control those genes exercise over the physiological network. Such change happens across a sequence of multiple changes—one change deriving from another in a chain of action and reaction—and it occurs over a longer period of time.

Here's a suggestion: Right now, sit down and make a list of your health issues. What are the things that really bother you, the things you really, really want to change? Maybe it's that you're tired of feeling this tired so much of the time, or maybe you're sick of taking four pills every morning with breakfast, or perhaps you want some improvement in—if not an end to—the joint pain you feel 24/7. Now rank these complaints for their severity on a scale of 1 to 5, with 5 being the least onerous and 1 being the very worst. Keep the piece of paper handy so you can remember where you started. Take another look at it twelve weeks after you initiate your personalized health-management program.

CHAPTER 12

Developing Your Baseline Program

In 2012, our research team at the Functional Medicine Clinical Research Center undertook a sixteen-month functional medicine–based intervention program in a group of 130 modestly overweight women and men. As you can imagine, in sixteen months of frequent visits, you get to know the participants in a study very well, and you come to appreciate their lives, their concerns, and who they are as people. So it was gratifying indeed that the study's preliminary results demonstrated the profound positive effects on health outcomes of certain fundamental actions taken in diet, lifestyle, and environment.

These actions constitute, in my view, a baseline program for helping every individual fulfill the WHO's definition of health—the perfect starting point for the development of a personalized health-management plan.

It works according to what I call the 80-20 principle. If these fundamental actions are built into an individual's life, that individual will be 80 percent along the way toward improving his or her health. The remaining 20 percent will come from building onto this baseline specific actions to address the individual's personal process imbalances, as we'll see in more detail in the next chapter.

I saw the 80 percent baseline effect in action back in the late 1990s, when a high-ranking army commander in the Desert Storm campaign came to our research center for a health consultation. Since his return from the war, he had not felt right. At the age of fifty-four, he was experiencing fatigue, severe and progressive muscle weakness, and—his key worry—a deteriorating memory. He knew of some family history of cardiovascular disease and exertion intolerance, but he had never experienced any such problems himself. In fact, he had been an Ironman athlete before Desert Storm and had served in previous military combat situations without any ill effects. The military doctors had put him through an extensive battery of tests for infectious diseases, poisoning, or a definitive diagnosis. To date, all had come up negative. The only medical assessment he had received was that he was suffering from post-traumatic stress disorder and needed rest and counseling.

Our researchers were aware that resilience studies on animals put under extreme physical and mental stress demonstrated the importance of overall health and basic nutrition in improving resilience, and we believed our commander was deficient in both. We further hypothesized that he may have had some type of genetic susceptibility to specific substances he may have been exposed to in the desert, where his unit was camped for many months. This led us to a twofold plan of action: the implementation of a baseline program to strengthen his overall health and refresh his capability for resilience, to be followed by a program aimed at strengthening the commander's detoxification and cellular energy processes.

What was most interesting was how quickly he recovered his strength after implementing the first steps of the baseline program—before he went on to the more complex components of his personalized program to restore process imbalances. Within six months, he had regained his resilience and was able to return to active duty.

For me, this example was a lesson in how important it is, when embarking upon a personalized health-management program, to take what might seem simple first steps. The health payoff can be enormous.

The functional medicine baseline program consists of recommendations for diet and dietary supplements, exercise, stress management, and management of your environment—the factors that interact with our genes to affect the balance of our seven core physiological processes.

Yet even as you follow the recommendations and make your own choices to develop your baseline program, it makes sense to be aware of what your family health history may tell you about your own genetic susceptibilities. Specifically, is there a history of any of the following in your family?

1. Heart disease
2. Diabetes
3. Cancer
4. High blood pressure
5. Depression or mental illness
6. Autoimmune or inflammatory disorders
7. Obesity
8. Osteoporosis
9. Dementia
10. Allergies, atopic dermatitis, or asthma
11. Alcoholism or drug abuse
12. Emotional or psychological burnout
13. Inborn genetic disease
14. Anemia
15. Eye diseases such as glaucoma or macular degeneration

Again, none of these conditions is strictly inherited, but a family history of any of them indicates an area of possible genetic sensitivity. Coupled with your responses to the Health Self-Assessment Questionnaire and the answers you gave to the questionnaires in Chapters 4 through 10, family health history can help the detective work as you look for the patterns that define your own health strengths and weaknesses. So many of us feel doomed to repeat the conditions we saw our parents or grandparents suffer through, or we are stunned when we receive a diagnosis that is unheard of in the family's previous experience. Yet studies of disease prevalence in identical twins confirm that inherited genes alone are not decisive in causing a health condition or averting it. Rather, our differing degrees of genetic susceptibility to various conditions can be modified by lifestyle, diet, and environment. After all, families share these three things—lifestyle, diet, and environment—just as they share genes. The genes don't change; lifestyle, diet, and environment may.

The functional medicine baseline program is a first step toward changes that may modify your genetic expression to cure a chronic illness or get you squarely on the path to a state of good health in which you achieve balance in all your core processes.

THE BASELINE DIET

By now, you are well versed in the power of nutrition to influence genetic expression; the way we eat is no longer the best-kept secret of good health. In support of this, Chapter 11 laid out the basic criteria for what a diet should and should not do to support proper balance in and between each of the seven core physiological processes. The underlying objective is to lower physiological stress and increase the delivery of nutrients to the cells, tissues, and organs that control healthy physiological function.

Basically, we're looking for foods that stabilize the balance of hormones and cellular mediators released into the bloodstream after eating and thus help turn on the expression of the health-promoting genes, not the alarm genes. Such a baseline diet will include a great diversity of foods, but as a group, the characteristics that pertain are these: fresh, minimally processed, organic, natural, whole-food, multicolored, low-sugar, and low in saturated fat. Where fish are concerned, "natural" means line-caught wild fish that contain omega-3 oils. Why should your diet be multicolored? The colors in fresh fruits, vegetables, and beans represent their phytonutrient content. A multicolored diet gives you a wide-ranging palette of phyto-nutrients, each of which has its own unique and beneficial effect on genetic expression.

The baseline diet stays away from common allergy-producing foods until you know more about what might be problem foods based upon your own genetic uniqueness. The common triggers of food allergy or sensitivity include gluten-containing grains, uncultured dairy products, shellfish, citrus, eggs, yeast, any food that has seen mold or fungus, peanuts, whole soy, and processed foods containing multiple additives.

The baseline diet also avoids fried or fat-laden foods, whether they are high in animal fat or vegetable oils. It recommends that foods be cooked at as low a temperature as possible. Longer cooking at a lower temperature prevents the formation of glycotoxins and is therefore preferable to high-temperature cooking for short periods of time.

Finally, of course, make sure your baseline diet contains digestion-friendly foods. Yogurt enriched with probiotics is highly recommended, but be sure also that you get enough soluble and insoluble fiber in your diet. A diet that is 60 to 70 percent plant-based foods and 30 to 40 percent animal products will fulfill that requirement.

Does this mean you can't be a vegetarian on this baseline diet? No. But a vegetarian diet needs to be approached with some care to avoid imbalances in such nutrients as iron, vitamin B12, and calcium. Obviously, the composition of the diet is also key; a diet of potato chips, soft drinks, and hard candy could be called vegetarian, but under no circumstances could it be called healthy—or sensible.

Want to see what a typical week of the baseline diet might look like? The full menu plan and the recipes for the various dishes are provided in Appendix A, but with breakfasts like homemade granola or spicy carrot muffins, lunches of salad or casserole or hash, and dinners ranging from chicken and broccoli stir-fry to sea scallops with Asian flavoring, I think you see how diverse and satisfying this kind of eating can be. Keep in mind that the meal plan in Appendix A is not meant to be prescriptive; it's just representative of kinds of food and of the diversity of foods in a baseline diet. In fact, it will also help you make good choices when you are eating in a restaurant or on the go. Note that the foods fulfill the criteria set forth above for achieving the baseline goals.

Note also that the recipes for these meals mostly produce from four to six servings. That is intentional. First, leftovers are useful.

Second, and more important, you probably live with a spouse or partner, a roommate, or a family, and what we've learned is that making a change in diet works better when your significant others are engaged as well. In fact, engagement can be key to making any and all changes in behavior. For one thing, others can serve as a support group. For another, the people you live with are going to be affected by your personalized health-management program, too, and if you share the experience so that all of you own it, they too may be influenced to undertake more healthy eating. It can make the whole experience not just a joint venture but a joint *ad*venture, encouraging shopping together for food and preparing meals together.

THE BASELINE DIETARY SUPPLEMENT PROGRAM

In 2009, the Nobel Prize in Physiology or Medicine was awarded to three scientists, Elizabeth Blackburn, Carol Greider, and Jack Szostak, for their discovery of telomeres and their pioneering work on the enzyme that produces them, telomerase. Telomeres are a unique piece of chemical structure at the end of each chromosome in our genome, and they're there to protect the chromosome—and the information it holds—from damage. But as part of doing this job, telomeres get shorter, and that renders the chromosomes vulnerable to harm, making the genome as susceptible to defacement as the pages of treasured books in a library in which vandals have been let loose. Defacement results in a loss of the integrity of our genetic code, which in turn alters the core physiological processes that we associate with health and resilience, so the bottom line of the shortening of the telomeres is an increased incidence of all the chronic illnesses we dread—including cardiovascular disease, diabetes, dementia, and cancer.

We now know that lifestyle, diet, and environment play a role in determining the length of the telomeres. Research in Europe examined telomere shortening over a five-year period in individuals consuming a nutrient-dense Mediterranean diet. The study showed that telomere length "significantly predicted" decreases in weight, body mass index, waist circumference, and waist-to-height ratio.

Conclusion: longer telomeres mean less obesity, and the Mediterranean diet can be a key differentiating factor in telomere length. Yet another study, this one tracking 5,862 women, found that those adhering to the kinds of diet and lifestyle regimen defined in the functional medicine baseline program had significantly longer telomeres. Studies by Dean Ornish and Nobel laureate Elizabeth Blackburn on men with prostate cancer found that an aggressive lifestyle and diet intervention increased the activity of the enzyme telomerase, which repairs the shortened telomeres. In 2013, the Ornish-Blackburn group reported in *The Lancet Oncology* that prostate cancer patients adhering to a comprehensive lifestyle and diet intervention program experienced a significant 10 percent increase in telomere length versus the control group, which experienced a 3 percent *decrease* in telomere length. The study also found that the greater the compliance with the lifestyle and diet intervention program, the greater the increase in the length of the telomeres. Bottom line: nutrition preserves and produces telomere length essential for good health.

We also know that vitamins B3 (niacin), folic acid, and B12 all play important roles in maintaining telomere length. Michael Fenech, a senior scientist in nutrition at the Commonwealth Scientific and Industrial Research Organisation (CSIRO), Australia's national research agency, has published numerous studies defining the roles that specific nutrients play in protecting our book of life against injury. The U.S. National Institute of Environmental Health Sciences published the compelling results of a study of 586 women, aged thirty-five to seventy-four, exploring the role that supplementary vitamins and minerals may have in protecting our telomeres. The telomeres were 5 percent longer in the women who took a multivitamin supplement daily than in those women who did not. Longer telomeres were also noted in women who supplemented daily with 3 grams of omega-3 fatty acids.

These are important observations about health. They tell us that the role of nutrients in cellular function goes beyond that of protecting us against vitamin deficiency diseases like scurvy, beriberi, pellagra, or rickets. The preservation of telomere length is a cellular measure of organ reserve, the key marker of biological age. It is now clear that a well-balanced multivitamin-mineral supplement and a fish oil supplement may do much more than just produce "expensive urine." These nutrients help protect our most precious asset, the DNA in our book of life, thus enhancing and extending our health span.

A prudent baseline dietary supplement program, therefore, is a reasonable component of any personalized health-management program. It should include the following daily doses:

- A multivitamin-mineral supplement with at least 1,000 IU of vitamin D
- 1,000 to 2,000 milligrams of vitamin C
- 2 to 3 grams of omega-3 oil containing EPA/DHA
- A probiotic supplement containing at least 3 billion live organisms.

THE BASELINE EXERCISE PROGRAM

Get yourself a pedometer. Really. Head for the nearest sporting goods store or, if you're digitally inclined, find the right app for your smartphone so you can track the number of steps you take as you walk. It is a great way to begin an exercise program; there are no barriers to getting started, no new equipment to buy apart from the pedometer or the app, no place you can't just start walking. Your goal is gradually to get to a point where you are walking a *minimum* of 10,000 steps per day.

Now that may seem like a lot of steps, but it's less than you think. I find that taking the dog out three times a day uses up about 6,000 steps each day, so you can see that the steps quickly add up. A fifteen-minute post-meal walk, which, as we'll show in Chapter 13, significantly improves blood sugar and insulin regulation, can typically take about 2,000 steps. So the 10,000-steps-per-day target is not unrealistic. Still, you will probably need to make a conscious effort at first to get there, because the amount of walking most of us tend to do often comes up short of the target.

That the effort is worth it, however, is not in doubt. Studies on university students who went from "sedentary" to 10,000 steps per day showed lowered blood pressure and improved cardiovascular fitness after only six weeks. In several other studies, achieving the target resulted in improved cardiovascular function, psychological well-being, and blood cholesterol and HDL levels.

Here's even more proof: Studies confirm that days after stopping a regular walking program, insulin sensitivity decreases, and angry fat starts to accumulate. The impairment in insulin sensitivity occurs before the accumulation of body fat—an indication yet again that it is not obesity alone that causes type 2 diabetes but the alteration in the cellular communications process from the altered physiological fitness. So walking 10,000 steps per day is definitely worth the effort. Don't stop.

What if you are already engaged in a regular activity program? Good! But make sure that you do it regularly and that you hit appropriate goals of intensity and duration. Specifically, you should get into your aerobic training zone—a pulse rate of approximately 180 minus your age in years—and stay there for twenty minutes at least five times per week. Or, think of it as engaging in an activity that puts you in your aerobic training zone for a minimum of 150 minutes per week.

The choice of activity is up to you; mix and match the aerobic and anaerobic, the cardiovascular fitness with the strengthening and flexibility as you find what is enjoyable for you and what fits into your daily routine. The key is to just do it.

THE BASELINE STRESS MANAGEMENT PROGRAM

In my view, just about everyone living in today's fast-paced, time-urgent global society could benefit from some form of stress management. We're all carrying too much allostatic load, which in turn diminishes our capability for resilience. The urgency to get things done now has become a prison, constraining our minds and oppressing our bodies.

Yet even a little bit of time reserved each day to listen to music, be out in nature, look at art, tend a garden, or remain still or quiet in reflection or prayer can create the genetic expression that renews core physiological processes—and instills a sense of peace.

A simple way to get started is with techniques of cognitive behavioral and mindfulness therapies. These combine traditional behavioral therapies with strategies of meditation to reduce stress and anxiety. Start by inventorying the events in your life that trigger a distress response, that create a sense of burden or anxiety. Prioritize them, and then create a mindful approach to controlling your body's response to them.

Creating such an approach is not easy. It requires practice to prepare yourself to think about how you will respond to stressors the next time you confront them. But the time spent in preparation through mindful contemplation or quiet introspection will pay dividends the next time you are exposed to the triggering event. Sometimes, the introspection itself might create a tension that you would like to avoid, but practice in confronting that tension is a key part of preparedness, and preparedness is the solution to the recurring distress you feel when you do confront those tension-making issues.

The skill of meditative relaxation can be learned; it can be developed, although getting good at it typically requires a safe, quiet spot and at least twenty minutes of time a day. At first the busy-mind syndrome takes over, but with practice in addressing in quietude how you will manage the response to issues, you learn to execute that response when issues in fact trigger your alarm reaction.

As skill in mindfulness-based cognitive therapy increases, individuals typically begin to reorder the balance of importance between things to do and ways to be. Our society rewards us for doing things, but some of the most important moments in our lives are about being present—without necessarily doing anything at all. Finding the right balance between doing and being is a key objective of mindfulness-cognitive therapy. It helps us fulfill Dr. Eliot's two rules from Chapter 11: don't sweat the small stuff, and anything that is going to kill us is the small stuff.

The health payoff from implementing a baseline stress management program has been demonstrated to be significant. One study found that mindfulness-based cognitive therapy, along with exercise, was the most promising treatment approach for chronic fatigue syndrome. Another showed that mindfulness-based cognitive behavioral therapy was effective in managing chronic illnesses associated with increased allostatic load in Gulf War veterans. A randomized controlled trial of mindfulness-based cognitive therapy in 130 men and women with significant chronic stress showed that the therapy significantly improved the subjects' social coping skills and reduced their alarm physiology.

One of the most interesting recent studies was done on patients suffering from severe post-traumatic stress disorder (PTSD). The study showed that the mindfulness-based cognitive therapy altered the genetic expression of a very important network of genes, regulated by the gene FKBP5, which controls coping with stress and the central nervous system's response to stress. The therapy increased the expression of FKBP5, which clinically improved the PTSD symptoms and enlarged the volume of the hippocampus, the region of the brain associated with mood, memory, and emotion. These results are powerful evidence of how trauma or stress signals from the environment can alter genetic expression in the physiology of alarm. They also demonstrate how mindfulness-based cognitive therapy can modify the imbalanced core physiological processes associated with traumatic stress.

So again, the work done gaining skill in responding to stress pays dividends. Find twenty minutes each day to practice your mindful introspection. Here's an idea: do it while walking some of your 10,000 steps to combine exercise and mindfulness, letting each bolster the other.

THE BASELINE ENVIRONMENTAL MANAGEMENT PROGRAM

We learned about a kind of benevolent hormesis back in Chapter 9—the idea that exposure to very small amounts of some things may have a much greater effect on our health than expected. There's also a malevolent version of hormesis—for example, in the way very low levels of the plasticizer BPA can alter genetic expression and cellular function with a subtle but significantly adverse impact on long-term health. We can put both versions of this principle to work in managing our environment when we remember Sidney Baker's wonderful instruction about how to address autism: "Take away the things that are a problem and provide the things that are missing." Put a bit more elaborately, we can say our aim is to take away the things that create genetic expression of the physiological alarm responses in our environment, and to provide the things that create genetic expression of the physiological resilience responses—and hope for a hormetic effect on both sides of the equation.

To this end, a baseline environmental management program should focus on ending exposure to persistent organic pollutants (POPs); to the toxic minerals lead, mercury, cadmium, and arsenic; to such forms of ionizing radiation as ultraviolet and X-ray; and to foods that have been exposed to biocides and herbicides.

What about nonionizing environmental energy pollution from the use of cellular telephones? My answer to this is to use a headset hardwired from the earpiece to the phone. This provides the minimum of exposure to the microwave frequencies that can interfere with the cellular communications process.

What about GMOs—genetically modified foods? This is a thorny issue. It is true that scientists have been studying the effects on animals of consuming genetically modified plants—and have found no unequivocal evidence that they cause any adverse health effects. But what is also true is that as scientists have developed new ways of observing subtle changes in genetic expression and its influence on cellular physiology, new questions have emerged.

The question most commonly raised is whether the genetic modification of plants by the insertion of foreign genes from other organisms could produce more allergenic proteins in the plant food. Studies analyzing the composition of proteins in genetically modified crops have so far found no definitive answers to this question.

Another question is if GMO varieties of plants could have different epigenomes from wild-growing varieties, and if so, if this could confer a different influence on people eating the plant.

Finally, we want to know whether studying the effects of feeding GMO plant foods to animals is a reliable marker for evaluating their long-term safety in humans. After all, rats and mice, the common test animals in these studies, live a very short life span compared with humans. The duration of their exposure to GMO products is thus also much shorter, so these studies may tell us very little about the effects of long-term usage.

One of the most controversial of GMO crops is rice—controversial because the majority of the world's population derives its calories from this plant. A number of animal studies by prominent researchers in China have all demonstrated the safety of specific strains of GMO rice. But many in the field are still not convinced that these studies offer sufficient proof of safety to be able to say that GMO rice makes no difference to human physiology.

In my view, the body of science evaluating both the long-term safety of GMO foods and their cellular effects is still in development. Questions continue to be raised as to why food-related allergies and sensitivities are on the rise throughout the world; could GMO varieties have any relationship to this rapid increase in allergies? A GMO potato is one into which the gene of a Brazil nut has been inserted; the same has been done to soybeans. In both cases, insertion of the Brazil nut genes increases the essential sulfur amino acid methionine level in the plant protein. And allergy testing of the GMO potato and the GMO soy confirmed that each is able to trigger brazil nut allergy.

In short, I think it is premature to render a final decision on the safety of GMO. It may prove safe and effective in improving the food crop in some cases and cause long-term adverse implications for health in other cases. For the moment, we must insist on full disclosure in the labeling of all GMO food products so that consumers can know what they're taking in if they choose the product. I'll add only that my personal preference is to eat organic foods that I can be sure are not derived from GMO plants or animals.

BUILDING ON THE BASELINE

Introduce a functional medicine baseline program into your life right now. You don't need to wait till you have analyzed your own specific core process imbalances or devised strategies for restoring balance. You have a pretty good idea by now in any event about what may be contributing to your specific chronic illnesses or problems. Getting going on a baseline program as soon as possible is a great first step toward addressing those causes. It's also the foundation onto which you will layer the very specific strategies for dealing with your very specific imbalances.

CHAPTER 13

Personalizing Your Health-Care Management Program

Over a period of five years, as best she could date the onset of her misery, Diana gained forty pounds, despite trying every diet known to man, and acquired doctors' prescriptions, one after the other, for a total of six medications per day. Asked how she felt, she could answer you in one word: "Lousy." She could also expand the answer to embrace a number of complaints, including no energy at all and a diminishing enthusiasm for life. Asked to what she attributed her weight gain, ill health, and depression, she offered another one-word answer: "Menopause."

After five years of decline, she caught the flu just as winter set in, and it knocked her down completely. Although the infection was eventually zapped by rest, fluids, and symptom-controlling medicines, Diana remained ill throughout the winter. Even spring offered no jump of resilience to snap her back. All the symptoms that had bothered her before the flu now simply seemed worse, and she despaired of ever feeling well again.

The straw that broke the camel's back and sent Diana to a functional medicine practitioner was that her hair started falling out. Fast. She couldn't help her reaction: Stupefied at finding herself clutching a handful of hair, she burst into tears. "What is happening to me?" she sobbed, "and why can't someone fix it?"

Diana sought out one of the physicians in our group at the Functional Medicine Clinical Research Center here in Seattle and was given a full functional medicine evaluation. The conclusion was that she had a significant imbalance in her detoxification and defense processes and needed a personalized program that would be layered onto the diet and dietary supplement components of the baseline program to address those core imbalances. Of particular importance also was the mindfulness-focused cognitive behavioral training; this was key to managing the stress that both Diana and her functional medicine practitioner felt was a significant contributor to her core imbalances. Here are some of the modifications in Diana's personalized plan.

- A low-allergy food plan with increased vegetable protein—plus a rice protein supplement—and increased levels of vegetables, especially of the cruciferous family, containing phytonutrients that specifically support detoxification
- Increased water intake of at least six 8-ounce glasses per day
- A supplement of sodium bicarbonate daily to augment alkaline reserve
- An inulin prebiotic and a high-potency probiotic
- A tailored nutritional supplement program delivering specified levels of vitamins, minerals, and phytonutrients to support the detoxification process, including:

    A balanced B-vitamin complement with increased amounts of folic acid, vitamin B12, pantothenic acid, biotin, and the trace mineral zinc

    A phytonutrient supplement composed of concentrates from broccoli and brussels sprouts as well as a supplement of N-acetylcysteine to support glutathione needs for the detoxification process

Diana saw and felt little progress in the first month of this program, and she questioned whether it was worth the effort. By the sixth week, however, she began to realize that she was feeling better; above all, she noticed that the hair loss had stopped and that new hair was growing back into places where it had thinned considerably. This was sufficient encouragement for her to stick with her program;

by twelve weeks she could record enough progress that she felt and looked like a "new woman"—her phrase.

She felt so much better, in fact, that she adhered to the program for six months in all. By then, she had lost more than thirty-five pounds, was taking only two daily medications, had a full head of hair, and was wearing clothes she had not worn for seven years. Her cloud of depression had also lifted; Diana felt a renewed zest for living.

She and her physician now adjusted her personalized health-management program to reflect her new condition, giving her greater latitude in her food choices and a lower level of nutritional supplementation. That was six years ago as I write this, and Diana remains a woman of high energy and great stamina, powers present in her genetic makeup that had been dampened by the specifics of her gene-environment interaction and that were unlocked by her personalized health management intervention and her ongoing health-management program.

No book can evaluate you and pinpoint your most significant process imbalance, as her physician did for Diana. No book can design a personalized health-management program for you to the level of detail of Diana's program. What this book can do—and what we will do in this chapter—is provide planning tools that can help shape your analysis so you can draw the right insights from your own observations and self-assessments. Just as you look for patterns in which you observe and assess, this chapter shows you some of the patterns typical of imbalances in each of the seven core physiological processes—and it suggests ways to restore balance to each system, and therefore to the body's systems network as a whole. A more detailed guide to additional resources—professional help from a practitioner trained in functional medicine, for example, or access to coaching, support, or additional information—will be provided in Appendix C, "Resources."

One of the tools that you may want to avail yourself of—and one that will be further discussed in Appendix C—is genetic testing, now available commercially, although not in all states. You basically submit a saliva sample and get back an analysis of your DNA. In getting to know your genes, you'll also find out where the risks are so that you can take steps now to avert or avoid those risks. This is a highly sophisticated and important tool, priced to be accessible, and well worth it.

WHERE'S THE IMBALANCE?

For now, however, it's time to turn to the self-assessment questionnaires and identify where your imbalances may be so that you can get to work doing something about them.

You'll begin by evaluating the answers you gave to the health self-assessment back in the Introduction. The aim is to get an idea of where the imbalances are and how bad they are.

This is not a diagnosis. That's a concept belonging to the "old" medicine of infectious disease. Diagnosis looks at symptoms in order to prescribe ways to combat them. What you're looking for in preparing your personalized health-management program is patterns in your physiological functioning—all together and process by process—so that you can begin to affect the underlying causes of the chronic illnesses that may be diminishing the quality of your life today or threatening your future health and well-being.

I would add one more important point—not so much a medical concept but equally important as a tenet of this new way to address your health. Precisely because what you are about to develop is a *personalized* health-management program, there is no room in it for any finding of blame or guilt in your interpretation of your self-assessments. The idea that we have "done something wrong" or "done this to ourselves" is foreign to every impulse of medicine and has no place in the world of health. Rather, what you're doing is seeking long-term improvement in health and function by applying revolutionary discoveries in health to your own needs, desires, and health status. It's a good thing to do.

So here again is the Health Self-Assessment Questionnaire you first saw in Chapter 1. See if your answers are still the same.

MY HEALTH SELF-ASSESSMENT

1. Do you feel that your health has gotten worse over the past two years?
2. Have you lost or gained more than 10 percent of your body weight over the past five years—even though you weren't intentionally dieting?
3. Do you have trouble going to sleep or staying asleep?
4. Does pain in your joints or muscles limit your physical activity or mobility?
5. Do you commonly feel fatigued for no apparent reason?
6. Are you frequently depressed or anxious?
7. Do you have problems with memory?
8. Is there a consistent ringing in your ears?
9. Do you feel that you are losing your strength?
10. Do you take more than two prescription medications?
11. How about over-the-counter medications? Do you commonly take any of these?

   a Anti-inflammatories
   b Antacids
   c Analgesics
   d Sleeping remedies

12. Do you suffer from allergies?
13. Do you occasionally have episodes of poor concentration or confusion?
14. Do you commonly suffer from shortness of breath or feel winded?
15. Have you lost any of your sense of taste or smell over the past few years?
16. Do you feel that you have lost significant amount of muscle mass over the past few years?
17. Have you heard from your doctor that you have any of the following?

a Elevated blood pressure
b Elevated blood cholesterol
c Elevated blood glucose

18. Has your dentist told you that you have gum or periodontal disease?
19. Do you frequently alternate constipation and diarrhea or feel pain or discomfort in your digestive area?
20. Have you been told that you have chronic bad breath?
21. Are you shorter than you used to be, or have you any evidence of calcium deposits?
22. Do you catch every cold and flu that's going around?

On a piece of paper, list the numbers of the questions to which you answered yes. If you answered yes to the majority of questions, it is likely you have multiple imbalances in your core physiological processes. Focus specifically on questions 1, 2, 3, 10, 11, 17, and 22. Did you answer yes to all or most of these? If so, that's a strong indication of multiple imbalances in your core physiological processes.

What is significant about these seven questions? Six of them—2, 3, 10, 11, 17, and 22—are fairly standard signals of lack of overall well-being and suggest you have some imbalances in your core physiological processes. Yet the very first question, asking if you feel your health has gotten worse over the past two years, has been identified in numerous studies to be one of the most important early-warning indicators of core imbalance. The reason? Most people are a lot more attuned to their health than they realize. While we may block out of our consciousness those issues we don't want to deal with—like signals of ill health—our subconscious keeps track of such issues, and the result is often a general feeling of deteriorating health.

Feelings need to be backed up by data, however, as the scientist in me rushes to add. The best way to pinpoint areas of imbalance before they become troublesome is to track the trajectory of your health, and the best way to do that is to record such standard blood biomarkers as cholesterol, PSA for men, blood sugar, hemoglobin A1c, uric acid, calcium, and triglycerides—among others—on an annual basis. Studies make it clear that it is when the values of blood biomarkers start to change rapidly that you're in trouble. A general feeling of malaise will show up in hard data, if you are conscientious about getting the tests done every year.

What do your other questionnaire answers tell us? Here is how the yes answers to the health self-assessment questions match up against the core physiological processes. If you checked even some of the yes answers for a core process, you are likely to have an imbalance in that process. If you checked all, you certainly do.

Yes Answers	Core Physiological Process
2, 4, 9, 12, 13, 15, 16, 19, 20	Assimilation-elimination
2, 3, 4, 7, 8, 12, 13, 20, 22	Detoxification
4, 6, 8, 12, 13, 16, 18, 19, 20, 22	Defense
2, 3, 4, 6, 15, 18, 22	Cellular communications
2, 3, 4, 6, 15, 17, 18, 21	Cellular transport
2, 4, 5, 7, 9, 13, 14, 16	Energy
2, 3, 4, 14, 16, 21	Structure

Now rank the process imbalances by the percentage of yes answers for each. Obviously, for example, four yes answers out of a possible six shows a worse imbalance than five yes answers out of a possible ten.

Of course, as you have learned, all the core physiological processes are interconnected in the network of systems that is your body, so an imbalance in one is likely to affect an imbalance in another. Nevertheless, pinpointing the most significant imbalance offers a starting point for the design of your personalized program. Think of it as a first cut at understanding your genome, a first draft of insight into the genes writing your book of life.

BEGINNING TO CHANGE THE MESSAGE

So now let's get specific. The core process self-assessments let you zero in on any and all processes where you show an imbalance. You'll want to consult with your functional medicine practitioner about specifics for dealing with your imbalance—depending on its severity and other factors—but here are some general recommendations for getting started.

ASSIMILATION-ELIMINATION

1. Do you alternate between constipation and urgency?
2. Do you get indigestion?
3. Does your stool have an oily appearance?
4. Do you suffer from frequent intestinal gas or bloating?
5. Is stomach or intestinal pain a regular occurrence?
6. Do you frequently get gastric reflux?
7. Are headaches a common occurrence?
8. Are you allergic or sensitive to many foods?
9. After eating, do you find you experience joint or muscle pain?
10. Do you have bad breath?
11. Are you depressed or subject to mood swings?
12. Do you have trouble keeping your weight under control even though you watch your diet?
13. Is your blood sugar elevated?
14. Do you suffer from kidney stones?
15. Is your blood pressure higher than it should be?

Five or more yes responses to the questionnaire for Chapter 4 suggest an imbalance in your core physiological process of assimilation-elimination. Restoring balance in the process is the precise aim of the Four R Program, which is a commonsense approach to most health problems in this area, but a number of specific conditions warrant particular mention.

Indigestion is certainly one of the most common complaints arising from an imbalance in this core process—an everyday occurrence that prompts those experiencing it to prowl drugstore aisles looking at shelf upon shelf of antacid medications. Indigestion may well have elicited a positive response to question 2 in your self-assessment questionnaire for this subject. Typically, what's at issue is an upper intestinal problem in the stomach associated with what is called gastroesophageal reflux disease, or GERD. If it is a frequent occurrence, chances are that particular foods are triggering the response, so identifying the trigger foods is essential.

Be aware, however, that indigestion could indicate an enzyme deficiency, easily resolved with a digestive enzyme supplement, or could even signal an infection from the food-borne bacteria *Helicobacter pylori*.

Oily stool, asked about in question 3, is an indication that the fats you ingest are not being well digested—possibly as a result of the pancreas secreting insufficient digestive enzyme or the gallbladder releasing insufficient bile—and you might want to lower the amount of fat in your diet. But be alert to the fact that both of these causative factors can be an early sign of gallstone formation and poor assimilation of essential fatty acids and fat-soluble vitamins. It's therefore a symptom to be taken very seriously.

If you answered yes to the questions concerning headaches, intestinal pain after eating, bad breath, or mood swings—7, 9, 10, 11—you may be sensitive to such foods as dairy products, grain products, sugared foods, and foods high in saturated fat or fried foods. If so, you probably want to consider solutions that help you maintain a healthy balance of enteric microflora.

Balance throughout your assimilation-elimination process also reestablishes proper immune balance—remember that the intestinal tract is the seat of your immune system—and this fact underlies the Four R Program. Keep in mind that while the four steps of the program can be executed simultaneously, it may take up to four weeks to experience the program's full benefits.

Here's a recap of the Four R Program: Remove, Replace, Reinoculate, Repair.

Start by identifying foods you may be sensitive or allergic to. The best way to do this is to eliminate a food you suspect for a period of two weeks to see if your symptoms improve. That may sound laborious, but studies show that most of us consume more than 80 percent of our calories in fewer than fifteen foods, so it's less laborious than you think. Then follow the first R of the program and remove these foods from your diet. In general, you probably would do well to avoid foods or beverages that contain high-fructose corn syrup sweetener as well as foods in which sugars, fat, and salt are key ingredients.

The second R, replace, seeks to put back into your core assimilation-elimination process what it needs to digest fat and protein easily. On a Mediterranean diet, this will be less of a problem since this way of eating is reasonably low in fats. If you seek a digestive enzyme supplement, look for those derived from porcine sources that are high in chymotrypsin and lipase activity; the former helps the breakdown and therefore the digestion of protein, the latter of fat.

Reinoculate, the third R of the program, means adding prebiotic and probiotic supplements to improve the assimilation-elimination process. The prebiotics act as food for the probiotics, which in turn help the digestive process—a perfect example of a symbiotic relationship from which your body benefits.

Finally, the fourth R repairs the process through the use of specific nutrients that strengthen the gastrointestinal barrier and support intestinal transport of water and thus elimination.

FOR AN IMBALANCE IN THE ASSIMILATION-ELIMINATION PROCESS

If You Answered Yes to...	Try This...
5 or more questions	Four R Program
Question 2	Identify trigger foods of GERD
Question 3	Less fat
Questions 7, 9, 10, 11	Supplements to balance microflora

DETOXIFICATION

1. Are you sensitive to fragrances and odors?
2. What about food—any sensitivities?

3. Sensitive to particular medications?
4. To alcohol?
5. Do you get a bad reaction from MSG—monosodium glutamate—in food?
6. Do you have sensitivity to caffeine?
7. Have you ever been sick from exposure to chemicals?
8. Does cigarette smoke bother you or make you sick?
9. Are you sensitive to smog or air pollution?
10. Do you sometimes wake up in the morning feeling as if you've been drugged?
11. Ever have unexplained skin rashes?
12. Do you ever experience brain fog?
13. Do you feel a tingling in your hands or feet?
14. Is there consistent ringing in your ears?
15. Do you experience unexplained muscle pain?

Your responses to the questionnaire in Chapter 5 measure your personal sensitivity to environmental exposures and reveal possible symptoms of chronic toxicity. Whether from outside the body or within, accumulating toxins burden the body's immune, nervous, and hormone-producing endocrine systems, so the symptoms of chronic toxicity are often seen as issues related to those systems. In addition, the more body fat, the greater the opportunity for storage of fat-soluble toxins; it means that body fat can contribute to chronic toxicity, which in turn connects to metabolic poisoning and increased risk of type 2 diabetes, cardiovascular disease, elevated blood pressure, kidney disease, neurodegenerative conditions like Parkinson's and Alzheimer's diseases, and certain forms of cancer.

If you scored high on this questionnaire, therefore, make it a priority to design a personalized health-management program that seeks to restore balance to your detoxification process. I wrote a book on the subject in 1999, *The 20-Day Rejuvenation Diet Program*, in which I described the results of a study of one hundred participants—with a range of chronic health complaints—who undertook a structured, twenty-day diet high in specific phytonutrients aimed at strengthening their detoxification process. In essence, this was a clean organic-foods diet comprising vegetable products—specifically, cruciferous vegetables, soluble fiber-rich legumes, and spices—and limited amounts of lean poultry and fatty fish. Eliminated were wheat products, caffeine, sugars, artificial sweeteners, chocolate, alcohol, synthetic colorings and flavorings, and preservatives. Monitored daily by our medical staff, the group experienced a greater than 40 percent decrease in such symptoms as low energy, sleep disturbances, fatigue, poor mental concentration, and chronic muscle pain.

In other words, dietary changes are a key path to restoring balance to your detoxification process. What are some key dietary supplements to support this process? They include the B-complex vitamins; the minerals iron, zinc, and magnesium; N-acetylcysteine; and phytonutrient concentrates from broccoli, brussels sprouts, green tea, pomegranate, watercress, turmeric, kudzu, red grape skins, and hops.

THE 20-DAY DIETARY DETOX

Yes	No
Organic vegetables	Wheat products
Lean poultry	Caffeine
Fatty fish	Sugars or artificial sweeteners
B-complex vitamins	Chocolate
Phytonutrient concentrates	Alcohol
	Synthetic colorings and flavorings
	Preservatives

DEFENSE

1. Do you tend to get every cold and flu that goes around?
2. Do you have sore joints that are made worse by modest exercise?
3. Ever get skin rashes of unknown origin?
4. Are you unusually sensitive to the sun?
5. Do your joints swell up?
6. Do you suffer chronic pain in your hands, wrists, ankles, or feet?

7. Is your grip getting weaker?
8. Are you losing muscle?
9. Do you have chronic sinus infections?
10. Are fungal infections—like athlete's foot, for example—a common occurrence?
11. Do you have frequent bladder or urinary tract infections?
12. Do you have chronic intestinal pain or discomfort?
13. Do you have dental problems associated with periodontal disease?
14. Does it feel to you that your leg or back pain is chronic?
15. Do you take anti-inflammatory medications regularly?
16. Do you frequently take prescribed antibiotics to get over an infection?
17. Have you ever been diagnosed with any of the following?

    a Epstein-Barr virus
    b Herpes virus
    c *Candida albicans*
    d Lyme disease (*Borrelia burgdorferi*)
    e A waterborne parasite like *Entamoeba histolytica* or *Cryptosporidium parvum*
    f HIV
    g Cytomegalovirus
    h Clostridium

The Chapter 6 questionnaire about the defense process is aimed at learning how often and how much you experience infection and inflammation. Frequent or severe infections over time indicate too little activity in your cell-mediated and humoral immune systems. Frequent or severe inflammation indicates too much activity in the two functional units of that system.

The solution is not to "boost" your immune system, as so many nutritional supplements claim to do. Rather, you need to restore balance to your defense process. It's a fallacy to suppose that the presence of an autoimmune disease means that you are allergic to yourself. There's no such thing. Your immune process has evolved over millions of years to protect you from infectious organisms and foreign substances. An imbalance in the process makes you overreact to exposure to substances your body's immune system sees as foreign or out of place; that's what causes the inflammation. The way to redress the imbalance is to both reduce the exposure to foreign substances and provide the things that the immune system needs to send the correct messages to the genes that control inflammation.

How do we do that? By taking away the immune-reactive substances and adding back the immune-stabilizing substances. And how do we take away immune-reactive substances? First, we have to determine what they are. Some of the more obvious possibilities are gluten, pollutants, xenobiotic chemicals, and even overuse of alcohol. Chronic infections of the mouth—for example, periodontal disease—can trigger an imbalance in the defense system, and vice versa: an imbalance in the defense system can increase the risk of periodontal disease. People who regularly visit the dentist to have their teeth cleaned and who regularly practice impeccable oral hygiene at home but who nevertheless have periodontal disease probably have an underlying imbalance in their defense process. That's the source of their infection. Also, if you're of a certain age, it's not impossible that mercury released from old mercury-amalgam tooth fillings may be burdening your defense process—something that has begun to show up a lot in members of the baby boom generation.

Immune-stabilizing foods and nutrients include mushrooms, vitamin C supplements of from 1 to 6 grams per day, and such botanical medicines as echinacea. In addition, some specific supplemental nutrients have been found to be of value in restoring balance to the defense process. Among these are zinc, vitamins E, A, and D, omega-3s, and a range of phytonutrients from spices—including curcumin from turmeric, allicin from garlic, and capsaicin from hot peppers.*

---

* Recommended daily doses for defense process intervention: zinc (10–30 mg), natural source vitamin E (400–800 IU), omega-3 EPA/DHA (3–5 grams), vitamin A (2,500 IU), vitamin D (1,000–5,000 IU), probiotics, green tea epigallocatechin gallate (100 mg), and curcumin (100 mg).

> ### FOR AN IMBALANCE IN THE DEFENSE PROCESS: DON'T "BOOST" YOUR IMMUNE SYSTEM; RESTORE IT
>
> 1 Identify and remove immune-reactive substances.
> 2 Add immune-stabilizing foods.
> 3 Use these supplements.
>   a Zinc
>   b Vitamins E, A, D
>   c Omega-3s
>   d Spices

CELLULAR COMMUNICATIONS

1. Do you suffer from arthritis-like pain or inflammation?
2. Do you have night sweats?
3. Does a change in the weather produce joint pain?
4. Do your joints swell after physical activities?
5. Do you suffer from a feeling of low energy in the morning that takes until noon to overcome?
6. Do the stresses of your life affect your health?
7. Do you feel "wired and tired"?
8. Is your libido low for your age?
9. Are you chronically depressed?
10. Are you concerned that you're more forgetful than you should be?
11. Is it difficult to get to sleep or stay asleep?
12. Do you have chronic infections of the sinuses, tonsils, intestines, skin, or mouth?
13. Do you routinely take anti–inflammatory medications, either over-the-counter or by prescription?
14. Are you on blood pressure medication?
15. Do you take antidepressants?

Five or more yes answers to the Chapter 7 questionnaire tell you that you have an imbalance in your cellular communications process and it is spreading alarm messages to cells, tissues, and organs around your body. All those thousands upon thousands of message substances are zooming every which way: the neurotransmitters that regulate nervous system functions, the cytokines that control inflammatory and immune system functions, the stress hormones that influence arousal and metabolic functions, sex steroid hormones that regulate reproductive and energy functions, adipokines from adipose tissue that regulate appetite and metabolic functions, hormones like insulin that regulate cellular energy function. An imbalance in the function of any one of these classes of cellular communication agents can alter physiological function in all the other processes—especially in the closely linked processes of assimilation–elimination, detoxification, and defense.

So if you scored high on the questionnaires for all three of those processes as well as for cellular communications, where should you start? In your assimilation–elimination process, the place where more than half your immune system is located and which can therefore trigger alteration in the cellular communication process. Begin with a plan to restore balance there. If there is no evidence of an imbalance in assimilation-elimination, your next priority is your detoxification process. Absent an imbalance there, then your primary focus should be on restoring balance to your cellular communications process first and foremost.

That means finding an approach that influences all the players within the cellular communications network. Menopause provides a good example, as a number of studies we pursued at the Functional Medicine Clinical Research Center made clear. Here's why:

Hormones are of course some of the most important cellular communications substances in the body, powerful modulators of genetic expression. Their influence on communicating messages that affect all the core physiological processes is significant. In fact, they affect every aspect of our function from muscle strength and integrity to mood and mental function, from reproductive health to how we manage stressful events and how we look and feel. Our study focused on menopausal women experiencing significant adverse symptoms—night sweats, sleep disturbances, hot flushing, mood swings. What we found was that their symptoms were due not just to the fact that their ovaries were no longer releasing the estrogen hormones, but also to the way estrogen was being metabolized in their bodies and how it was being influenced by the imbalance in such other hormones as the stress hormone cortisol, the sex hormone progesterone, and insulin. In other words, it wasn't just the cessation of ovarian activity that was causing the women's symptoms; it was the imbalances in a number of related cellular communications substances—all networking together in their influence on health and vitality. What this told us was that, to alleviate the women's discomforts, we needed to manage the imbalances within this system, not just focus on trying to improve the effects of estrogen.

The program we designed called for a diet plan with specified phytonutrient supplements, an exercise program, and relaxation-mindfulness training. The diet focused on lean protein from chicken and fish, the elimination of sugar-rich foods and beverages, increased fiber-rich vegetables and beans, soy-based products, increased intake of cruciferous vegetables known to improve the metabolism of estrogen, and a supplement containing an extract of Siberian rhubarb (*Rheum rhaponticum*) containing the phytonutrient rhaponosides, identified as a modulator of the estrogen cellular communication process. An extract of indole-3 carbinol (I3C) and its relative diindolylmethane (DIM), both found in cruciferous vegetables, helped improve estrogen-related symptoms, while black cohosh extract (*Cimicifuga racemosa*) and the soy phytonutrients genistein and daidzein helped manage estrogen-related cellular communication imbalances. The outcomes for the women in the study were highly positive.

The same story applies to cellular communications imbalances in men, and a similar dietary plan, using a different group of phytonutrient extracts, had an equally positive effect. The most common male symptom of cellular communications imbalance is benign prostatic hyperplasia, or BPH—an enlargement of the prostate gland deriving from an alteration in testosterone metabolism coupled with an increase in activity of inflammatory messenger substances. The phytonutrient beta-sitosterol proved effective in improving cellular communications in the prostate, as did the cruciferous vegetable phytochemicals I3C, DIM, and lycopene, the red phytonutrient pigment in tomatoes.

Does this suggest that there may be a place in medical treatment for selective bioidentical hormone replacement therapy? By "bioidentical," I mean hormones that are identical to natural hormones at the molecular level—what Linus Pauling would have called "orthomolecular." In my view, BHRT should be one of the tools available to be used in a personalized health-management program—but only when administered by a physician trained in the discipline. It should be remembered that hormones are very potent modulators of cellular function, and whereas a little replacement may be good, more can be dangerous.

Finally, it's important to remember the role of allostatic load in designing a personalized intervention for cellular communications imbalance. It is why a primary objective of such an intervention should be a relaxation-mindfulness practice. In addition, some phytonutrient-rich botanical medicines can be of great help when increased allostatic load is an issue—among them, Siberian ginseng and *Rhodiola rosea*, or golden root, and Ashwagandha, or Indian ginseng; they have a long history of use as adaptogens working at the cellular level to normalize imbalanced cellular communications associated with the stress response. An adaptogen acts as a dual agonist-antagonist: When cellular communications activity is low, the adaptogen stimulates reaction; when activity is excessive, it antagonizes the activity and diminishes its function. It is thus a natural balancer of the process.

FOR AN IMBALANCE IN CELLULAR COMMUNICATIONS: DON'T SHOOT THE MESSENGER; IDENTIFY WHAT'S CREATING THE MESSAGE

1 Underlying inflammation?

2 Insulin resistance?

3 Poor fitness?

4 Toxicity?

5 Gastrointestinal imbalance?

CELLULAR TRANSPORT

1. Do you frequently experience brain fog and find it hard to focus?
2. Is your blood sugar count higher than it should be?
3. Do you frequently suffer from digestive problems if you eat high-protein foods?
4. Do you feel sleepy from time to time, especially after meals?
5. Have you gained weight—especially around the middle of your body?
6. Have your blood triglyceride levels gone up?
7. Do you have high blood pressure?
8. Have you noticed a loss of muscle over the last few years?
9. Is your LDL cholesterol higher than it should be?
10. Do you take a statin drug?
11. Have you been told that you have low albumin or hematocrit levels in your blood?
12. Has your doctor told you to cut back on the amount of cholesterol in your diet?
13. Have you been told that you have reduced kidney function?
14. Is your vision as sharp as it once was?
15. Do you have any concerns about the health of your heart and blood vessels?

The fifteen questions of the Chapter 8 questionnaire revolve around cellular transport of the critical nutrients protein, fat, and carbohydrate as well as of vitamins. If you answered yes to question 6, 9, 10, 12, or 15, you may have fat transport imbalances. If you answered yes to question 1, 2, 4, 5, or 13, you likely have a carbohydrate transport imbalance with specific issues in managing the transport of the carbohydrate glucose. If you answered yes to question 3, 7, 8, or 11, you potentially have protein transport imbalances.

An imbalance in the transport of protein can be related to either a dietary protein insufficiency or insufficient dietary intake of what is called quality protein. Protein in the diet is essential for health, of course, but the quality of the protein is also important, where "quality" refers to the makeup of the amino acids in the protein and whether the protein is digestible. Digestibility is important; after all, shoe leather is made up of protein, but trying to eat it to fulfill our protein needs would not be satisfactory.

As to amino acids, they are the building blocks of proteins. There are twenty amino acids in all, of which eight are called essential amino acids. "Essential" means that these eight cannot be made from anything else in the body; instead, they have to be ingested directly from our diet if we are to meet our needs to build the body's proteins. These essential amino acids are transported through the bloodstream as part of the blood protein albumin. Low levels of albumin in the blood—or of hematocrit, another key marker of protein insufficiency—can therefore reflect imbalances in amino acid availability and transport.

A high-quality dietary protein provides a proper balance of essential amino acids. In general, animal proteins from meat or milk have higher levels of essential amino acids than do vegetable proteins. This is why vegetarian diets were once thought to be unable to provide adequate protein. But then along came Frances Moore Lappé with her classic 1971 book, *Diet for a Small Planet*, debunking this idea by showing that a combination of grains and legumes provides a balance of essential amino acids that is equivalent to that of proteins of animal origin. Lappé cited all those cultures that do just that—corn and beans in Central America, rice and soy across Asia.

If dietary protein is not properly digested and the amino acids don't get absorbed, transported, and utilized in protein synthesis in the cells, then you will see signs of protein deficiency. On the other hand, a very high-protein diet can result in an overload of the transport process and result in kidney dysfunction. That's why people with chronic kidney disease are often told to consume less protein; it takes the stress off a kidney that might be working too hard to transport excessive protein. In this as in all things in the body, not too much and not too little is what works: balance!

If your issue is a problem of transport of the blood sugar glucose—yes answers to question 1, 2, 4, or 14—then you want to modify your diet to include more protein, slightly lower carbohydrate content, and modest fat intake in the form of omega-3 and omega-9 oils from fish and virgin olive oil, respectively. This is of course the essence of the Mediterranean diet.

Defects in glucose transport and utilization show up first as insulin resistance—that is, the body's inability to use the insulin it produces effectively, so that glucose builds up in the blood instead of being transported to the cells. That of course affects many core physiological processes and leads to metabolic syndrome from which follows a range of chronic illnesses from cardiovascular disease to arthritis to type 2 diabetes.* It is, in a way, the physiological imbalance of our age, and it is so critical that the staff of the Functional Medicine Clinical Research Center has long believed it warrants regular testing for such biomarkers as hemoglobin A1c, oral glucose tolerance, uric acid in the blood, high-sensitivity CRP (hs-CRP), and the ratio of blood triglycerides to HDL to catch it early.

For as we saw back in Chapter 1 in reviewing the work of Dr. Dean Ornish, changes in diet and lifestyle behaviors can literally correct cellular transport imbalances severe enough to cause even major blockage of the arteries to the heart.

A friend of mine, Joseph Piscatella, is living proof of that. I met

---

* Not to mention obesity, dementia, osteoporosis, blindness, kidney disease, and certain forms of cancer.

Joe in 1983 shortly after he had published the *Don't Eat Your Heart Out Cookbook*, written with the renowned heart surgeon Dr. Denton Cooley. Joe is arguably the longest living "recipient" of coronary bypass surgery. At the age of thirty-four—lean, fit, a nonsmoker, with a young family—he was diagnosed as being on the verge of a massive heart attack. At the time—the late 1970s—such a diagnosis would have doomed him to an early death. Instead, Joe became one of the first people to undergo a coronary bypass operation, after which he committed himself to a personalized program for restoring and maintaining his cellular transport process. It is to this that he credits what is now a long and healthy life—still going strong.

Dietary changes that may correct cellular transport imbalances include a lessening of carbohydrate intake to lower the amount of glucose in the blood—the body metabolizes carbohydrates into glucose—or, more specifically, eating the right kind of carbohydrate in the right amount. The right kind are unrefined starches—whole-grain bread, pastas, and cereals, for example—which release glucose slowly into the bloodstream. Avoiding carbs altogether can be problematic because the body functions most efficiently when proper amounts of glucose are available for transport, but reducing your intake of white starch and sugar and increasing your intake of whole grains and minimally processed vegetables and beans—all low-glycemic-index foods—will have little impact on blood glucose levels.

What about rice? With its high glycemic index, white rice is not good at managing blood sugar levels—that is, glucose. But the story is more complicated than that. After all, until recently, countries that were historically dependent on rice experienced minimal diabetes. One answer is that there are two varieties of rice, amylose and amylopectin. Amylose starch from long-grain rice is chemically more packed together in its architecture and therefore takes longer to break down in the intestinal tract; it's a timed-release carb with less impact on blood glucose levels than the short-grain, amylopectin sticky rice. Historically, in these rice-eating societies, the eating of long-grain rice cooled the metabolic conversion of food to energy, while the eating of animal foods high in saturated fats heated it up—the yin and yang mirrored in eating as in all aspects of culture.

In addition to taking care with carbohydrates, a diet supporting cellular transport will focus on phytonutrients from such foods and spices as cinnamon, bitter melon, garlic, sage, oregano, hops, soy, salmon, nuts, avocado, oats, garbanzos, lentils, and kidney beans. Soluble fibers will also slow the release of glucose into the blood.

Equally effective for cellular transport is regular daily exercise. Study upon study confirms this. One at the George Washington School of Medicine found that a fifteen-minute walk on level ground at normal walking speed after each meal significantly lowered blood glucose levels in people with metabolic syndrome or prediabetes. This finding is in accord with the fascinating work of James A. Levine, professor of medicine at the Mayo Clinic and a world-renowned expert on obesity, who has demonstrated that the most effective way for people to implement a fitness program is by taking a twenty-minute walk after meals. Even what Dr. Levine calls NEAT—non-exercise activity thermogenesis, or fidgeting—can help lower blood sugar levels (and shed pounds) by supporting cellular transport.

Measured in time, the threshold for a significantly beneficial effect on glucose transport—as evidenced by improved biomarkers like hemoglobin A1c levels—is approximately 25 minutes a day or a total of 150 total minutes per week. It's not too much time to spend to keep a balance in this core physiological process.

One important note: The connection between cellular transport imbalances and imbalances in the detoxification process is a close one. It has been our experience at the research center that if a low-glycemic-load diet plus an exercise program do not together correct an insulin resistance issue, the next step is to intervene in the detoxification processes. Our research shows that programs to restore detox balance also improve blood sugar, insulin, and triglyceride levels—a validation of the idea that persistent organic pollutants stored in fat tissues in the body can release toxic substances that poison the energy powerhouses of the cell, the mitochondria, and reduce insulin production and cellular action. The resulting defect in glucose transport can of course progress to insulin resistance, metabolic syndrome, type 2 diabetes, cardiovascular disease, and a host of other chronic illnesses.

One more thing: your answer to question 14, about vision, offers insight into the very complex transport process that nourishes the eyes. Central to the process is the macula of the eye, the only tissue in the body that purposely concentrates a pigment from the diet into the tissue. The pigment is lutein, and it is found in dark green leafy vegetables. A healthy macula contains enough concentrated lutein to color the tissue yellow. During an eye exam, your doctor will check out the color of the macula; a loss of color, representing either a deficiency in dietary intake of lutein or an imbalance in the transport of nutrients to the eye, could lead to damage to the retina. Age-related macular degeneration (AMD), more common than glaucoma, is the main cause of blindness in adults, affecting older adults in particular and often resulting in a loss of vision in the center of the visual field—the macula—because of the damage to the retina. It is increasing at an alarming rate. So a yes answer to this question may be an important early-warning signal to which you clearly want to pay attention.

ZEROING IN ON YOUR TRANSPORT IMBALANCE

If You Answered Yes to . . .	Your Transport Imbalance Is Likely in . . .
Questions 6, 9, 10, 12, 15	Blood cholesterol and triglycerides
Questions 1, 2, 4, 5, 13, 14	Blood sugar glucose and insulin control
Questions 3, 7, 8, 11	Dietary protein intake, digestion, or utilization

ENERGY

1. Do you routinely feel a fatigue you can't explain or justify?
2. Are eight hours of sleep not enough for today?
3. Do you get muscle pain after even moderate exercise or activity?
4. Often feel brain fog?
5. Do you have trouble walking comfortably up a flight of stairs? Are you excessively winded when doing so?

6. Do you lack ambition or have low energy?
7. Ever find that you just can't tolerate disturbances around you that you used to be able to ignore or dismiss or manage?
8. Do you worry about undertaking an activity that incorporates exercise because you know you won't feel good afterward?
9. Are you often bone-weary?
10. Do you feel you just don't have the energy to cope with the issues of daily living?
11. Do you frequently get headaches for no known reason?
12. Have your senses of smell and taste gotten worse?
13. Are you forgetting things you shouldn't be forgetting?
14. Do you feel older than your age?
15. Does a regular old cold wipe you out for a prolonged period of time?

A breakdown in the function of the cellular energy powerhouses, the mitochondria, first affects those tissues with the highest level of mitochondrial activity—the brain, the muscles, and the heart. The questions you answered in Chapter 9 are designed to show if you have the memory issues, mood problems, exercise intolerance, chronic pain, or poor cardiovascular tone and function that may reflect an imbalance in your core energy process.

If so, a program of mitochondrial resuscitation can restore the balance. This requires going beyond the obvious question of maternally inherited mitochondrial DNA to factors within your control that can cause mitochondrial dysfunction. If you answered yes to the majority of questions 1, 2, 3, 4, 9, 10, 12, and 13, then there is a strong likelihood that you are suffering from an imbalance in energy processes; mitochondrial resuscitation can be a great help.

It means taking much larger quantities of substances that support mitochondrial function than would be found normally even in a well-balanced diet. Basically, these are levels of nutrients used for children with severe inborn mitochondrial DNA mutations, and they are orders of magnitude greater than the amounts recommended for a usual need.

HERE'S WHAT AN ADVANCED PROGRAM OF MITO-CHONDRIAL RESUSCITATION MIGHT INCLUDE:

- CoQ10 50–200 mg
- N-acetylcysteine 500–3,000 mg
- N-acetyl carnitine 200–2,000 mg
- Lipoic acid 200–2,000 mg
- Niacin (B3) 50–1,000 mg (caution about flushing reaction at higher doses)
- Pyridoxine (B6) 10–50 mg
- Riboflavin (B2) 50–200 mg
- Thiamine (B1) 50–200 mg
- Folic acid 800–3,000 mcg
- Cobalamine (B12) 50–1,000 mcg
- Selenium 50–200 mcg
- Zinc 10–30 mg
- Ascorbic acid (vitamin C) 1,000–3,000 mg
- Mixed tocopherols (natural vitamin E) 100–800 IU
- Vitamin D3 1,000–5,000 IU
- Resveratrol (grapes) 50–200 mg
- Curcumin (turmeric) 50–200 mg
- Epigallocatechin gallate (green tea) 50–200 mg

Paul was the founder and president of a small business. It was a success, but Paul worried that he wasn't as sharp as he used to be and that his competitors might be getting the better of him. It bothered him. He was bothered too by the fact that his tolerance for exercise had gone out the window. He could barely play nine holes of golf these days, even using a golf cart. He also ached all over; he swallowed ibuprofens like they were peanuts, but he still had sore muscles. Paul also had sleep apnea, so his physician had put him on a machine that forced him to wear a mask all night. Although this helped him get some sleep, he still didn't feel good, and the machine was not exactly helpful to his marriage. He felt he was losing his edge in every sphere of his life.

Paul's conditions were classic collective evidence of oxidative injury and mitochondrial dysfunction, deriving primarily from a diet consisting of too much of too little; he was simply undernourished in what was necessary for his proper bioenergetics. His personalized program was easy: to a Mediterranean diet was added a group of nutrient supplements geared to his mitochondrial resuscitation, primarily antioxidants and vitamins, which Paul took on a daily basis.* Improvement came quickly and kept growing. Within eight weeks, Paul was able to stop using the sleep machine; his apnea was gone. He awoke refreshed and felt that his brain was working well again. Although he had begun a modest daily walking program at the start of his program, he now embraced a serious fitness plan; he joined the local health club and took a class at least three times a week. By the following summer, he was back to doing what he had done as a young man—hiking the Rockies in Wyoming. He said he felt like a young man again too.

Paul's eight-week response to his program of mitochondrial resuscitation was rapid; it's safe to say it may take up to six months to feel the full benefits of such a program. But as implementation proceeds, you will typically begin to notice improved endurance, better sleep patterns, diminished fatigue, and greatly reduced muscle pain after exercise. Once full benefits have been reached and you feel you have completed the therapeutic phase of the program, it makes sense to transition to a maintenance program with lowered amounts of the supplemental nutritional support. The goal is to be able to sustain your endurance and mitochondrial function by maintaining a phytonutrient-rich food plan and a regular strength and conditioning exercise program. Also, once a person has undergone a successful detoxification program, it is much easier to sustain mitochondrial

---

* N-acetylcysteine (2,000 mg), lipoic acid (2,000 mg), coenzyme Q10 (50 mg), methyl-cobalamin (a form of vitamin B12; 500 mcg), folic acid (800 mcg), vitamin B1 (50 mg), vitamin B2 (50 mg), vitamin B3 (100 mg), vitamin B6 (25 mg).

function with diet and exercise. You can then personalize the level of supplemental nutrients required to support your mitochondrial function by reducing your intake of the mitochondrial support nutrients and seeing how each reduction makes you feel.

In Paul's case, as in so many cases, the detective work was a matter of looking at things in a new way and connecting the dots into a pattern of health and disease, rather than simply a list of symptoms. Even people who should be able to see the patterns don't always, as was made very clear to me some years ago in Dallas, where I was giving a seminar for doctors. Following a three-hour session on mitochondrial bioenergetics and toxic substances, one of the docs cornered me; he was waving a file containing laboratory data. *His* laboratory data, as it turned out, because he was suffering the very symptoms of energy deficit I had just described. Yet as far as he could see, nothing in the data in his lab report pointed to mitochondrial function as the source of his troubles. "Take a look," he offered.

What I saw was in fact the precise model of what I had been lecturing about: an elevated body mass index with insulin resistance, elevated inflammation markers, and elevated GGTP enzyme level in his blood. Remember GGTP? It produces glutathione in the body, possibly in order to detoxify a buildup of chemicals causing mitochondrial imbalance. But this doctor, trained to look at data from an "old medicine" perspective, simply could not apply a new paradigm of understanding to his own information; he just couldn't see it any other way.

I went through it with him, and he soon got it. And once he had it, he ran with it, putting together his own personalized program combining detoxification and mitochondrial resuscitation measures. The first step toward change is often to see the picture in a fresh light.

STRUCTURE

1. Do you feel you're getting shorter over time?
2. Have any back problems?
3. Do you frequently get a sore neck?
4. Are you a frequent cell phone user?

5. Have you been told that you have elevated hemoglobin A1c?
6. Do charbroiled foods show up frequently in your diet?
7. Any memory problems?
8. Do you have a weight problem even though you watch your calories like a hawk?
9. Is your waist-to-hip ratio greater than 1?
10. Do you eat a lot of foods and drinks stored in plastic containers?
11. Are you one of those people who are "cold all the time"?
12. Have you been told you have reduced bone mass?
13. Are you menopausal?
14. Do you pretty much avoid dairy products?
15. Do you eat proportionally way more animal protein than vegetables?

For an extreme example of the relationship between structure and function, I can think of nothing more searing than the shocking evidence I once saw of what happened over time to a group of drug abusers. The evidence was in the form of photographs of eight individuals—four men, four women—in their late twenties and early thirties, all of them arrested for selling and using drugs.

The initial pictures showed eight normal, attractive people. The next batch was taken a few years later, after a subsequent arrest for continued drug use. The difference was overwhelming. Although only a few years had passed, all eight individuals looked decades older. Their faces were so distorted it was hard to recognize that they were the same people as in the initial photographs. It made me wonder what their organs, tissues, cells, and subcellular structures looked like. I knew that they too would have aged unrecognizably, and that the deterioration in structure would be reflected in deteriorated health and function.

So-called recreational drugs illustrate how exposure to foreign substances can produce profound imbalances in our core physiological processes, effecting change in the overall structure and function of the individual. It's an extreme example; the genes of the people in the photographs had spoken so loudly and with such hostility to these foreign invaders that they completely distorted their genetic expression, causing these radical changes in all aspects of the addicts' structure and function.

Structural imbalances can also occur much more subtly and not as severely through injuries, poor posture, or lack of proper muscle-strengthening activities or flexibility. The effects on physiological function may not be as profound as those seen in the group of drug abusers, but nevertheless influence the other core physiological processes.

If many of your answers to the Chapter 10 questionnaire indicate an imbalance in your core structural process, your health and function are also at risk. Today, the most prevalent structural imbalance is central obesity. Unfortunately, most weight-loss remedies are ineffective. If they succeed at all, it is only temporarily before the dieter swings back to an even higher weight. The reason is that these weight-loss diets focus too heavily on managing calorie intake and not enough on controlling the type of information in the message a specific calorie delivers to the genes. Calories perceived by the body to be foreign or hostile turn on the genes that store food as fat; this angry fat produces adipokines that trigger inflammation, which can lead to chronic illness.

Our research center has published study after study—as have many other researchers—demonstrating how a food plan comprising foods that send friendly messages to the genes produces proper appetite control and results in a new, healthy set-point weight and leaner body composition, one that is minus the angry fat that is the biggest risk for disease. Moreover, studies have shown how and why severely obese patients, most on various medications for various ailments, who undergo gastric bypass bariatric surgery are typically able to eliminate their meds within days of the surgery. Well before they lose any substantial weight, the rerouting of their digestive tract has begun to send different messages to their genes, calming their angry fat. Again, the structure of the body connects directly with its function through genetic expression. Yes, you can do it with surgery, but that is a lot riskier—a lot costlier in so many ways—than doing it through changes in lifestyle, diet, and environment.

In short, the priority in the design of a personalized program to restore structural balance is to harness the genes themselves to do the work of reshaping the body's structure and function—simply by sending them the right information from our diet, lifestyle, and environment. Such a plan will combine an eating plan that sends the right messages to the genes—resulting in the loss of angry fat and the activation of mitochondrial energetics in the muscle—with an exercise program for long-term control of energy processing.

If your imbalance is structural at the whole-body level—that is, if you answered yes to question 1, 2, 3, or 12, your whole-body structure has been compromised, and physical medicine may be the answer. Osteopathy, chiropractic, therapeutic massage, or acupuncture can be an important first step in improving health. Be aware that structural imbalances resulting from sports injury or trauma probably require rehabilitation, not physical medicine.

Be aware also that adequate amounts of calcium and vitamin D are important for your skeletal health; if you undertake weight-bearing exercises as part of your personalized program for restoring structural balance, these should be taken as supplements. But take them *only* if you engage in weight-bearing exercise. Astronauts at zero gravity for extended periods of time lose bone despite ingesting calcium and vitamin D supplements. It requires resistance, like gravity, for exercise movement to incite our genes to express the necessary proteins to capture calcium and build bone. Without the resistance, the specific genes for bone formation remain at rest, and bone loss results.

FOR AN IMBALANCE IN STRUCTURE, ADDRESS BOTH THE PHYSIOLOGICAL AND THE PHYSICAL

For weight loss (physiological):	A food plan that sends friendly messages to the genes in order to control appetite and create a new set point for a healthy body weight.
For whole-body issues (physical):	Physical medicine and/or exercise, with calcium and vitamin D supplements when you are doing weight-bearing exercise.

CHAPTER 14

Your Health-Care Revolution

At the beginning of this book, I promised you a revolution in health care comparable in its impact to that of the bacteriological revolution at the beginning of the last century. That prior revolution led to the conquest—or at least the control—of infectious diseases. This one will empower us to get a handle on the chronic illnesses that are burdening our increasing longevity.

In the first revolution, the main players were the physicians, clinical researchers, and pharmaceutical companies devising medication after medication to zap our infections and palliate our symptoms. In this revolution, the main players are us. The breakthroughs in our understanding of how lifestyle, diet, and the environment influence genetic expression and determine how we look, act, and feel make each one of us part of the transformation in health care. It's up to us to work with our health-care professionals to develop our own personalized health-management program. As I wrote early on, we have both the opportunity and the power to realize our optimum genetic potential.

The transformation cannot happen soon enough. Globally, the rise in the prevalence of chronic illness, striking people of all ages, both genders, and all races, is exponential. It is reminiscent of, if not equivalent to, the infectious disease epidemics of earlier centuries. But if we are confronting a de facto plague of chronic illness, we have the knowledge and technologies to both prevent and manage the progressively harmful health conditions the plague brings us.

It starts with our new understanding of how the human genome is read and with the application of a systems biology view of the body as a network of interaction among seven core physiological processes. We see that the expression of each individual's unique set of genes can be edited by environmental factors and by the individual's nutritional habits and lifestyle behaviors. Those revisions to the book of life may cause imbalances in one or more of our core physiological processes, starting us on the path to illness. In Shakespeare's words, the fault "is not in our stars, but in ourselves"—not rigidly fixed in our genes, but capable of being re-edited and re-revised by our subsequent actions and shifts in behavior. This both gives the lie to genetic determinism and makes it clear that if we change environment, diet, and lifestyle in certain ways, we can restore balance to our core processes and thereby affect our personal pattern of health and disease.

THE REVOLUTION IS HAPPENING

We see it happening all over—in clinical research and in on-the-ground evidence about one chronic illness after another. Again, not a moment too soon: the World Health Organization 2011 Summit on the global economic burden of noncommunicable diseases estimated that the cost of chronic disease would hit $47 trillion by 2030—due mostly to heart disease, metabolic diseases like type 2 diabetes, chronic respiratory diseases like asthma, chronic kidney disease, cancer, and dementia.

This last, dementia, may be the most costly of all—both in dollars and in its impact on the sufferers of dementia and their families. In the United States as of 2012, dementia has been costing more than either cancer or heart disease—more than $200 billion in 2012 alone. We have as yet found no effective drugs for the management of dementia, but a variety of clinical studies indicate that lifestyle changes can improve mental functioning. At the famous Karolinska Institutet in Sweden, a study found that changes in diet and exercise improved cognitive function and reduced dementia. A study at the Mayo Clinic concluded that early intervention with lifestyle medicine could delay the onset of dementia, although it was not sufficient to treat later stages of Alzheimer's dementia. But numerous studies have indicated that a Mediterranean diet can lower the incidence of both Alzheimer's and non-Alzheimer's dementia.

Similarly compelling evidence supports personalized lifestyle changes in addressing insulin resistance and type 2 diabetes—specifically with health-management programs to improve glucose transport and insulin signaling. Because insulin resistance disturbs sleep and collaterally damages so many tissues, potentially damaging the eyes, kidneys, nerves, heart and arteries, and brain, such programs can have a major impact on health.

Where cardiovascular disease is an issue, personalized programs of health management, particularly through diet, have shown clear and profound benefits as they signal the genes to reduce inflammation and improve fat transport. A 2013 study in the *New England Journal of Medicine* calculates the significant impact of a Mediterranean diet rich in virgin olive oil and nuts in reducing the incidence of major cardiovascular events—including heart attack. Some of my own research, including that performed in collaboration with Deanna M. Minich and published in *Nutrition Reviews* in 2008, shows the value of certain phytonutrients serving as selective kinase response modulators (SKRMs) to influence genetic expression and lower the risk of cardiovascular disease. Multiple research studies confirm the point: phytonutrients in a well-designed diet plan do indeed speak to our genes.

Stress is another key driver of core imbalances leading to a range of chronic illnesses—as well as a contributor to infectious disease—and the research continues to show how a personalized health-management program can reduce the allostatic load associated with excess stress. Allostatic load can come both from psychological distress and from exposure to xenobiotic substances. Whatever the origin of the allostatic load, the research is clear that restoring balance to detoxification processes can reduce the burden on our defense systems and thereby lessen the chance of inflammatory responses causing autoimmune diseases.

Much research has also focused on the role of healthy gut microflora in sending healthy messages to our genes—and the impact on our genes if the microflora are adversely affected by a poor-quality diet. We know that high-fat, high-sugar foods increase the risk of metabolic endotoxemia—that is, the release of toxic substances from the intestinal tract into the blood, adding to the total load of alarm message our genes pick up from the environment, compounding "bad" communication with the fat cells and making them angry, augmenting the risk of disease. A personalized diet program can restore balance to the enteric microflora and change the signals our genes receive.

I offer this not to repeat what has been said in the previous chapters but as a reminder that the functional medicine revolution—anchored in the idea of personalized health management—is now accessible to all. From head to heart to gut to toe, from cognitive impairment to stress to that spare tire around the middle, scientists are showing how individuals can change the course of events that lead to chronic disease. That means you.

YOUR MOVE

The good news is that just at a time when we need a new, fresh approach to managing the growing burden of chronic disease, the solution has emerged. It derives from the genetic uniqueness we each have and the recognition that there is no such thing as a one-size-fits-all therapy.

The human genome evolved over several million years, shaped by numerous environmental factors. Your particular human genome is distinguished by unique skills and capabilities written into your book of life. The question is: How will you adjust your lifestyle, diet, and environment to realize the potential of that uniqueness?

You now have the tools to create a personalized health-management program to help you do just that. Building on the baseline program presented in Chapter 12, you can follow the guidelines set forth in Chapter 13 and begin to design your own plan.

The resources for helping you do so continue to multiply, and many key websites—a font of information—are listed in Appendix C. They will tell you how to find a functional medicine practitioner, learn more about ongoing research, get answers to your personal questions, connect with other health-conscious consumers, locate a lab for your own genetic testing, and more.

My aim in this book has been nothing less than to create a global population that is better informed about today's health-care revolution—one reader at a time, starting with you. I hope it leads you to make some changes in the interest of your own good health today and in the future, and I know that's not easy. Changing customary behaviors and ingrained habits never is, even when it's as worthwhile as it can be for you.

And there's no book of rules telling you how to do it or enforcing compliance. Guidelines and suggestions on how to personalize your program are just that, and they are only as valuable as the commitment to apply them. In other words, you need to own your own program and find your own way to apply the guidelines in your own life. The good news is that the more committed you are, the more positive your health outcomes will be, and the better your health outcomes, the greater the reinforcement of your commitment.

You don't need much in the way of accessories. You might want a tape measure so you can track your waist-to-hip ratio—less than 1 is the goal. A portable machine to measure blood pressure might be a good idea as well. And a pedometer, whether on your belt or on your smartphone, is a definite recommendation as you measure your daily quota of 10,000 steps. Moreover, as you'll see in Appendix C, there is a burgeoning industry in mobile apps for tracking health and fitness, and these can certainly be useful in keeping you aware of the intimate relationship between your actions and your genetic expression. You can also go to our website at www.plminstitute.org, where you'll find more information and answers to most of your questions.

The promise of future technologies is very exciting indeed, but equally exciting in my mind is how the new ideas born of the genomic era are reframing old observations and are prompting a melding of the best knowledge and practical experience from many perspectives—East and West, traditional and futuristic, the laboratory and the village.

Most exciting of all, I think, are the broader social implications of the functional medicine revolution. Darwin published *On the Origin of Species* in 1859, and his description of evolution and natural was a game-changer for the way people have looked at life ever since. Simplified—often to the point of a simplistic slogan, "survival of the fittest"—Darwin's analysis of evolution got boiled down to the notion that some people are just born more fit than others. Those people had won the gamble of genetic roulette, and everyone else was out of luck—stuck with an inferior genetic profile. Most tragically, this social Darwinism, as it was called, eventually became a catchall justification for some of the most tainted ideologies of all time—the pseudoscience of eugenics, racism, imperialism, and Nazism.

Now, however, thanks to the genomic revolution, social Darwinism must give way to the new biology of genetic expression and epigenetics—and therefore to a new model of genetic plasticity. Biological bigotry—the idea that some are born more fit and therefore more worthy—is dead and buried. Long live the new reality of genetic uniqueness and taking charge of your own pattern of health. Now we have scientific certainty that differentiating function on the basis of "genetic fitness" is as phony and as empty as differentiating function on the basis of race or gender. All are simply unacceptable. There are no superior genes. There are only superior diet, lifestyle, and environment, and we all have an equal genetic opportunity to create them for ourselves.

The Baseline Seven-Day Eating Plan

SUGGESTED RECIPES

Day 1 Breakfast
Nutri-Ola Cereal or Breakfast Bar

2 cups arrowroot, buckwheat flour, or finely ground filberts, walnuts, or sesame seeds

1 cup filberts or walnuts, coarsely ground

1 cup whole sesame seeds

1 cup finely chopped dried apples, papaya, or raisins

½ cup honey or concentrated frozen fruit juice or fruit puree

½ cup sesame, walnut, or soy oil

2 tsp pure vanilla extract

Preheat oven to 275 degrees. Use a blender or food processor to grind the arrowroot, the nuts, and the seeds to desired consistency. Mix all this in a large bowl. Mix with fruit and sweetener, oil, and vanilla. Pour over the dry mixture and stir lightly. Spread mixture into a lightly oiled baking pan (15" × 10" × 1"). Bake for 1 hour, stirring every 15 minutes. Cool. Break into small pieces for cereal or large chunks for snacks. **10 SERVINGS.**

Day 1 Breakfast
Baked Apples

6 cooking apples, cored

⅓ cup golden raisins

2 Tbsp unsweetened apple cider
1½ cups water
¼ cup frozen unsweetened apple juice concentrate
2 tsp pure vanilla extract
1 tsp cinnamon
1 tsp arrowroot

Remove peel from top third of each apple. Arrange apples in a small baking dish. In a medium saucepan, combine other ingredients and bring to a boil, stirring frequently. Reduce heat and simmer 2–3 minutes until slightly thickened. Distribute raisins, filling centers of the apples. Pour sauce over apples. Bake, uncovered, at 350 degrees 1 to 1½ hours, basting occasionally, until apples are easily pierced with a fork. Remove the dish from the oven and allow to cool somewhat. Spoon juice over apples. Serve warm. **SERVES 6.**

Day 1 Lunch
MARINATED TUNA AND VEGETABLES
2 large carrots cut into 2" julienne strips
½ small head cauliflower, separated into florets
1 package (10 oz) frozen peas
½ cup thinly sliced celery
¼ cup sliced green onion
1 can (6½ oz) water-packed tuna, well drained
1 Tbsp balsamic vinegar
3 Tbsp olive oil

Steam carrots and cauliflower together in a basket, 10 minutes. Add peas. Cook 5 minutes more, or until vegetables are tender-crisp. Combine cooked vegetables, celery, and green onion in a medium bowl. Add tuna, vinegar, and oil. Toss, cover, and chill before serving. **SERVES 2.**

Day 1 Dinner
RED CABBAGE SALAD
1 medium head red cabbage, coarsely chopped
10 radishes, sliced
3 Granny Smith or other tart apples, diced
2 green onions, chopped
1 stalk celery, chopped
¼ cup chopped walnuts
1–2 Tbsp lemon juice
Dash garlic powder
2 Tbsp olive oil
1 Tbsp balsamic vinegar

Mix everything in a bowl and let sit for an hour, stirring once or twice. **SERVES 4.**

From *The Territorial Seed Company Garden Cookbook,* edited by Lane Morgan

Day 1 Dinner
SPLIT PEAS AND RICE
2 tsp curry powder
2 onions, finely chopped
1 green bell pepper, finely chopped
4 Tbsp olive oil
2 cups brown rice
6 cups water
1 cup yellow split peas

In a large heavy pot, sauté the curry, onions, and green pepper in 3 tablespoons oil until onions are tender. Stir in the rice and continue to cook 5 minutes or until rice begins to turn white. Add water and bring to a boil. Cook, covered, over low heat 20 minutes. Sauté yellow split peas in remaining oil. Add split peas to the cooking rice and cook 30 minutes more. **SERVES 4.**

Day 2 Breakfast
EGGLESS COUNTRY SCRAMBLE
1 pound regular tofu, drained and crumbled

2 Tbsp tamari

2 Tbsp olive oil

½ cup chopped onion

2 red potatoes, diced

½ cup sliced fresh mushrooms

½ cup chopped green bell pepper

1 clove garlic, minced

½ tsp thyme

½ tsp caraway seeds

½ tsp red pepper flakes

1 tomato cut in wedges for garnish

In a small bowl, blend tofu with tamari. Set aside. Heat oil in large, nonstick skillet over medium heat. Sauté onion and potatoes about 5 minutes until onion is translucent and potatoes are golden brown. Add mushrooms, green pepper, garlic, and spices and cook 3–5 minutes longer, until peppers and mushrooms are soft. Transfer vegetables to a bowl. Return skillet to low heat and sauté tofu until dry, about 3 minutes. Add vegetables to tofu, scramble well, and cook just until vegetables are heated through. Serve immediately with wedges of tomato. **SERVES 4.**

From the *Delicious! Collection,* edited by Sue Frederick

Day 2 Lunch
MANDARIN ALMOND SALAD
Lettuce—whatever type you prefer (red leaf, Bibb, romaine, radicchio) and as much as you want

1 cup (or more) chopped celery

1 Tbsp minced parsley

11 ounces drained mandarin oranges (or fresh ones) or drained juice-packed pineapple

Dressing

½ cup tarragon vinegar or lemon juice

1 tsp tarragon leaves

⅛ tsp fresh ground pepper

1 tsp honey

½ tsp Dijon mustard

½ cup flaxseed oil

½ cup sunflower oil

¼ cup toasted sliced almonds

Places spices and vinegar or lemon juice in a small bowl or blender and mix. Add oil slowly, mixing continuously until dressing is a light creamy color. Refrigerate for 1 hour before serving over salad. Garnish with almonds. **DRESSING MAKES ENOUGH FOR 8 TO 12 SALADS AND KEEPS WELL IN THE REFRIGERATOR.**

From *Guilt-Free Indulgence*

Day 2 Dinner

CHICKEN AND BROCCOLI SKILLET

2 whole medium chicken breasts, split, boned, and cut into ½" strips, all visible skin and fat removed.

⅛ tsp black pepper

¼ cup chopped onion

2 Tbsp olive oil

1 package (10 oz) frozen cut broccoli, thawed (or 1 pound fresh), separated into small florets

1 tsp fresh lemon juice

¼ tsp dried thyme

3 medium tomatoes cut into wedges

Season chicken strips with pepper. In medium skillet, cook chicken and onion quickly in the oil until chicken is done. Stir in broccoli, lemon juice, and thyme. Cook, covered, 6 minutes. Add tomato wedges. Cook, covered, 3–4 minutes longer. **SERVES 4**

Day 3 Breakfast

MUESLI

3 cups puffed rice

1 cup organic brown rice dry cereal

3 cups cornflakes

1 cup roasted soy nuts, peanuts, or almonds

1 cup sunflower seeds

1 cup each of any two of the following: currants or raisins, dried
   date bits, dried cherries or apples, dried peach or apricot bits

Toss all ingredients together and store in airtight containers.
**MAKES 10 CUPS. (THIS RECIPE MAKES A QUICK, TASTY BREAKFAST OR SNACK, AND
IT'S GREAT TO TAKE WITH YOU WHEN YOU TRAVEL.)**
From *The Gluten-Free Gourmet,* by Bette Hagman

Day 3 Lunch

QUICK QUINOA CASSEROLE

1 cup quinoa (pronounced keen-wa)

2 medium potatoes, peeled (or scrubbed) and chopped

2 carrots, trimmed and cut into rings

2 onions, chopped

1 cup brown lentils

2 cups vegetable stock or tomato juice

1 tsp chili powder (or to taste)

½ tsp cumin (or to taste)

1½ tsp tamari

Put quinoa in a bowl and cover with water. Swirl bowl and drain in a
fine sieve or a colander lined with cheesecloth. Repeat several times,
until the water runs clear. Put quinoa and all other ingredients in
Dutch oven and bring to a boil. Reduce heat and simmer until carrots are tender, about 30 minutes. Stir several times during cooking,
adding more liquid if necessary. **SERVES 4.**

Day 3 Dinner

RISI E BISI

1¾ cups fat-free chicken broth (or one 14½-oz can)

1 cup long-grain brown rice

8 oz canned no-salt tomatoes in juice

3 cloves garlic, finely chopped

1 cup peas, fresh or frozen

1 tsp Italian seasoning blend

Dash white pepper (optional)

½ cup finely chopped green onion

In a medium saucepan bring broth to a boil over high heat. Add rice, cover, and reduce heat to low. Cook for 50 minutes, or until rice is tender and liquid is absorbed. While rice is cooking, cut up canned tomatoes, reserving ¼ cup juice. Combine tomatoes, ¼ cup juice, garlic, peas, and seasoning in a large skillet. Sauté over medium-high heat 5–7 minutes or until garlic and peas are at desired doneness. When rice is tender, stir into skillet. Heat until rice mixture is hot, approximately 5 minutes. Remove from heat, sprinkle with green onion, and serve. **3 SERVINGS.**

From *Cooking Without Fat,* by George Mateljan

Day 4 Breakfast

BANANA SHAKE

1 frozen banana

⅔ cup vanilla-flavored almond milk

Combine in blender and process until smooth. **SERVES 1**

Day 4 Breakfast

SPICY CARROT MUFFINS

1 cup white-rice flour

⅓ cup potato starch flour

3 Tbsp tapioca flour

½ cup rice bran

1 tsp cinnamon
¾ tsp baking soda
2 tsp baking powder (nonaluminum)
¼ tsp nutmeg
1 cup shredded carrots
⅔ cup orange juice
⅓ cup raisins
¼ cup vegetable oil
¼ cup brown sugar
Egg replacer to equal 2 eggs

In a large bowl combine flours, bran, cinnamon, baking soda, baking powder, and nutmeg. Mix well. Combine carrots, orange juice, raisins, oil, brown sugar, and egg replacer. Add to dry mixture, mixing until dry ingredients are moistened. Grease 10 medium muffin cups or line them with paper liners. Fill about ⅔ full of batter. Let stand for 5 minutes. Bake in preheated 425-degree oven for 20 minutes. **MAKES 10 MUFFINS.**

From *The Gluten-Free Gourmet*

Day 4 Lunch
HEAVENLY QUINOA HASH

1 cup raw quinoa (pronounced keen-wa)
2 cups water
¼ tsp salt-free herb blend
2 cooked potatoes, diced
1 onion, sliced
2 cloves garlic
1 green or red bell pepper, diced
¼ cup minced parsley
1 Tbsp olive oil

Rinse quinoa according to directions given in recipe for Quick Quinoa Casserole (Day 3 Lunch). Bring water to a boil. Stir in quinoa, cover, and simmer 15 minutes until grains become translucent and pop open. Drain immediately. Combine quinoa with remaining ingredients, except oil. Taste and adjust seasonings. Sauté hash in oil until warmed thoroughly and lightly browned. **SERVES 6.**

Day 4 Dinner
STIR-COOKED CHICKEN AND VEGETABLES
1 whole chicken breast, skin, bones, and all visible fat removed
1 onion, chopped
2 Tbsp olive oil
1 green or red bell pepper (or a combination) cut in strips
2 cups broccoli florets
1 cup Chinese edible pea pods
Tamari sauce

Cut chicken into thin strips, about 2" long and ½" wide. In a wok or large frying pan stir-cook onion in 1 tablespoon oil until it is translucent. Add the other tablespoon oil and the chicken. Quickly cook over medium-high heat until the chicken is thoroughly cooked. Remove chicken from pan and set aside. Quickly brown vegetables, adding pea pods only during final 2 minutes. Add chicken last and serve over rice. Season with tamari sauce. **SERVES 2.**

Day 5 Breakfast
OVEN-BAKED POTATO PANCAKES
2 large baking potatoes (1½ pounds), peeled
1 tsp oregano
½ tsp chili powder
¼ tsp salt
⅛ tsp pepper
½ small onion, minced
2 Tbsp potato flour
1 Tbsp olive oil
Rice vinegar to taste

Coarsely grate potatoes. Rinse in colander under cold water. Press out as much moisture as possible. Place grated potatoes in medium bowl. Combine seasonings, onion, and flour. Work mixture evenly into potatoes, pressing into 8 flat circles. Preheat oven to 450 degrees. Rub 1½ tsp oil onto cookie sheets. Bake 10 minutes, then press each pancake down with a spatula and bake 2–5 minutes more. Loosen around each pancake with spatula and carefully flip over. Return to oven and bake until crisp (5–6 minutes). Serve immediately, sprinkled with rice vinegar. **MAKES 8 PANCAKES.**

Day 5 Lunch
TORTILLA CHIPS
12 soft corn tortillas, thawed in bag

Preheat oven to 275 degrees. Cut tortillas into four quarters. Lay pieces in a single layer on two dry baking sheets.

Bake 20–30 minutes until crisp. **SERVES 6**

To serve soft: After allowing to thaw in bag, remove and wrap in foil or place in covered baking dish. Heat in warm oven for a few minutes. Serve warm. Optional: Before baking, sprinkle tortillas with onion powder, garlic powder, or chili powder.

From *The McDougall Plan,* by John A. McDougall, MD, and Mary A. McDougall

Day 5 Lunch
LENTIL LUST SOUP
2 large carrots, chopped
1 onion, chopped
2 stalks celery, chopped
7½ cups pure water or vegetable broth
2 cloves garlic, minced
1½ cups lentils (red, green, or combination)
Pinch of thyme
Dash of paprika
2 Tbsp tamari

Salt-free seasoning to taste

Cumin or chili powder to taste (optional)

Coarsely chop carrots, onion, and celery. Add to water or broth along with minced garlic and lentils. (If you use red lentils add them 25 minutes after green lentils, because they need only a short time to cook.) Bring soup to a boil and add thyme, paprika, and tamari. If you prefer a spicy soup add a few pinches at a time of cayenne, chili powder, curry powder, and/or cumin. Reduce heat to medium-low and simmer covered 45 minutes to 1 hour until lentils are soft. For a creamy consistency, puree about half of the soup in a blender and return to soup pot. **SERVES 4.**

From *Guilt-Free Indulgence*

Day 5 Dinner
SPICY BLACK BEANS AND TOMATOES
½ onion, chopped

2 cloves garlic, minced

1 tsp olive oil

1 can chopped stewed tomatoes (or 2–3 fresh chopped)

1 small (4-oz) can diced green chilies

1 can black beans, drained (or 1½ cups cooked dry beans)

½ tsp cumin

½ tsp ground red pepper

¼ tsp chili powder

1 Tbsp chopped fresh cilantro (substitute parsley if you can't find cilantro in the market)

Sauté onion and garlic in olive oil over medium heat until tender. Add tomatoes and green chilies. Reduce heat and cook uncovered 6–8 minutes until thickened. Stir in beans and remaining ingredients. Cover and heat 5 minutes. **SERVES 8.**

Day 6 Breakfast

OATMEAL

1 cup water or vanilla-flavored almond milk
½ cup natural whole-grain old-fashioned oatmeal

Boil water or milk. Stir in oats. Cook about 5 minutes over medium heat, stirring occasionally.

Day 6 Breakfast

RASPBERRY RICE MILK SMOOTHIE

½ banana
1 handful of frozen raspberries
Few drops of lemon juice
1 cup rice milk

Peel banana and cut into slices. Put the raspberries, banana, and lemon juice into the blender. Mix until you obtain a puree, and then add the rice milk. Mix until the mixture becomes frothy. Serve chilled.

Day 6 Lunch

SANTA FE CORN SALAD

3 cups fresh corn, cooked (or one 17-oz can whole kernel corn, drained)
1 can (10 oz) kidney beans, drained
½ cup sliced celery
1 red bell pepper, chopped
1 green bell pepper, chopped
3 green onions finely chopped (include green tops)
½ cup cilantro, chopped (optional)
1 Tbsp canola oil
¼ cup salsa
½ tsp chili powder

In a large bowl toss all ingredients together. Chill for at least 30 minutes before serving. **SERVES 8.**

Day 6 Lunch

HUMMUS SPREAD OR DIP

1½ cups dry garbanzo beans (or 2 cans, drained)

¾ cup liquid from garbanzos, or pure water

4 cloves garlic, minced

1 Tbsp tamari

2 tsp cumin

1 tsp coriander

¼ cup fresh lemon juice

¼ cup flax oil

¼ cup tahini (sesame butter)

Sort dry garbanzos, rinse, cover with pure water, and soak overnight. Drain, rinse, and bring to a boil in a pot of pure water. Reduce heat and simmer 2 hours, stirring occasionally and adding more water as needed. When garbanzos are tender (or if using canned beans) drain and place in blender with ¾ cup liquid. Process with garlic, tamari, and spices until smooth, scraping down sides a few times. Add lemon juice, oil, and tahini. Process until thoroughly blended. Refrigerate and use as needed. It will keep well several days. Hummus can be thick or thin, depending on what you want to use it for. It will thicken when it is chilled. **MAKES 4 CUPS.**

From *Guilt-Free Indulgence*

Day 6 Lunch

VEGETARIAN CHILI

3 Tbsp olive oil

1 medium onion, coarsely chopped

4 cloves garlic, minced

½ pound mushrooms, chopped

2 cups cauliflower pieces

1 large potato, peeled (or scrubbed) and chopped

1 large green pepper, seeded and chopped

2 large carrots, peeled (or scrubbed) and chopped

3 cups fresh or frozen corn kernels

1 (28-oz) can plum tomatoes, chopped, including juice

1 (15-oz) can pinto or kidney beans including liquid

1 cup tomato juice

1 Tbsp ground cumin

2 Tbsp chili powder

1 tsp paprika

1½ tsp salt-free herbal blend

⅛ tsp cayenne

2 Tbsp tomato paste

3 Tbsp red wine vinegar

Heat olive oil in Dutch oven over medium heat. Add onion and garlic and sauté until onion is translucent, about 5 minutes. Add mushrooms and sauté another 10 minutes. Stir in cauliflower, potato, green pepper, carrots, corn, tomatoes, beans, tomato juice, cumin, chili powder, paprika, salt-free herbs, cayenne, tomato paste, and vinegar. Bring mixture to a boil. Reduce heat to simmer. Cover and cook, stirring occasionally, until vegetables are tender, about 30 minutes. **SERVES 6.**

From *Guilt-Free Indulgence*

Day 6 Dinner

SPICY GARBANZO CURRY

2 Tbsp olive oil

1 large onion, chopped

1 large green bell pepper, chopped

4 cloves garlic, minced

3½ cups chicken broth

6 medium thin-skinned potatoes, scrubbed and cut into chunks

2 (15-oz) cans garbanzo beans, drained (or 4 cups cooked garbanzo beans)

1 (6-oz) can tomato paste

1 Tbsp curry powder

1 Tbsp cayenne

3 cups hot cooked rice

Chopped green onion

In Dutch oven over medium heat combine oil, onion, bell pepper, and garlic. Stir occasionally and cook until vegetables are tender, about 7 minutes. Stir in broth, potatoes, garbanzos, tomato paste, curry powder, and cayenne. Cover and simmer until potatoes are tender, 30–40 minutes. Spoon over rice. Top with chopped green onion. **SERVES 6**

Day 7 Breakfast
STRAWBERRY-BANANA SMOOTHIE
1 fresh or frozen ripe banana
4 strawberries
½ cup apple cider
½ cup pure water

Combine in blender or processor until smooth. **SERVES 1.**

Day 7 Lunch
RICE SUMMER SALAD
½ cup cider vinegar or wine vinegar
¼ tsp dry mustard
1 tsp tarragon, dried (or 1 Tbsp fresh, chopped)
4 cups cooked brown rice
6 green onions, finely chopped
2 stalks celery, chopped
1 large green bell pepper, chopped
1 cup cauliflower
1 cup broccoli
1 large tomato, chopped
1 cup cooked green peas
4–5 Tbsp diced pimiento
¼ cup chopped parsley
1 cucumber, chopped (optional)
Freshly ground pepper to taste

Mix vinegar, mustard, and tarragon. Pour over cooked rice. Mix well. If rice is warm, let cool to room temperature before adding remaining ingredients. When rice is cool, add remaining ingredients. Toss gently. Cover and refrigerate at least 2 hours before serving. **SERVES 8.**

Day 7 Dinner
ORIENTAL SCALLOPS
12 oz sea scallops
2 Tbsp tamari
1 Tbsp fresh lemon juice
½ tsp ground ginger
¼ tsp dry mustard
8 cherry tomatoes
1 medium green bell pepper, cut into 1" pieces

Thaw scallops, if frozen. Place in shallow glass dish. Combine tamari, lemon juice, ginger, and dry mustard. Pour over scallops. Cover and let stand at room temperature for 1 hour. Drain, reserving marinade. On four skewers, alternate scallops, tomatoes, and green pepper. Place on rack of broiler. Broil 5" from heat, 7–8 minutes per side, basting with marinade. **SERVES 2.**

Glossary of Scientific Terminology

Acute: An illness or injury that often has rapid onset or a single cause and can be resolved with medical intervention.

Adaptogen: A substance that helps the body adapt to a changing environment or stressful situation.

Adenosine triphosphate (ATP): A chemical compound produced in the mitochondria of the cell that is related to energy production.

Adipocytes: Cells that make up fat tissue, which is also called adipose tissue.

Adipokines: A family of messenger substances manufactured and secreted into the bloodstream by adipocytes.

Adrenaline: A key stress hormone that is involved in many processes in the human body, including mitochondria bioenergetics and insulin balance.

Advanced glycation end-products: Protein structures formed through the process of glycation that can stimulate an immune inflammatory response.

Adverse drug reaction (ADR): An atypical or toxic metabolic response to a drug approved for use.

Albumin: A blood protein manufactured in the liver that can be a marker of protein sufficiency and amino acid balance.

Allostasis/Allostatic load: A concept developed by researcher Bruce McEwen that refers to a process by which the human organism makes adjustments to maintain homeostasis.

Alzheimer's disease: A progressive neurodegenerative disorder that is the most common cause of dementia in the elderly.

Amino acids: Amino acids are the building blocks of proteins. There are twenty amino acids, of which eight are essential.

Amylase: An enzyme secreted in saliva that is involved in the process of digestion.

Amylopectin: The short-grain variety of rice, which has a greater impact on glucose levels.

Amylose: The long-grain variety of rice, which has lesser impact on glucose levels.

Anemias: Hematological aberrations, various forms of which are nutrient-related.

Ankylosing spondylitis: An inflammatory immune condition, also called "bamboo spine," that may affect individuals who carry a unique histocompatibility gene. One of the more than eighty autoimmune diseases.

Antibiotics: Proteins that are produced by the immune system and are highly selective in their action against the causes of specific infectious diseases.

Antioxidants: Molecules generally consumed in the diet to reduce damaging oxidative processes and produce cellular redox balance (the reduction/oxidation potential of the cell). This activity has a profound effect on signal transduction and intracellular communication.

Apolipoprotein E gene (ApoE): A genetic variant that has been linked to a higher incidence of Alzheimer's disease and heart disease.

Arthritis: A systemic inflammatory condition affecting the joints. One of the more than eighty autoimmune diseases.

Ashwagandha: An adaptogenic herb that has a history of medicinal use. Often called "Indian ginseng."

Asthma: A chronic inflammatory condition of the lungs in which swelling of the airways leads to wheezing and difficulty breathing.

Atopy: Allergic reaction that may be hereditary and results in skin rashes and asthma.

Attention deficit disorder: A condition in which the brain is hyperstimulated and unable to stay on task.

Autism: A neuropsychiatric disorder with symptoms that relate to behavior, social interaction, and cognitive ability.

Autistic spectrum disorder: A group of developmental disorders that have in common impairments in social interaction, communication, imagination, and behavior, but can be found together with any level of ability, from profound general learning disability to average or even superior cognitive skill.

Autoimmune diseases: A variety of conditions that result when the body—for unknown reasons—generates an immune response against its own cells and tissues.

Ayurvedic medicine: A traditional philosophy of medicine that originated in India.

B cells: Immune system cells that neutralize toxins by secreting antibodies against them. These are known as the antibody-producing cells.

Benign prostatic hyperplasia (BPH): An enlargement of the prostate gland deriving from an alteration in testosterone metabolism coupled with an increase in activity of inflammatory messenger substances.

Biochemical individuality: A concept developed by Dr. Roger Williams in which health and disease are linked to genetic and environmental uniqueness.

Bioenergetics: A term used to describe the constellation of cellular processes related to the physiological energy of an organism; how energy is harnessed, made available, used, and transformed to support physiological processes.

Bioidentical hormone replacement therapy (BHRT): A therapy using hormones that are identical to natural hormones at the molecular level.

Biological aging: The rate of speed at which the human body loses organ reserve.

Biomarkers: Physiological indicators of health status.

Bisphenol-A (BPA): A synthetic molecule, persistent and not easily degraded, that has been used in the production of plastic for several decades. Significant levels of BPA are now found in the environment, and ongoing research has demonstrated an association between exposure and increased prevalence of disease.

Body mass index (BMI): An approximation of body composition, or percent body fat, using a measurement of height and weight. BMI is often coupled with the waist-to-hip ratio; together they can provide an estimate of visceral adipose tissue (VAT), fat tissue that accumulates around the abdomen.

Bone density: Bone mass or reserve, which is directly related to maintenance of bone integrity and resistance to fracture.

Boswellia serrata: The gum resin extract known as frankincense, which has been demonstrated to have anti-inflammatory properties.

Bovine spongiform encephalopathy (BSE): Also called mad cow disease, a neurodegenerative disease causing spongy degeneration in the brain and spinal cord in cattle.

BRCA mutation: A genetic mutation linked to higher risk of breast cancer.

Caloric restriction (CR): Generally a 30 percent reduction in calorie intake, a dietary approach that has been demonstrated to significantly increase life expectancy in animals.

Cancer: A constellation of diseases that can occur as the result of cellular malfunction and abnormal cellular division—oncogenesis—which reflects a systemic alteration that is the body's response to genetic triggers, environmental influences, or in many cases a combination of the two.

Candida albicans: A yeast generally present in the gastrointestinal tract that can cause illness or dysfunction in the event of overgrowth.

Carbohydrate: A nutritional molecule made up of the sugar glucose in long chains that can impact the body in a variety of ways depending on type and source.

Catalase: An enzyme involved in the body's system of cellular detoxification and antioxidation.

Celiac disease: A disorder in which the lining of the small intestine is damaged by a family of proteins called gluten, found in cereal grains. The intestinal damage prevents nutrients from being absorbed, and it is associated with a range of digestive symptoms as well as dementia.

Chelation: The binding of minerals by substances like the sulfur amino acid cysteine.

Cholecystokinin: A neurotransmitter hormone produced in the intestinal tract that has been linked to appetite.

Cholesterol: A molecule manufactured in the liver that is a precursor to hormones and bile acids. Cholesterol is necessary for proper fat digestion and metabolism and as a critical component of membranes. Cholesterol status is used as a biomarker for potential risk of heart disease and stroke.

Chromosome: The DNA molecule that carries the genetic code of an organism. Humans have twenty-three pairs, with half of each pair provided by the biological mother through her egg and the other half provided by the biological father through his sperm.

Chronic: Conditions, ailments, and illnesses that do not have a single cause, treatment, or cure. With a chronic health concern, the patient lives with the disease and the efforts at treatment for an indefinite time period.

Chronic fatigue syndrome (CFS): A syndrome characterized by bone-weary fatigue, muscle weakness, swollen glands, brain fog, intolerance of exercise that was previously well tolerated, and the desire to sleep through the day.

Chyme: Partially digested food.

Circulatory system: The heart and blood vessels, which pump blood throughout the body.

Clostridium: A bacterium normally present in the human gastrointestinal tract that can cause illness or dysfunction in the event of overgrowth.

Coenzyme Q10: A nutritional agent that has a relationship to mitochondrial energy production, cardiac function, and cardiomyopathies and is a member of the antioxidant family of substances.

Compression of morbidity: A theory of aging developed by Dr. James Fries that states that natural aging does not have to be accompanied by increased disability and functional impairment.

Conjugases: A family of enzymes principally found in the liver that are involved with cellular detoxification.

Creutzfeldt-Jakob disease: The human variant of bovine spongiform encephalopathy, which is transmitted to humans through contaminated animal products in the food supply.

Cryptosporidium: A parasite associated with a high risk of waterborne disease.

Cyclooxygenase (COX): An enzyme in cells associated with inflammation.

Cytochrome P450 (CYP450): An enzyme supersystem composed of more than fifty different kinds of enzymes, each with its own gene, that is involved with detoxifying toxins and metabolizing substances native to all living cells.

Cytokines: Proteins made by the immune cells that control cellular communication, including the communication of inflammation among organs.

Cytomegalovirus: A viral infection that may be connected to atherosclerosis.

Daidzein: A phytonutrient in soy connected to management of estrogen-related cellular communication imbalances.

Dementia: A loss of cognitive function associated with aging.

Depression: A mood disorder that may be linked to alterations in brain chemistry due to myriad variables, including environment.

Detoxification: Physiological processes occurring primarily in the liver that convert toxic substances into nontoxic by-products that are eliminated from the body via the kidneys and intestines.

Diabetes: A chronic condition in which an individual has elevated blood sugar levels. Type 1 diabetes is due to an autoimmune response that destroys the islets of Langerhans cells so that the pancreas simply cannot secrete insulin. Type 2 diabetes, which constitutes nearly 80 percent of the global incidence of this disease, stems from an imbalance in glucose transport that is affected by an individual's diet, lifestyle, and environment.

Diagnosis: Historically, doctors define a disease according to a cluster of symptoms; through clinical, laboratory, and pathological findings; and through clinical knowledge and judgment. The concept of diagnosis is driven by an assumption that the patient has a disease, an assumption that may or may not be true.

Digestive system: The cells, receptors, bacteria, tissues, and organs in the body working together to promote the digestion of food, absorption of nutrients, and elimination of waste.

Diindolylmethane (DIM): A phytochemical produced by digestion of cruciferous vegetables.

Dimercaptosuccinic acid (DMSA): A chelating agent.

Docasahexaenoic acid (DHA): An omega-3 fatty acid found in cod liver oil and other nutritional oils that has anti-inflammatory properties.

Down syndrome: Also called trisomy 21, a genetic condition associated with the mutation of one chromosome.

Duodenal ulcer: A condition of the gastrointestinal tract that may be associated with *Helicobacter pylori* infection.

Dysbiosis: A microbial imbalance of the gut.

Eicosapentaenoic acid (EPA): An omega-3 fatty acid found in cod liver oil and other nutritional oils that has anti-inflammatory properties.

Electrocardiogram (EKG): A diagnostic test to measure electrocardiac rhythm.

Endocrine system: The body's hormonal messaging system.

Endosymbiotic theory: A concept developed by Dr. Lynn Margulis that suggests mitochondria were originally bacteria that millions of years ago infected a host human cell, adapted to being there, and have remained there ever since because of a mutually beneficial symbiosis.

Endothelial dysfunction (ED): Blood vessel response to chronic insult or injury. In cardiovascular medicine, a noninvasive test for ED is sometimes used as a marker for predicting stroke, heart attack, coronary heart disease, congestive heart failure, and renal disease.

Endotoxemia: The release of toxic substances from the intestinal tract into the blood; also known as leaky gut syndrome.

Entamoeba histolytica: A waterborne parasite.

Enteric microflora: Collectively refers to the many types of bacteria found in the intestines, including symbiotic, commensal, and parasitic.

Epigenetics: The prefix *epi-*, from Greek, signifies something over and above. Epigenetics refers to things that reside above the control of the expression of the genome. Epigenetic events are heritable alterations in gene function that are mediated by factors other than changes in primary DNA sequence.

Epstein-Barr virus: A chronic viral illness linked to the herpes family that causes profound fatigue.

Erythromelalgia: A rare autoimmune disease that periodically causes the ankles and feet or hands and arms to swell, turn red, and become hot to the touch.

Essential fatty acids: Nutritional substances that transport fats and cholesterol in the blood and play a vital role in human metabolism.

Extracellular matrix: A network of nerves found in the connective tissue below the skin that acts as a whole-body signaling system.

Fat: Adipose tissue. Fat cells (adipocytes) are metabolically active and elaborate their own messenger molecules.

Fibromyalgia: A complex condition involving myalgic pain, fatigue, sleep disturbances, cognitive dysfunction, and immunological suppression.

Flavin adenine dinucleotide (FADH): A key substance derived from vitamin B2 that is involved in cellular energy production and metabolism.

Flavonoids: Phytochemicals that play a role in cellular detoxification.

Folate: Folic acid (vitamin B5), vitamin B12, vitamin B6, and betaine are all very important for support of the folate cycle. The folate cycle is the cycle that generates active methyl groups through S-adenosylmethionine.

Food allergy/food sensitivity: A food allergy produces an immuno-inflammatory cascade within the body. With food sensitivity, individuals may experience symptoms of imbalance when consuming foods they previously tolerated, but these foods do not trigger a measureable immune response.

Free radicals: Oxygen molecules that can have a damaging effect on mitochondria, which is theorized to contribute to cellular aging.

Fructans: Fibers from plant foods that seem to be the preferred food of the symbiotic and commensal families of bacteria in the intestine.

Functional medicine: A medical approach that is related to determining the imbalances in physiological, physical, and mental function that result in chronic disease.

Gaia hypothesis: The Gaia hypothesis, developed by Dr. Lynn Margulis, suggests that it is cooperation rather than competition—networking rather than the struggle of the unfit against the fit—that is the true driving force of evolution.

Gamma-glutamyl transpeptidase (GGT or GGTP): Elevated levels of this enzyme in the blood have historically signaled liver injury due to alcohol or drug toxicity, but are now also linked to toxic exposure, obesity, and diabetes.

Gastric reflux: A reflux of gastric contents up into the esophagus that can be a combination of acid and also bio- and pancreatic enzymes, all of which can degrade the esophageal mucosa and create gastrointestinal symptoms and complications.

Gastrin: A hormonal messenger molecule involved in communication between the gut and the brain.

Gaucher's disease: A genetic metabolism disease involving the accumulation of fatty substances.

General adaptation syndrome (GAS): The clinical model of stress as developed by Dr. Hans Selye and encompassing three stages of response: arousal, adaptation, and exhaustion.

Genes: The carriers of the genetic code—the book of life—present in each cell. Within the human species, genes can be very similar in the larger sense, but small differences encoded within genes (single nucleotide polymorphisms) account for more than 3 million variants in gene expression.

Genetic determinism: The belief that genes alone determine the pattern of disease and dysfunction in the life of an individual.

Genetic expression: The concept that environment and lifestyle can influence the expression of genes, and therefore also disease and health patterns.

Genetically modified organisms (GMOs): Crops that have been altered at the genetic level and introduced into the food supply, sparking debate about safety and disclosure practices.

Genistein: A phytonutrient in soy connected to management of estrogen-related cellular communication imbalances.

Genome: The whole of an individual's genetic information.

Genomics: The study of genetic sequencing as well as the influence of epigenetic factors on gene expression.

Genotype: Genotype is our genetic makeup, the potential of various traits to develop in us.

Germ theory: The breakthrough understanding that submicroscopic organisms cause infectious diseases.

Ghrelins: Hormonal messenger molecules involved in communication between the gut and the brain.

Ginger: A root that has traditional medicinal applications.

Glucagon-like peptide 1 (GLR-1): A hormone that raises blood sugar levels.

Glucose: A carbohydrate that is absorbed directly into the bloodstream during digestion and is extremely important in human metabolism.

Glucose test: A challenge that can help measure organ reserve. The subject drinks a sugar solution containing a specified amount of sugar. The level of glucose in the subject's blood is then monitored periodically over the next three to six hours to measure the subject's ability to properly metabolize the sugar load.

Glucosinolates: Nutrients found in the cabbage family that play a role in cellular detoxification.

Glucuronidation: A detoxification process in the body that can be influenced by nutritional substances.

Glutathione: A nutrient of central importance in human physiology because of its roles in mitochondrial function, redox potential, and cellular detoxification.

Gluten: A family of proteins found in cereal grains that cause celiac disease in genetically susceptible individuals.

Glycemic load: A dietary calculation relative to the level of sugar in the blood after eating certain foods.

Glycotoxins: Advanced glycation end-products produced by high-heat cooking resulting in the chemical combination of sugars with protein that have been linked to inflammatory response and chronic disease.

Gout: An autoimmune condition caused by an imbalance of uric acid leading to inflammation.

Hashimoto's thyroiditis: An autoimmune disease of the thyroid featuring alternating bouts of hypothyroidism and hyperthyroidism, with symptoms that can affect the entire body. This is one of the eighty autoimmune diseases.

HDL cholesterol: High-density lipoproteins—often referred to as "good" cholesterol. HDL cholesterol is a protein carrier whose task is to pick up the cholesterol from the artery wall and take it back to the liver to be broken down and excreted.

Health span: The length of time an individual lives a disease-free life.

Helicobacter pylori (H. pylori): Food-borne bacteria that cause infection of the gastrointestinal tract.

Hematocrit: A blood marker of protein insufficiency.

Hemoglobin A1c: A hemoglobin protein used clinically as a measurement of diabetes.

High blood pressure: A condition that arises from hypertension, a complex shift in our metabolic function that gives rise to changes in vascular endothelial compliance, leading to less vasorelaxation and more vasoconstriction.

High-fructose corn sweeteners: Sweeteners derived from high-fructose corn syrup and used in the manufacture of many processed foods.

High-sensitivity C-reactive protein (hs-CRP): A blood biomarker that is an indicator of chronic inflammation linked to several chronic diseases.

Homocysteine: A blood biomarker used as an indicator of vascular disease.

Hormone replacement therapy (HRT): A combination of equine estrogens and synthetic progesterone used to treat the symptoms of menopause in women for several decades that has now been linked to an increased risk of heart disease and dementia.

Hormones: Chemicals native to human physiology that maintain optimal health and function.

Human Genome Project: A project to map the human genome initiated in 1990 under the direction of Dr. Francis Collins and successfully completed in 2000 with the additional involvement of Dr. Craig Venter.

Humulones: Phytonutrient compounds derived from hops.

Hypochlorite: A caustic form of oxygen that makes up the chemical structure of bleach and promotes oxidation.

Immune system: The complex surveillance system of the human body that has the primary task of fighting infection. In the case of imbalance in the immune system—which can result from myriad causes: infection, toxic exposure, stress, hormonal imbalance, activity patterns, or nutrient intake—autoimmune disease and chronic conditions can result.

Indole-3-carbinol (I3C): A substance derived from cruciferous vegetables that can support processes of detoxification.

Inflammation: A natural immune response in the body. The presence of chronic inflammation in the body has been linked to altered cellular communication and the development of chronic disease.

Inflammatory bowel disease: A collective term embracing both ulcerative colitis and Crohn's disease. These disabling conditions are characterized by diarrhea, pain, bleeding, and other intestinal symptoms, and by lifelong relapses. Ulcerative colitis is confined to the mucosal layer of the large bowel, whereas Crohn's disease can affect any portion of the intestinal tract. The pathogenesis of inflammatory bowel disease is complex, but it appears to involve interaction between three essential components: host genotype, the community of intestinal bacteria, and the gut mucosal immune response.

Innate immunity: The presence of specialized white cells within the human organism that exist for the purpose of ingesting and killing foreign molecules in the body.

Insulin: A hormone produced by the pancreas that plays a significant role in human metabolism.

Insulin resistance: An imbalance in glucose transport that impairs glucose tolerance and is linked to the cluster of conditions known as metabolic syndrome.

Ischemic heart disease: Heart disease due to hardened arteries that reduce the blood supply to the heart.

Islets of Langerhans: Specialized cells in the pancreas that secrete insulin into the bloodstream.

Junk DNA: Noncoding regions of the human genome that were thought to have no function in genetics, but now are found to contain information that controls genetic expression.

Kinase: Substance that acts as a cellular signaling messenger.

Kupffer cells: Specialized immune cells found in the liver that transmit messages of inflammation.

Lactic acid: A waste product made by the body that results when activity exceeds the capacity of the mitochondria to produce the necessary level of energy, resulting in pain.

L cells: Specialized cells in the small intestine. Bitter-tasting foods can stimulate the L cells to release glucagon-like peptide-1 and in turn help to manage blood sugar and insulin levels

LDL cholesterol: Low-density lipoprotein—often referred to as "bad" cholesterol. LDL cholesterol is transported from the liver on a specific protein carrier whose job is to deliver it to the artery wall.

Life span: The total amount of time spent living, regardless of health status.

Lipoic acid: A substance produced by metabolism and used as a nutritional supplement that has been shown to improve insulin sensitivity and glucose transport.

Lyme disease (*Borrelia burgdorferi*): Lyme disease, at least in the chronic stages, is a multisymptom, multisystem disorder caused by the bite of the tick *Ixodes scapularis*. The bacterium is injected into the skin, travels very quickly into the bloodstream, and disseminates quite rapidly into the central nervous system, often causing neurological symptoms. The hallmark of the illness is a bull's-eye rash that can occur within a couple of days of contact with the tick.

Lymphatic system: The network that connects the glands of the body and across which lymphatic fluid transports hormones and other substances.

Macular degeneration: The most common cause of blindness in older individuals. Dietary variables appear to play a role in the loss of the fovea and detachment of the macula. This has to do with insufficiencies of dietary intake of carotenoids, particularly the lutein family of orange or yellow type pigments.

Maillard reaction: A glycosylation reaction where the aldose form of a reducing sugar, like glucose, reacts with the lysine amino group and a protein to make a glycosylation product. In cooking, glycosylation makes crusty bread. In plasma, glucose can react with proteins to form "crusty" proteins floating in the blood. These are called advanced glycation end-products, or AGEs. Accumulation of AGEs is associated with biological aging.

Mediterranean diet: The Mediterranean diet, which emphasizes consumption of whole grains, fresh vegetables and fruits, and healthy fats, has been associated with greater longevity and quality of life in many epidemiological studies.

Menopause: A normal transition that most women go through in their fifth decade of life, but timing can vary widely. Symptoms influencing physiological, cognitive, mental, and physical functioning can result as a consequence of fluctuating hormone values.

Metabolic syndrome: A cluster of conditions first identified by Dr. Gerald Reaven that include a high level of triglycerides in the blood, low HDL levels, elevated blood pressure, high levels of blood glucose, and what is called central obesity—meaning an apple-shaped body that is significantly overweight or obese. All of these conditions result from insulin resistance and an imbalance in glucose transport that impair glucose tolerance.

Metallothioneins: A family of proteins found in virtually every cell of the body that bind minerals very tightly and conduct their exit from the body via elimination in the stool or urine.

Methylenetetrahydrofolate reductase (MTHFR) polymorphism: A single-nucleotide polymorphism that is extremely influential in controlling the metabolism of the important B vitamin known as folic acid.

Microvilli: Millions of tiny folds that line the surface of the intestinal tract and through which nutrients are absorbed across the intestinal lining.

Minerals: Substances—calcium, magnesium, and potassium are examples—native to the human body and important for maintaining function.

Mitochondria: Structures within human cells that are called the "energy powerhouses." Mitochondria provide energy for the way we function—the way we derive our spark in order to keep our biochemical engines running. Maintenance of mitochondrial function is extraordinarily important for the prevention of oxidative stress.

Mitochondrial DNA: Mitochondrial DNA is inherited only from one's mother.

Monosodium glutamate (MSG): A form of delivery of glutamic acid that is perceived as "umami" in terms of taste. Sensitivity to MSG is a widespread issue.

MPTP: A powerful neurotoxin produced by the pesticide paraquat when heated and thought to contribute to Parkinson's-like symptoms.

Mucopolysaccharides: A unique class of substances found in mushrooms and other vegetables that are thought to support immune system function.

Multiple sclerosis: An inflammatory autoimmune disease of the nerve cells in the brain and spinal cord. MS has been shown to have a gradient of prevalence with latitude, a finding that has been theorized to link to vitamin D deficiency, which is more common in the northern hemisphere.

N-acetylcysteine: A nutrient that is the precursor of glutathione in the mitochondria, which has been shown to be anti-inflammatory. It is often termed NAC.

Natural selection: A theory popularized by Charles Darwin, who suggested evolution favored "survival of the fittest."

Nervous system: The body's communication system composed of the brain, spinal cord, and nerves.

Neurotransmitter: Messaging substances that carry information throughout the body.

Nicotinamide dinucleotide (NADH): A substance derived from vitamin B3 (niacin) that is used in cellular energy production and metabolism.

Noncoding DNA: At one time called junk DNA, noncoding DNA contains the information that controls the expression of our genes.

Nonsteroidal anti-inflammatory drugs (NSAIDs): Nonnarcotic, nonaddictive medications used to influence inflammation, including aspirin, ibuprofen, indomethacin, and ketoprofen.

Nutraceutical: Specific nutrients used in therapeutic doses to remedy imbalances in core physiological processes.

Nutrigenomics: A new field of research aimed at determining the correct intake of specific nutrients to meet the genetically determined needs of an individual.

Obesity: An increased waist-to-hip ratio where the fat stores of the body are concentrated around the waist as intra-abdominal fat. This type of excess fat accumulation is associated with increased incidence of such chronic illnesses as type 2 diabetes, heart disease, stroke, dementia, kidney disease, and both breast and prostate cancers.

Obesogen: A substance that can promote obesity, and a term that has been used to describe the presence of persistent organic pollutants (POPs) in the body.

Obstructive pulmonary disorder: A chronic and progressive condition of the lungs that may be connected to inflammation.

Organ reserve: The amount of organ function that is available to manage physiological demand under stress.

Orthomolecular medicine: A term coined by Dr. Linus Pauling and based upon the Greek prefix for "upright" or "correct," used in the general sense to describe a medicine that would mix and match substances native to human physiology—vitamins, minerals, nutrients, hormones, metabolites, and cellular building blocks—to the right levels for an individual's optimal health and function.

Osteocalcin: Signaling substances produced by bone cells that influence insulin activity and blood sugar levels.

Osteoporosis: A metabolic bone disease characterized by a defect in bone remodeling and the loss of normally mineralized bone.

Osteoprotegerin: Signaling substances produced by bone cells that influence insulin activity and blood sugar levels.

Oxidative stress: A general shift in cellular function that damages cellular membrane constituents and mitochondria and causes DNA strand breaks and DNA oxidation. Oxidative stress can be affected by numerous factors, including diet, lifestyle, and activity pattern. High oxidative stress is linked to aging and chronic illness.

Paradigm shift: A term popularized by Thomas Kuhn in his book *The Structure of Scientific Revolutions*. History has witnessed many changes in the field of medicine as a result of paradigm shift, and the dynamics in today's health-care system also reflect a period of great change.

Paraquat: A defoliant that has been widely used as a pesticide. It has been implicated in producing Parkinson's-like symptoms in individuals who consumed contaminated marijuana.

Parkinson's disease: A degenerative neurological disease affecting movement and characterized by persistent tremor.

Perimenopause: The time period in a woman's life that immediately precedes menopause. The World Health Organization has defined perimenopause as the period from which abnormalities associated with hormone changes begin to occur to one year after the last menstrual period.

Periodontal disease: A chronic infection of the mouth that can trigger immune response.

Persistent organic pollutant (POP): Endocrine-disrupting chemical that is fat-soluble and can accumulate in tissues, and, in so doing, can modify physiological function in such a way as to set in motion a process that leads to obesity and type 2 diabetes.

Phagocyte: Cell of the immune system that engulfs and destroys foreign substances.

Pharmaceutical: Drug developed to address the identifiable cause or agent of a disease.

Pharmacology: The science of studying chemical agents and their effect on human physiology.

Phenotype: Phenotype is what happens when our genotype interacts with the environment, realizing the potential of particular traits and thereby giving rise to observable characteristics in the way we look, act, feel, and perform.

Phenylalanine: An amino acid in protein that must be controlled in the diet of an individual with phenylketonuria.

Phenylketonuria (PKU): One of the most common genetically linked diseases of infancy. Developmental disability and early death can be avoided if the child is fed a controlled diet low in phenylalanine, an amino acid in protein.

Phytochemical: Plant-derived substance and botanical medicine that has been shown to alter cellular communications.

Phytosterols: A class of phytonutrients; some have been found to lower LDL cholesterol and others to support insulin sensitivity and balance glucose transport.

Plaque: A deposit of fat clinging to an artery wall and causing blockage. Plaque can be measured using positron emission tomography (PET).

Polypharmacy: Use by an individual of several drugs together in order to address the different symptoms arising from a range of causative factors.

Postmenopause: The years of a woman's life following menopause. The change in the hormonal environment following menopause requires attention to specific areas of health risk, including bone loss, cardiovascular disease, and dementia.

Potassium citrate: An alkaline salt that can affect the acid-alkaline balance of the body.

Prebiotics: Compounds that are not digested in the upper part of the gastrointestinal tract. They are fermented by specific types of bacteria in the gut, and therefore they modulate the endogenous population of the gut microbiota.

Prions: A combination of the words "protein" and "infection," the term was coined by Dr. Stanley Prusiner to describe natural proteins that had undergone a post-translational modification of their shape

Probiotics: Bacteria that tend to be given orally (in the diet or as a supplement) and remain viable within the gastrointestinal tract. It has been known for a long time that some bacteria can have beneficial effects on physiology in human bodies.

Promoter regions: A term that replaced "junk DNA" and is used to describe regions in the genome that control translation of genotype into phenotype.

Prostate-specific antigen (PSA): A prognostic marker for both benign prostate hypertrophy and prostate cancer that is used to track relative risk, prognosis, and follow-up on intervention in at-risk individuals.

Protein: A nutrient necessary for many essential physiological functions that has generated debate about protein quantity (percent calories as protein) and quality (vegetable, animal, dairy, and egg sources). Proteins are made up of long chains of amino acids that are ordered in a specific manner depending upon the specific protein. The order of the amino acids in protein is determined by the organism's genes.

Psychoneuroimmunology (PNI): A physiological supersystem—nervous, endocrine, and immune—that operates as a team to translate outside messages to inside function.

Recommended dietary allowance (RDA): Minimum levels of nutrients needed to maintain health as established by the Food and Drug Administration.

Reductionism: A philosophy of compartmentalization, where the individual parts are viewed separately from the whole.

Reproductive system: The respective male or female organ systems involved in reproductive processes.

Respiratory system: The lungs, bronchi, and larynx and their collective activities to move oxygen throughout the body.

Resveratrol: A phytonutrient derived from red grapes and peanut skins that influences mitochondrial function and cellular signaling related to gene expression.

Rheumatoid arthritis: An autoimmune disease involving inflammation of the joints.

Sarcopenia: A medical term describing loss of muscle mass.

Schizophrenia: A family of conditions associated with altered brain chemistry that can produce delusions and paranoia. Schizophrenia has been linked to excessive dopamine activity in certain brain regions, although antipsychotic drugs, which often block dopamine receptors, are not always helpful in managing the condition.

Scrapie: A neurodegenerative condition caused by a structurally modified protein that affects sheep and goats.

Secretin: A hormonal messenger molecule involved in communication between the gut and the brain.

Selective kinase response modulators (SKRMs): Phytochemicals that influence genetic expression by their ability to modulate genetic expression through effects on the kinase regulatory network.

Selective serotonin reuptake inhibitors (SSRIs): A class of pharmaceutical antidepressants that increase serotonin levels in the nervous system.

Serotonin: A hormonal messenger molecule released directly from nerve terminals in the brain's central nervous system. Serotonin is commonly described as the mood-elevating neurotransmitter.

Sickle-cell anemia: A cellular disease resulting from a genetic alteration in one part of the hemoglobin protein molecule; in consequence, the hemoglobin has a "sickle" shape.

Single nucleotide polymorphisms (SNPs): The alteration in the genetic code that relates to the substitution of one of the four DNA building blocks (nucleotides) for another. There are more than 3 million potential variations that have been identified in human genes and that account for variability in things like disease susceptibility.

Sodium butyrate: The sodium salt of the simple 4-carbon fatty acid butyric acid; when administered intravenously to patients with sickle-cell characteristics, it has been shown to prevent the hemoglobinopathies associated with the genetic disorder.

Somatostatin: A hormonal messenger molecule involved in communication between the gut and the brain.

Statin: A family of pharmaceutical drugs approved for lowering high levels of cholesterol in the blood by blocking the manufacture of cholesterol in the liver.

Stress: The physiological response to a change in environment. The term, borrowed from physics, was first applied to human physiology by Dr. Hans Selye.

Stroke: A cardiovascular event that results in blood loss to the brain and may be linked to defects in fat transport.

Sulforaphane: A phytonutrient found in cruciferous vegetables that has been found to play a role in cellular detoxification.

Superoxide dismutase (SOD): An antioxidant enzyme produced within the mitochondrial cell specifically to defuse damaging forms of oxygen before they can cause injury.

Systemic lupus erythematosus (SLE): An autoimmune disease that has higher prevalence in women and therefore may relate to androgen-estrogen balance and estrogen metabolism.

Systems biology: An approach to medicine that views the body as a network of interactions among core physiological processes.

Tay-Sachs disease: A genetic disease of infancy that causes progressive deterioration of nerve cells and usually results in death.

T cells: Specialized cells of the immune system that control immediate response to foreign materials and are involved in what is known as innate immunity.

Telomerase: The enzyme that repairs damaged telomeres.

Telomeres: Unique pieces of chemical structure at the end of each chromosome in our genome that are present to protect the chromosome. Telomeres get shorter during replication, which leaves the chromosome vulnerable to damage. Lifestyle, diet, and environment have been shown to play a role in determining the length of the telomeres

Thyroid: The thyroid is the environmental sentinel gland. It senses the outside environment in terms of various substances to which the organism is exposed.

Tinnitus: The medical term that describes a persistent ringing in the ears.

Tocotrienols: Relatives of vitamin E that are found in high levels in palm oil and act as antioxidants.

Traditional Chinese medicine (TCM): TCM holds an important position in primary health care in rural areas of China. It is also appreciated in urban and well-developed areas for its 5,000-year-old tradition. The Chinese government has undertaken enormous efforts to modernize TCM by investing in scientific and clinical research and trying to better understand its underlying principles. Western interest in TCM stems from the hope that it might complement western medicine by providing different tools for different applications. Medicinal herbs play a very important role in TCM.

Transglutaminase: The autoantigen enzyme associated with celiac disease.

Triglycerides: A form of fat in the blood that, when elevated, is a marker of metabolic syndrome, type 2 diabetes, and heart disease risk.

Turmeric: A spice that has been demonstrated to have anti-inflammatory properties due to the presence of the phytochemical curcumin.

Umami: The taste activated by monosodium glutamate (MSG).

Uric acid: A natural material in the blood often associated with gout. Elevated uric acid may be a response to oxidative stress, and it may actually be an important antioxidant.

Vitamins: Chemical compounds whose importance to health was first identified in diseases connected to nutritional deficiencies. Vitamins are now found to influence gene expression and cellular function.

VLDL cholesterol: Very-low-density lipoprotein. Low-density lipoprotein comes from VLDL as a breakdown product.

Women's Health Initiative (WHI): A large-scale study initiated by the National Institutes of Health in 1991 on the use of hormone replacement therapy to treat the symptoms of menopause. The HRT trial was halted in 2003 when it was determined the therapy may actually increase risk of breast cancer and heart disease, an announcement that caused concern, confusion, and controversy. HRT therapy had been considered a safe and effective treatment for several decades prior to the findings of the WHI.

Xenobiotics: From the Greek *xenos*, "stranger," and *bios*, "life." These are foreign and potentially toxic molecules not native to the human body.

Resources

PRINCIPAL RESOURCE WEBSITE
Personalized Lifestyle Medicine Institute www.plminstitute.org

FUNCTIONAL MEDICINE PRACTITIONER REFERRAL
Institute for Functional Medicine www.functionalmedicine.org

PERSONALIZED MEDICAL LABORATORY SERVICES
WellnessFx www.wellnessfx.com

LIFESTYLE, PERSONALIZED HEALTH, AND INDIVIDUALS
Blue Zones www.bluezones.com
Continuum Center for Health and Healing healthandhealingny.org
Institute for Functional Medicine (IFM) www.functionalmedicine.org
Personalized Lifestyle Medicine Institute www.plminstitute.org
TEDMED www.tedmed.com
Townsend Letter www.townsendletter.com
Dr. Bethany Hays—True North Health Center www.truenorthhealthcenter.org
Dr. David Perlmutter www.drperlmutter.com
Dr. Deanna Minich—Food and Spirit www.foodandspirit.com
Dr. Dean Ornish www.ornishspectrum.com
Dr. Frank Lipman—Be Well www.drfranklipman.com
Dr. Mark Hyman—The UltraWellness Center www.drhyman.com
Dr. Mehmet Oz www.doctoroz.com
Dr. Mimi Guarneri—Pacific Pearl La Jolla Center for Health & Healing
   www.mimiguarnerimd.com
Dr. Sara Gottfried www.saragottfriedmd.com
Dr. Susan Blum—Blum Center for Health www.blumcenterforhealth.com

Research Institutes and Educational Resources

Bastyr University www.bastyr.edu

Broad Institute www.broadinstitute.org

Buck Institute for Research on Aging www.buckinstitute.org

Center for Integrative Medicine, University of Maryland School of Medicine
www.compmed.umm.edu

Center for Mind-Body Medicine www.cmbm.org

Children's Hospital Oakland Research Institute (CHORI) www.chori.org

Cleveland Clinic www.clevelandclinic.org

Cochrane Collaboration www.cochrane.org

Cold Spring Harbor Laboratory www.cshl.edu

Commonwealth Scientific and Industrial Research Organisation (CSIRO)
www.csiro.au

Environmental Health Trust www.ehtrust.org

Environmental Working Group www.ewg.org

Fred Hutchinson Cancer Research Center www.fhcrc.org

GeneImprint www.geneimprint.com

Institute for Health Metrics and Evaluation www.healthmetricsandevaluation.org

Institute for Systems Biology www.systemsbiology.org

Institute of Molecular Medicine www.immed.org

Institutes for the Achievement of Human Potential www.iahp.org

Johns Hopkins Bloomberg School of Public Health www.jhsph.edu

Linus Pauling Institute at Oregon State University lpi.oregonstate.edu

Mayo Clinic www.mayoclinic.com

Monell Chemical Senses Center www.monell.org

National Institutes of Health www.nih.gov

Preventive Medicine Research Institute www.pmri.org

Samueli Institute www.samueliinstitute.org

Scripps Center for Integrative Medicine http://www.scripps.org/services
/integrative-medicine

TRANSCEND Research Program www.nmr.mgh.harvard.edu/transcend/

United States National Library of Medicine (PubMed) www.ncbi.nlm.nih.gov
/Pubmed

Van Andel Institute www.vai.org

Awareness and Advocacy Organizations

Autism Research Institute www.autism.com

Cancer Treatment Centers of America www.cancercenter.com

Center for Celiac Research and Treatment www.celiaccenter.org

Defeat Autism Now (DAN) www.defeatautismnow.net

Donna Karan Urban Zen Foundation www.urbanzen.org

Harmony Hill Cancer Retreat Center www.harmonyhill.org
HealthCorps www.healthcorps.org
National Foundation for Celiac Awareness www.celiaccentral.org
Patients Like Me www.patientslikeme.com
Slow Food USA www.slowfoodusa.org
Vitamin Angels www.vitaminangels.org

PROFESSIONAL ORGANIZATIONS AND HEALTH-CARE POLICY
American College of Nutrition (CBNS) www.americancollegeofnutrition.org
American Botanical Council (ABC) http://abc.herbalgram.org/site/PageServer
Clinton Foundation www.clintonfoundation.org
National Center for Complementary and Alternative Medicine www.nccam
.nih.gov
Personalized Medicine Coalition www.personalizedmedicinecoalition.org
United Natural Products Alliance www.unpa.com

NUTRITION AND WEIGHT MANAGEMENT RESOURCES
CDC Obesity www.cdc.gov/obesity
Center for Human Nutrition (UCLA) www.cellinteractive.com/ucla/
Functional Medicine Clinical Research Center (FMCRC) www.metagenics.com
HBO: The Weight of the Nation theweightofthenation.hbo.com/
Interleukin Genetics weight management www.inherenthealth.com
Organic Trade Association www.ota.com
Self-Health Network www.selfhealthnetwork.com
Tufts University Friedman School of Nutrition Science and Policy www.nutri
tion.tufts.edu
Tufts University Jean Mayer USDA Human Nutrition Research Center on
Aging www.hnrca.tufts.edu
USDA Nutrient Database www.ndb.nal.usda.gov

LABORATORY SERVICES AND BIOMARKER ANALYSIS
23andMe www.23andme.com
Cleveland Heart Lab www.clevelandheartlab.com
Genova Diagnostics www.gdx.net
Interleukin Genetics www.ilgenetics.com
Pathway Genomics www.pathway.com
WellnessFx www.wellnessfx.com

ONLINE TOOLS, DEVICES, AND APPS

Cure Together www.curetogether.com/

Fit Bit www.fitbit.com

Jaw Bone Fitness www.jawbone.com

Human: Move 30 minutes or more Apple and Android app stores

Pill Advised www.pilladvised.com

Notes

CHAPTER 1: THE DISEASE DELUSION AND THE CHRONIC-ILLNESS CONUNDRUM

19　Today, almost half of adult Americans: National Center for Chronic Disease Prevention and Health Promotion. *The Power of Prevention. Chronic Disease . . . The Public Health Challenge of the 21st Century.* Atlanta, GA, 2009.

19　Among Medicare beneficiaries: Thorpe KE, Howard DH. The rise in spending among Medicare beneficiaries: the role of chronic disease prevalence and changes in treatment intensity. *Health Aff (Millwood).* 2006;25(5):w378–88. (Epub 2006 Aug 22.)

19　A 2011 study by the: Bloom DE, Cafiero ET, Jané-Llopis E, Abrahams-Gessel S, Bloom LR, et al. *The Global Economic Burden of Noncommunicable Diseases.* Geneva: World Economic Forum, 2011.

19　Actually, a study published: Murray CJ, Vos T, Lozano R, Naqhavi M, Flaxman AD, et al. Disability-adjusted life years (DALYs) for 291 diseases and injuries in 21 regions, 1990–2010: a systematic analysis for the Global Burden of Disease Study 2010. *Lancet.* 2012;380(9859):2197–223.

20　Diabetes, meanwhile, has become a: Pradeepa R, Prabhakaran D, Mohan V. Emerging economies and diabetes and cardiovascular disease. *Diabetes Technol Ther.* 2012;14 Suppl 1:S59–67.

25　And Avandia, the anti-diabetic: Nissen SE, Wolski K. Effect of rosiglitazone on the risk of myocardial infarction and death from cardiovascular causes. *N Engl J Med.* 2007;356(24):2457–71.

26　The study found that for many women: Rossouw JE, Anderson GL, Prentice RL, LaCroix AZ, Kooperberg C, et al. Risks and benefits of estrogen plus progestin in healthy postmenopausal women: principal results from the Women's Health Initiative randomized controlled trial. *JAMA.* 2002;288(3):321–33.

26　The study found that for many women: Shumaker SA, Legault C, Rapp SR, Thel L, Wallace RB, et al. Estrogen plus progestin and the incidence of dementia and mild cognitive impairment in postmenopausal women: the Women's Health Initiative Memory Study: a randomized controlled trial. *JAMA*. 2003;289(20):2651–62.

29   In a watershed 1980 paper: Fries JF. Aging, natural death, and the compression of morbidity. *N Engl J Med*. 1980;303(3):130–35.

30   The results of the study confirmed: Vita AJ, Terry RB, Hubert HB, Fries JF. Aging, health risks, and cumulative disability. *N Engl J Med*. 1998;338(15):1035–41.

32   Before 1940, the incidence of breast cancer: King MC, Marks JH, Mandell JB; New York Breast Cancer Study Group. Breast and ovarian cancer risks due to inherited mutations in BRCA1 and BRCA2. *Science*. 2003 Oct 24;302(5645):643–46.

33   Using the sophisticated diagnostic tool: Gould KL, Ornish D, Scherwitz L, Brown S, Edens RP, et al. Changes in myocardial perfusion abnormalities by positron emission tomography after long-term, intense risk factor modification. *JAMA*. 1995;275(11):894–901.

34   The Ornish group's conclusion: Ornish D, Scherwitz LW, Billings JH, Brown SE, Gould KL, et al. Intensive lifestyle changes for reversal of coronary heart disease. *JAMA*. 1998;280(23):2001–2007.

39   No wonder one of the: Conner, Steve, "Glaxo Chief: Our Drugs Do Not Work on Most Patients." *The Independent* 8 Dec 2003. http://independent .uk.co. Web. 2013 Apr. 26.

40   Holman articulated and advocated: Holman H, Lorig K. Patient self-management: a key to effectiveness and efficiency in care of chronic disease. *Public Health Rep*. 2004;119(3):239–43.

CHAPTER 2: THE BIOLOGICAL BREAKTHROUGH THAT IS CHANGING EVERYTHING

44   Florence Nightingale, dispatched to the Crimean War: Keith JM. Florence Nightingale: statistician and consultant epidemiologist. *Int Nurs Rev*. 1988 Sept–Oct;35(5):147–50.

47   Half a century later, in the mid-1960s: Sagan L. On the origin of mitosing cells. *J Theor Biol*. 1967 Mar;14(3):255–74.

47   In this view, evolution is: Lovelock JE, Margulis L. Homeostatic tendencies of the earth's atmosphere. *Orig Life*. 1974 Jan-Apr;5(1):93–103.

50   As the deciphering went on, we learned: Varki A, Altheide TK. Comparing the human and chimpanzee genomes: searching for needles in a haystack. *Genome Res*. 2005 Dec;15(12):1746–58.

51   People who carry the variant SNPs of the MTHFR gene: Trimmer EE.

Methylenetetrahydrofolate reductase: biochemical characterization and medical significance. *Curr Pharm Des*. 2013;19(14):2574–93.

51   People who carry the variant SNPs of the MTHFR gene: Klerk M, Verhoef P, Clarke R, Blom HJ, Kok FJ, et al. MTHFR 677CT polymorphism and risk of coronary heart disease: a meta-analysis. *JAMA*. 2002 Oct 23–30;288(16):2023–31.

51   People who carry the variant SNPs of the MTHFR gene: Gorgone G, Ursini F, Altamura C, Bressi F, Tombini M, et al. Hyperhomocysteinemia, intima-media thickness and C677T MTHFR gene polymorphism: a correlation study in patients with cognitive impairment. *Atherosclerosis*. 2009 Sep;206(1):309–13.

52   Back in 1950, renowned biochemist Dr. Roger Williams: Williams RJ, Beerstecher E, Jr, Berry LJ. The concept of genetotrophic disease. *Lancet*. 1950 Feb 18;1(6599):287–89.

53   It was in this 1949 paper that Pauling first: Pauling L, Itano HA, et al. Sickle cell anemia, a molecular disease. *Science*. 1949 Apr 29;109(2835):443.

53   Pauling advanced this concept further in 1968: Pauling L. Orthomolecular psychiatry. Varying the concentrations of substances normally present in the human body may control mental disease. *Science*. 1968 Apr 19;160(3825):265–71.

53   Among people with the MTHR SNP: Morris DW, Trivedi MH, Rush AJ. Folate and unipolar depression. *J Altern Complement Med*. 2008 Apr;14(3):277–85.

53   Among people with the MTHR SNP: Taylor MJ, Camey S, Geddes J, Goodwin G. Folate for depressive disorders. *Cochrane Database Syst Rev*. 2003;(2):CD003390.

57   In the case of the sickle-cell trait: Perrine SP. Fetal globin stimulant therapies in the beta-hemoglobinopathies: principles and current potential. *Pediatric Ann*. 2008 May;37(5):339–46.

57   It is now known that both: Alexander D. The National Institute of Child Health and Human Development and phenylketonuria. *Pediatrics*. 2003 Dec;112(6 pt 2):1514–15.

57   The Center for Disease Control and Prevention (CDC) now report: Blumberg SJ, Bramlett MD, Kogan MD, Schieve LA, Jones JR, Lu MC. Changes in prevalence of parent-reported autism spectrum disorder in school-aged US children: 2007 to 2011–2012. National Health Statistics Reports. 2013 Mar 20;65:1–12. Retrieved from: http://www.cdc.gov/nchs/data/nhsr/nhsr065.pdf.

58   The CDC and the American Academy of Pediatrics: Centers for Disease

Control. 2007. Autism A.L.A.R.M. Guidelines. http://www.cdc.gov/ ncbddd/autism/hcp-recommendations.html. Accessed 15 Jul 2013.

58   Already, this extensive genetic screening: Baudoin SJ, Gaudias J, Gerharz S, Hatstatt L, Zhou K, et al. Shared synaptic pathophysiology in syndromic and nonsyndromic rodent models of autism. *Science*. 2012 Oct 5;338(6103):128–32.

59   He wrote the classic: Rimland, Bernard. *Infantile Autism: The Syndrome and Its Implications for a Neural Theory of Behavior*. New York: Appleton-Century-Crofts, 1964.

60   The paper, in the February 28 issue: Wakefield AJ, Murch SH, Anthony A, Linnell J, Casson DM, et al. Ileal-lymphoid-nodular hyperplasia, nonspecific colitis, and pervasive developmental disorder in children. *Lancet*. 1998 Feb 28;351(9103):637–41.

61   The inquiry prompted a retraction: Horton R. A statement by the editors of The Lancet. *Lancet*. 2004 Mar 6;363(9411):820–21.

61   Among these are gluten-containing grains: Lau NM, Green PH, Taylor AK, Hellberg D, Ajamian M, et al. Markers of celiac disease and gluten sensitivity in children with autism. *PLoS One*. 2013 Jun 18;8(6):e66155. Print 2013.

61   Among these are gluten-containing grains: Kaminski S, Cielinska A, Kostyra E. Polymorphism of bovine beta-casein and its potential effect on human health. *J Appl Genet*. 2007;48(3):189–98.

62   It is also the conclusion articulated: Tuchman RF. Deconstructing autism spectrum disorders: clinical perspective. *Rev Neurol*. 2013 Feb 22; 56 Suppl 1;S3–S12.

62   For example, her team has identified: Frye RE, Sequeira JM, Quadros EV, James SJ, Rossignol DA. Cerebral folate receptor autoantibodies in autism spectrum disorder. *Mol Psychiatry*. 2013 Mar;18(3):369–81.

62   It is historically noteworthy: Rimland B. Controversies in the treatment of autistic children: vitamin and drug therapy. *J Child Neurol*. 1988;3 Suppl:S68–S72.

63   Herbert is a remarkably talented researcher: Herbert, Martha, and Karen Weintraub. *The Autism Revolution: Whole-Body Strategies for Making Life All It Can Be*. New York: Ballantine Books, 2012.

63   People who have this gene: Kotze MJ, van Rensburg SJ. Pathology supported genetic testing and treatment of cardiovascular disease in middle age for prevention of Alzheimer's disease. *Metab Brain Dis*. 2012 Sep;27(3):255–66.

64   Simply put, a person with the ApoE4 gene: Hanson AJ, Bayer-Carter JL,

Green PS, Montine TJ, Wilkinson CW, et al. Effect of apolipoprotein E genotype and diet on apolipoprotein E lipidation and amyloid peptides: randomized clinical trial. *JAMA Neurol.* 2013 Jun 17:1–9.

64 Simply put, a person with the ApoE4 gene: Head D, Bugg JM, Goate AM, Fagan AM, Mintun MA, et al. Exercise engagement as a moderator of the effects of APOE genotype on amyloid deposition. *Arch Neurol.* 2012 May;69(5):636–43.

65 Specifically, people whose diets encourage poor control: Cholerton B, Baker LD, Craft S. Insulin resistance and pathological brain ageing. *Diabet Med.* 2011 Dec;28(12):1463–75.

65 "Our results suggest," Craft wrote: Bayer-Carter JL, Green PS, Montine TJ, VanFossen B, Baker LD, et al. Diet intervention and cerebrospinal fluid biomarkers in amnestic mild cognitive impairment. *Arch Neurol.* 2011 Jun;68(6):743–52.

69 In 1975, Holliday and Pugh had found: Holliday R, Pugh JE. DNA modification mechanisms and gene activity during development. *Science.* 1975 Jan 24;187(4173):226–32.

69 Jirtle and Waterland published their findings: Waterland RA, Jirtle RL. Transposable elements: targets for early nutritional effects on epigenetic gene regulation. *Mol Cell Biol.* 2003 Aug;23(15):5293–5300.

70 The first evidence of this alarming trend: Olshansky SJ, Passaro DJ, Hershow RC, Layden J, Carnes BA, et al. A potential decline in life expectancy in the United States in the 21st century. *N Engl J Med.* 2005 Mar 17;352(11):1138–45.

71 Drs. Szyf and Meaney have taken our understanding: Szfy M, McGowan P, Meaney MJ. The social environment and the epigenome. *Environ Mol Mutagen.* 2008 Jan;49(1):46–60.

71 More and more, we are seeing that nutrition: Skinner MK, Manikkam M, Guerrero-Bosagna C. Epigenetic transgenerational actions of environmental factors in disease etiology. *Trends Endocrinol Metab.* 2010 Apr;21(4):214–22.

CHAPTER 3: THE FUNCTIONAL MEDICINE REVOLUTION

75 That is because it is one of those pockets of healthy longevity: Buettner, Dan. *The Blue Zones: Lessons for Living Longer from the People Who've Lived the Longest.* Washington, DC: National Geographic, 2008.

83 A once-powerful Native American tribe: Knowler WC, Pettitt DJ, Saad MF, Bennett PH. Diabetes mellitus in the Pima Indians: incidence, risk factors and pathogenesis. *Diabetes Metab Rev.* 1990 Feb;6(1):1–27.

84   That's what I mean when I describe Pima genes: Knowler WC, Pettitt DJ, Bennett PH, Williams RC. Diabetes mellitus in the Pima Indians: genetic and evolutionary considerations. *Am J Phys Anthropol.* 1983 Sep;62(1):107–114.

CHAPTER 4: ASSIMILATION AND ELIMINATION

104   One antidote is probiotics: Behnsen J, Derihu E, Sassone-Corsi M, Raffatellu M. Probiotics: properties, examples, and specific applications. *Cold Spring Harb Perspect Med.* 2013 Mar 1;3(3):a010074.

104   Since adequate stomach acid secretion: Greene W. Drug interactions involving cimetidine—mechanisms, documentation, implications. *Q Rev Drug Metab Drug Interact.* 1984;5(1):25–51.

106   In fact, some of the toxic microflora: Kim KB, Kim JM, Cho SH, Oh HS, Choi NJ, Oh DH. Toxin gene profiles and toxin production ability of *Bacillus cereus* isolated from clinical and food samples. *J Food Sci.* 2011 Jan–Feb;76(1):T25–T29.

106   In fact, some of the toxic microflora: Sun X, Savidge T, Feng H. The enterotoxicity of *Clostridium difficile* toxins. *Toxins (Basel).* 2010 Jul;2(7):1848–80.

106   Dubbed "the second brain": Gershon, Michael. *The Second Brain: The Scientific Basis of Gut Instinct and a Groundbreaking New Understanding of Nervous Disorders of the Stomach and Intestines.* New York: Harper, 1998.

107   It may calm the brain: Manocha M, Khan WI. Serotonin and GI disorders: an update on clinical and experimental studies. *Clin Transl Gastroenterol.* 2012 Apr 26;3:e13.

107   The answer is yes: Rizzoli R, Cooper C, Reginster JY, Abrahamsen B, Adachi JD, et al. Antidepressant medications and osteoporosis. *Bone.* 2012;51(3):606–13.

108   At one point, he and his research team focused: Huque T, Brand JG, Rabinowitz JL, Metabolism of inositol-1,4,5-triphosphate in the taste organ of the channel catfish, *Ictalurus punctatus. Comp Biochem Physiol B.* 1992 Aug;102(4):833–9.

108   At one point, he and his research team focused: Nomura T, Kurihara K. Similarity of ion dependence of odorant responses between lipid bilayer and olfactory system. *Biochim Biophys Acta.* 1989 Oct 17;1005(3):260–4.

108   Later research went even further: Schiffman SS. Taste and smell losses in normal aging and disease. *JAMA.* 1997 Oct 22–29;278(16):1357–62.

109   And indeed, certain foods that contain: Dotson CD, Zhang L, Xu H, Shin YK, Viques S, et al. Bitter taste receptors influence glucose homeostasis. *PLoS One.* 2008;3(12):e3974.

112   So as Andrew Scull relates: Scull, Andrew. *Madhouse: A Tragic Tale of*

Megalomania and Modern Medicine. New Haven, CT: Yale University Press, 2007.

113 We now see a cause-and-effect relationship: Hadjivassiliou M, Sanders DS, Grünewald RA, Woodroofe N, Boscolo S, et al. Gluten sensitivity: from gut to brain. *Lancet Neurol.* 2010 Mar;9(3):318–30.

114 A number of clinical studies: Rodrigo L, Hernández-Lahoz C, Fuentes D, Alvarez N, López-Vázquez A, González S. Prevalence of celiac disease in multiple sclerosis. *BMC Neurol.* 2011 Mar 7;11:31.

114 A number of clinical studies: Batur-Caglayan HZ, Irkec C, Yildirim-Capraz I, Atalay-Akyurek N, Dumlu S. A case of multiple sclerosis and celiac disease. *Case Rep Neurol Med.* 2013;2013:576921.

114 A good friend and colleague: Perlmutter, David, and Kristin Loberg. *Grain Brain: The Surprising Truth About Wheat, Carbs, and Sugar—Your Brain's Silent Killers.* New York: Little, Brown, 2013.

114 Research gastroenterologists call it: Pendyala S, Walker JM, Holt PR. A high-fat diet is associated with endotoxemia that originates from the gut. *Gastroenterology.* 2012 May;142(5):1100–1101.

114 Research gastroenterologists call it: Moreira AP, Texeira TF, Ferreira AB, Peluzio Mdo C, Alfenas Rde C. Influence of a high-fat diet on gut microbiota, intestinal permeability and metabolic endotoxaemia. *Br J Nutr.* 2012 Sep;108(5):801–9.

CHAPTER 5: DETOXIFICATION

125 It's scary enough to contemplate: Lazarou J, Pomeranz BH, Corey PN. Incidence of adverse drug reactions in hospitalized patients: a meta-analysis of prospective studies. *JAMA.* 1998 Apr 15;279(15):1200–1205.

127 In the United States, acetaminophen: Armstrong TM, Davies MS, Kitching G, Waring WS. Comparative drug dose and drug combinations in patients that present to hospital due to self-poisoning. *Basic Clin Pharmacol Toxicol.* 2012 Nov;111(5):356–60.

127 but while consuming alcohol: Hawton K, Simkin S, Gunnell D, Sutton L, Bennewith O, Turnbull P, Kapur N. A multicentre study of coproxamol poisoning suicides based on coroners' records in England. *Br J Clin Pharmacol.* 2005 Feb;59(2):207–12.

127 but while consuming alcohol: Schiødt FV, Rochling FA, Casey DL, Lee WM. Acetaminophen toxicity in an urban county hospital. *N Engl J Med.* 1997 Oct 16;337(16):1112–17.

129 Such a book for me was *Silent Spring*: Carson, Rachel. *Silent Spring.* Boston: Houghton Mifflin Company, Riverside Press, 1962.

130 Their work demonstrated also: Heafield MT, Fearn S, Steventon GB,

Waring RH, Williams AC, Sturman SG. Plasma cysteine and sulphate levels in patients with motor neurone, Parkinson's and Alzheimer's disease. *Neurosci Lett.* 1990 Mar 2;110(1–2):216–20.

130 Paraquat, it was learned: Landrigan PJ, Powell KE, James LM, Taylor PR. Paraquat and marijuana: epidemiological risk assessment. *Am J Pub Health.* 1983 Jul;73(7):784–88.

131 Such a conclusion is in keeping: Todd G, Noyes C, Flavel SC, Della Vedova CB, Spyropoulos P, et al. Illicit stimulant use is associated with abnormal substania nigra morphology in humans. *PLoS One.* 2013;8(2):e56438.

133 In 2008, a paper in the prestigious: Lang IA, Galloway TS, Scarlett A, Henley WE, Depledge M, et al. Association of urinary bisphenol A concentration with medical disorders and laboratory abnormalities in adults. *JAMA.* 2008 Sep 17;300(11):1303–10.

133 Four years later, a subsequent research paper: Melzer D, Osbourne NJ, Henley WE, Cipelli R, Young A, et al. Urinary bisphenol A concentration and risk of future coronary artery disease in apparently healthy men and women. *Circulation.* 2012 Mar 27;125(12):1482–90.

133 If that weren't enough: Trasande L, Attina TM, Blustein J. Association between urinary bisphenol A concentration and obesity prevalence in children and adolescents. *JAMA.* 2012 Sep;308(11):1113–21.

138 She knew about the Spanish cooking oil: Fournier E, Efthymiou ML, Lecoursier A. Spanish adulterated oil matter. An important discovery by Spanish toxicologists: the toxicity of anilides of unsaturated fatty acids. *Toxicol Eur Res.* 1982 Mar;4(2):107–112.

138 Specifically, these "cross-bearing" plants: Staack R, Kingston S, Walliq MA, Jeffery EH. A comparison of the individual and collective effects of four glucosinolate breakdown products from brussels sprouts on induction of detoxification enzymes. *Toxicol Appl Pharmacol.* 1998 Mar;149(1):17–23.

138 A Rockefeller University professor: Talang NT, Katdare M, Bradlow HL, Osborne MP, Fishman J. Inhibition of proliferation and modulation of estradiol metabolism: novel mechanisms for breast cancer prevention by the phytochemical indole-3-carbinol. *Proc Soc Exp Biol Med.* 1997 Nov;216(2):246–52.

139 Talalay attributes the protective power: Zhang Y, Kensler TW, Cho CG, Posner GH, Talalay P. Anticarcinogenic activities of sulforaphane and structurally related synthetic norbornyl isothiocyanates. *Proc Natl Acad Sci USA.* 1994 Apr 12;91(8):3147–50.

141 Needleman had just published: Needleman HL, Gunnoe C, Leviton A, Reed R, Peresie H, et al. Deficits in psychologic and classroom performance of children with elevated dentine lead levels. *N Engl J Med.* 1979 Mar 29;300(13):689–95.

CHAPTER 6: DEFENSE

151 Yes, says Dr. Fasano: Catassi C, Fasano A. Celiac disease. *Curr Opin Gastro-enterol.* 2008 Nov;24(6):687–91.

156 Now that it has been reported: American Autoimmune Related Diseases Association and National Coalition of Autoimmune Patient Groups. *The Cost Burden of Autoimmune Disease: The Latest Front in the War on Healthcare Spending.* Eastpointe, MI, 2011. Retrieved August 5, 2013 from: http://www.aarda.org/pdf/cbad.pdf.

157 To begin with, I must confess: Pauling, Linus. *Vitamin C and the Common Cold.* New York: W. H. Freeman, 1970.

158 Stone proclaimed the vitamin C intake: Stone I. *Homo sapiens ascorbicus,* a biochemically corrected robust human mutant. *Med Hypotheses.* 1979 Jun;5(6):711–21.

158 If the person is ill, however: Levine M, Padayatt SJ, Espey MG. Vitamin C: a concentration-function approach yields pharmacology and therapeutic discoveries. *Adv Nutr.* 2011 Mar;2(2):78–88.

159 Yet, as Dr. Robert Heaney: Heaney RP. Long-latency deficiency disease: insights from calcium and vitamin D. *Am J Clin Nutr.* 2003 Nov;78(5):912–19.

159 For example, although these illnesses: Heaney RP. Functional indices of vitamin D status and ramifications of vitamin D deficiency. *Am J Clin Nutr.* 2004 Dec;80 (6 Suppl):1706S–09S.

159 For example, although these illnesses: Ifergan I, Assaraf YG. Molecular mechanisms of adaptation to folate deficiency. *Vitam Horm.* 2008;79:99–143.

160 Dr. Meydani's group has demonstrated: Pae M, Meydani SN, Wu D. The role of nutrition in enhancing immunity in aging. *Aging Dis.* 2012 Feb;3(1):91–129.

160 A study of women: Mahalingam D, Radhakrishnan AK, Amom Z, Ibra-him N, Nesaretnam K. Effects of supplementation with tocotrienol-rich fraction on immune response to tetanus toxoid immunization in normal healthy volunteers. *Eur J Clin Nutr.* 2011 Jan;65(1):63–69.

160 Similar results were achieved: Han SN, Meydani SN. Vitamin E and infectious diseases in the aged. *Proc Nutr Soc.* 1999 Aug;58(3):697–705.

162 According to Holick: Grant WB, Holick MF. Benefits and requirements of vitamin D for optimal health: a review. *Altern Med Rev.* 2005 Jun;10(2):94–111.

162 Holick also points out: Hossein-nezhad A, Holick MF. Optimize dietary intake of vitamin D: an epigenetic perspective. *Curr Opin Clin Nutr Metab Care.* 2012 Nov;15(6):567–79.

162 His particular expertise in the field of: Stamets, Paul. *Mycelium Running: How Mushrooms Can Help Save the World.* Berkeley, CA: Ten Speed Press, 2005.

163 The National Institutes of Health: Miller S, Stagl J, Wallerstedt DB,

Ryan M, Mansky PJ. Botanicals used in complementary and alternative medicine treatment of cancer: clinical science and future perspectives. *Expert Opin Investig Drugs*. 2008 Sep;17(9):1353–64.

163   The National Institutes of Health: Abrams DI, Couey P, Shade SB, Kelly ME, Kamanu-Elias N, Stamets P. Antihyperlipidemic effects of *Pleurotus ostreatus* (oyster mushrooms) in HIV-infected individuals taking antiretroviral therapy. *BMC Complement Altern Med*. 2011 Aug 10;11:60.

163   For good reason: studies have shown: Grube BJ, Eng ET, Kao YC, Kwon A, Chen S. White button mushroom phytochemicals inhibit aromatase activity and breast cancer cell proliferation. *J Nutr*. 2001 Dec;131(12):3288–93.

163   For good reason: studies have shown: Jeong SC, Koyyalamudi SR, Jeong YT, Song CH, Pang G. Macrophage immunomodulating and antitumor activities of polysaccharides isolated from *Agaricus bisporus* white button mushrooms. *J Med Food*. 2012 Jan;15(1):58–65.

163   And Dr. Meydani's group at Tufts: Wu D, Pae M, Ren Z, Guo Z, Smith D, Meydani SN. Dietary supplementation with white button mushroom enhances natural killer cell activity in C57BL/6 mice. *J Nutr*. 2007 Jun;137(6):1472–77.

CHAPTER 7: CELLULAR COMMUNICATIONS

168   It's pretty pervasive in daily speech: Selye, Hans. *The Stress of Life*. New York: McGraw-Hill, 1956.

169   The term refers to that process by which: McEwen BS, Stellar E. Stress and the individual. Mechanisms leading to disease. *Arch Intern Med*. 1993 Sep 27;153(18):2093–2101.

171   Women feel the loss of estrogen: Alexander JL, Dennerstein L, Woods NF, McEwen BS, Halbreich U, et al. Role of stressful life events and menopausal stage in wellbeing and health. *Expert Rev Neurother*. 2007 Nov;7(11 Suppl):S93–S113.

171   Women feel the loss of estrogen: Woods NF, Mitchell ES. Symptom interference with work and relationships during the menopausal transition and early menopause: observations from the Seattle Midlife Women's Health Study. *Menopause*. 2011 Jun;18(6):654–61.

171   Some scientists—notably physicians Paul Ridker: Danik JS, Paré G, Chasman DI, Zee RY, Kwiatkowski DJ, et al. Novel loci, including those related to Crohn disease, psoriasis, and inflammation, identified in a genome-wide association study of fibrinogen in 17,686 women: the Women's Genome Health Study. *Circ Cardiovasc Genet*. 2009 Apr;2(2):134–41.

171   Some scientists—notably physicians Paul Ridker: Libby P, Ridker PM,

Maseri A. Inflammation and atherosclerosis. *Circulation*. 2002 Mar 5;105(9):1135–43.

172 The level of hs-CRP in the blood: Ridker PM. High-sensitivity C-reactive protein, inflammation, and cardiovascular risk: from concept to clinical practice to clinical benefit. *Am Heart J*. 2004 Jul;148(1 Suppl):S19–S26.

172 Levels of this blood biomarker above: Onat A, Can G, Herqenc G. Serum C-reactive protein is an independent risk factor predicting cardiometabolic risk. *Metabolism*. 2008 Feb;57(2):207–14.

172 Once the cytokines are released: Libby P. Inflammation in atherosclerosis. *Arterioscler Thromb Vasc Biol*. 2012 Sep;32(9):2045–51.

173 Since more than 100,000 people per year: Singh G. Recent considerations in nonsteroidal anti-inflammatory drug gastropathy. *Am J Med*. 1998 Jul 27;105(1B):31S–38S.

177 As scientists do, we of course gave a name: Desai A, Konda VR, Hall A, Bland J, Tripp M. Comparison of anti-inflammatory activity of two selective kinase response modulators (SKRMs), rho-iso-alpha acids (RIAA) and tetrahydro-iso-alpha acids (THIAA), in lipopolysaccharide (LPS) mediated inflammation in RAW 264.7 macrophages. *FASEB*. 2007;21:702.5.

178 And the many publications from scientists: Konda VR, Desai A, Darland G, Bland JS, Tripp ML. Rho iso-alpha acids from hops inhibit the GSK-3/NF-kappaB pathway and reduce inflammatory markers associated with bone and cartilage degradation. *J Inflamm (Lond)*. 2009 Aug 27;6:26.

178 And the many publications from scientists: Babish JG, Pacioretty LM, Bland JS, Minich DM, Hu J, Tripp ML. Antidiabetic screening of commercial botanical products in 3T3-L1 adipocytes and db/db mice. *J Med Food*. 2010 Jun;13(3):535–47.

178 And the many publications from scientists: Desai A, Darland G, Bland JS, Tripp ML, Konda VR. META060 attenuates TNF-α-activated inflammation, endothelial-monocyte interactions, and matrix metalloproteinase-9 expression, and inhibits NF-κB and AP-1 in THP-1 monocytes. *Atherosclerosis*. 2012 Jul;223(1):130–36.

181 From 2005 through 2012, a series: Desai A, Konda VR, Darland G, Austin M, Prabhu KS, et al. META060 inhibits multiple kinases in the NF-kappaB pathway and suppresses LPS-mediated inflammation in vivo and ex vivo. *Inflamm Res*. 2009 May;58(5):229–34.

181 From 2005 through 2012, a series: Holick MF, Lamb JJ, Lerman RH, Konda VR, Darland G, et al. Hop rho iso-alpha acids, berberine, vitamin D3 and vitamin K1 favorably impact biomarkers of bone turnover in postmenopausal women in a 14-week trial. *J Bone Miner Metab*. 2010 May;28(3):342–50.

182 In the study participants with osteoarthritis: Hall AJ, Babish JG, Darland GK, Carroll BJ, Konda VR, et al. Safety, efficacy and anti-inflammatory activity of rho iso-alpha-acids from hops. *Phytochemistry.* 2008 May;69(7):1534–47.

184 Dr. Kenneth Kornman and his colleagues: Kornman K, Rogus J, Roh-Schmidt H, Krempin D, Davies AJ, et al. Interleukin-1 genotype-selective inhibition of inflammatory mediators by a botanical: a nutrigenetics proof of concept. *Nutrition.* 2007 Nov–Dec;23(11–12):844–52.

CHAPTER 8: CELLULAR TRANSPORT

192 Much has been learned, and among the results: Kannel WB, Dawber TR, Friedman GD, Glennon WE, McNamara PM. Risk factors in coronary heart disease. An evaluation of several serum lipids as predictors of coronary heart disease: the Framingham study. *Ann Intern Med.* 1964 Nov;61:888–99.

193 Studies show a correlation between: Huang TL, Wu SC, Chiang YS, Chen JF. Correlation between serum lipid, lipoprotein concentrations and anxious state or major depressive disorder. *Psychiatry Res.* 2003 May 30;118(2):147–53.

193 Studies show a correlation between: Olié E, Picot MC, Guillaume S, Abbar M, Courtet P. Measurement of total serum cholesterol in the evaluation of suicidal risk. *J Affect Disord.* 2011 Sep;133(1–2):234–38.

194 Studies on competitive athletes confirm: Sqouraki E, Tsopanakis A, Kioussis A, Tsopanakis C. Acute effects of short duration maximal endurance exercise on lipid, phospholipid and lipoprotein levels. *J Sports Med Phys Fitness.* 2004 Dec;44(4):444–50.

195 From this unlikely discovery: Li, Jie Jack. *Triumph of the Heart: The Story of Statins.* New York: Oxford University Press USA, 2009.

195 Yes, medical studies confirm that people: Gutierrez J, Ramirez G, Rundek T, Sacco RL. Statin therapy in the prevention of recurrent cardiovascular events: a sex-based meta-analysis. *Arch Intern Med.* 2012 Jun 25;172(12):909–19.

195 In women, who suffer a different type: Mercuro G, Deidda M, Bina A, Manconi E, Rosano GM. Gender-specific aspects in primary and secondary prevention of cardiovascular disease. *Curr Pharm Des.* 2011;17(11):1082–90.

196 Statins may also produce adverse side effects: Parker BA, Gregory SM, Lorson L, Polk D, White CM, Thompson PD. A randomized trial of co-enzyme Q10 in patients with statin myopathy: rationale and study design. *J Clin Lipidol.* 2013 May–Jun;7(3):187–93.

197 Trials at the Center for Human Nutrition: Heber D, Yip I, Ashley JM, Elashoff DA, Elashoff RM, Go VL. Cholesterol-lowering effects of a proprietary Chinese red-yeast-rice dietary supplement. *Am J Clin Nutr.* 1999 Feb;69(2):231–36.

197 Trials at the Center for Human Nutrition: Li P, Yang Y, Liu M. Xuezhikang, extract of red yeast rice, inhibited tissue factor and hypercoagulable state through suppressing nicotinamide adenine dinucleotide phosphate oxidase and extracellular signal-regulated kinase activation. *J Cardiovasc Pharmacol.* 2011 Sep;58(3):307–18.

198 Well-known cholesterol researcher Daniel Steinberg, who tracked: Steinberg D. The LDL modification hypothesis of atherogenesis: an update. *J Lipid Res.* 2009 Apr;50 Suppl:S376–S81.

198 It is also recognized that vitamin B3: Hochholzer W, Berg DD, Giugliano RP. The facts behind niacin. *Ther Adv Cardiovasc Dis.* 2011 Oct;5(5):227–40.

198 It is also recognized that vitamin B3: Goldberg AC. Clinical trial experience with extended-release niacin (Niaspan): dose escalation study. *Am J Cardiol.* 1998 Dec 17;82(12A):35U–38U.

198 Elevated levels of very-low-density lipoprotein: Ooi EM, Ng TW, Watts GF, Barrett PH. Dietary fatty acids and lipoprotein metabolism: new insights and updates. *Curr Opin Lipidol.* 2013 Jun;24(3):192–97.

198 There is an interesting addendum to this: Reboul E, Borel P. Proteins involved in uptake, intracellular transport and basalateral secretion of fat-soluble vitamins and carotenoids by mammalian enterocytes. *Prog Lipid Res.* 2011 Oct;50(4):388–402.

198 What emerges from this added knowledge: Carrero JJ, Fonolla J, Marti JL, Jiménez J, Boza JJ, López-Huertas E. Intake of fish oil, oleic acid, folic acid, and vitamins B-6 and E for 1 year decreases plasma C-reactive protein and reduces coronary heart disease risk factors in male patients in a cardiac rehabilitation program. *J Nutr.* 2007 Feb;137(2):384–90.

198 What emerges from this added knowledge: Houston MC, Fazio S, Chilton FH, Wise DE, Jones KB, et al. Nonpharmacologic treatment for dyslipidemia. *Prog Cardiovasc Dis.* 2009 Sep–Oct;52(2):61–94.

201 A body at rest is a body: Oz MC, Roberts CS, Lemole GM. Role of lymphostasis in accelerated atherosclerosis in transplanted hearts. *Am J Cardiol.* 1987 Aug 1;60(4):430.

203 In 1949, Dr. Harold Himsworth: Himsworth HP. The syndrome of diabetes mellitus and its causes. *Lancet.* 1949 Mar 19;1(6551):465–73.

204 In 1968, Drs. John Farquhar and Gerald Reaven: Reaven G, Miller R.

Study of the relationship between glucose and insulin responses to an oral glucose load in man. *Diabetes*. 1968 Sep;17(9):560–69.

204 In 1968, Drs. John Farquhar and Gerald Reaven: Stern MP, Farquhar JW, Silvers A, Reaven GM. Insulin delivery rate into plasma in normal and diabetic subjects. *J Clin Invest*. 1968 Sep;47(9):1947–57.

204 All of these characteristics: Reaven GM. Banting lecture 1988. Role of insulin resistance in human disease. *Diabetes*. 1988 Dec;37(12):1595–1607.

205 By 2011, a study reported: Mozumdar A, Liquori G. Persistent increase of prevalence of metabolic syndrome among U.S. adults: NHANES III to NHANES 1999–2006. *Diabetes Care*. 2011 Jan;34(1):216–19.

205 The Mediterranean-style diet, as you probably know: Esposito K, Ciotola M, Giugliano D. Mediterranean diet and the metabolic syndrome. *Mol Nutr Food Res*. 2007 Oct;51(10):1268–74.

207 We believe this was the first clinical trial: Lerman RH, Minich DM, Darland G, Lamb JJ, Schiltz B, et al. Enhancement of a modified Mediterranean-style, low glycemic load diet with specific phytochemicals improves cardiometabolic risk factors in subjects with metabolic syndrome and hypercholesterolemia in a randomized trial. *Nutr Metab (Lond)*. 2008 Nov 4;5:29.

207 Babish's tests confirmed: Babish JG, Pacioretty LM, Bland JS, Minich DM, Hu J, Tripp ML. Antidiabetic screening of commercial botanical products in 3T3-L1 adipocytes and db/db mice. *J Med Food*. 2010 Jun;13(3):535–47.

CHAPTER 9: ENERGY

216 Dr. Harman suggested that aging: Harman D. Aging: a theory based on free radical and radiation chemistry. *J Gerontol*. 1956 Jul;11(3):298–300.

218 What we have now learned is: Daussin FN, Zoll J, Dufour SP, Ponsot E, Lonsdorfer-Wolf E, et al. Effect of interval versus continuous training on cardiorespiratory and mitochondrial functions: relationship to aerobic performance improvements in sedentary subjects. *Am J Physiol Regul Integr Comp Physiol*. 2008 Jul;295(1):R264–72.

219 Did you know that a common form of headache: D'Andrea G, Leon A. Pathogenesis of migraine: from neurotransmitters to neuromodulators and beyond. *Neurol Sci*. 2010 Jun;31 Suppl 1:S1–S7.

221 In a number of extreme adventure racing: Kim YJ, Kim CH, Shin KA, Kim AC, Lee YH, et al. Cardiac markers of EIH athletes in ultramarathon. *Int J Sports Med*. 2012 Mar;33(3):171–76.

221 We've also learned, through the extraordinary work: Ames BN. Dietary carcinogens and anticarcinogens. Oxygen radicals and degenerative diseases. *Science*. 1983 Sep 23;221 (4617):1256–64.

222 They found that the brain cells: Lin MT, Beal MF. Mitochondrial

dysfunction and oxidative stress in neurodegenerative diseases. *Nature.* 2006 Oct 19;443(7113):787–95.

222 Further exploration of the ApoE4 gene: Miyata M, Smith JD. Apolipoprotein E allele-specific antioxidant activity and effects on cytotoxicity by oxidative insults and beta-amyloid peptides. *Nat Genet.* 1996 Sep;14(1):55–61.

222 Further exploration of the ApoE4 gene: Jolivalt C, Leininger-Muller B, Bertrand P, Herber R, Christen Y, Siest G. Differential oxidation of apolipoprotein E isoforms and interaction with phospholipids. *Free Radic Biol Med.* 2000 Jan 1;28(1):129–40.

222 Ongoing research confirms these conclusions: Hanson AJ, Bayer-Carter JL, Green PS, Montine TJ, Wilkinson CW, et al. Effect of apolipoprotein E genotype and diet on apolipoprotein E lipidation and amyloid peptides: randomized clinical trial. *JAMA Neurol.* 2013 Aug 1;70(8):972–80.

222 Remember the work directed by: Cholerton B, Baker LD, Craft S. Insulin, cognition, and dementia. *Eur J Pharmacol.* 2013 Nov 5;719(1–3):170–79.

223 Too potent by far: Additional research has found: Jansson ET. Alzheimer disease is substantially preventable in the United States—review of risk factors, therapy, and the prospects for an expert software system. *Med Hypotheses.* 2005;64(5):960–67.

224 At the end of the twelve weeks, the biomarkers: Rigden S, Barrager E, Bland J. Evaluation of the effect of a modified entero-hepatic resuscitation program in chronic fatigue syndrome patients. *J Advancement Med.* 1998;11(4):247–62.

225 Pall culled all the research he could find: Pall ML. Chronic fatigue syndrome/myalgic encephalitis. *Br J Gen Pract.* 2002 Sep;52(482):763–64.

226 Instead of the effect of the treatment increasing: Calabrese EJ, Iavicoli I, Calabrese V. Hormesis: its impact on medicine and health. *Hum Exp Toxicol.* 2013 Feb;32(2):120–52.

226 Instead of the effect of the treatment increasing: Cornelius C, Perrotta R, Graziano A, Calabrese EJ, Calabrese V. Stress responses, vitagenes and hormesis as critical determinants in aging and longevity: mitochondria as "chi." *Immun Ageing.* 2013 Apr 25;10(1):15.

226 When it comes to mitochondrial protection: Mattson MP. Dietary factors, hormesis and health. *Ageing Res Rev.* 2008 Jan;7(1):43–48.

227 In this case, however: Nicolson GL, Ellithorpe R. Lipid replacement and antioxidant nutritional therapy for restoring mitochondrial function and reducing fatigue in chronic fatigue syndrome and other fatiguing illnesses. *Journal of Chronic Fatigue Syndrome.* 2006;13(1):57–68.

228 That calorie restriction could be a way to preserve health: McCay CM. Effect of restricted feeding upon aging and chronic diseases in rats and dogs. *Am J Public Health Nations Health.* 1947 May;37(5):521–28.

228 The conclusion was again evident: Yamada Y, Colman RJ, Kemnitz JW, Baum ST, Anderson RM, et al. Long-term calorie restriction decreases metabolic cost of movement and prevents decrease of physical activity during aging in the rhesus monkeys. *Exp Gerontol*. 2013 Aug 13. (Epub ahead of print.)

228 The genetic expression of the calorie-restricted group: Anderson RM, Weindruch R. Metabolic reprogramming, caloric restriction and aging. *Trends Endocrinol Metab*. 2010 Mar;21(3):134–41.

229 An added point of interest to the calorie restriction effect: Burzynski SR. Aging gene silencing or gene activation? *Med Hypotheses*. 2005;64(1):201–8.

CHAPTER 10: STRUCTURE

233 In 1951, the proceedings of the august National Academy of Sciences: Pauling L, Corey RB. Atomic coordinates and structure factors for two helical configurations of polypeptide chains. *Proc Natl Acad Sci USA*. 1951 May;37(5):235–40.

233 In 1951, the proceedings of the august National Academy of Sciences: Pauling L, Corey RB. The structure of synthetic polypeptides. *Proc Natl Acad Sci USA*. 1951 May;37(5):241–50.

233 In 1951, the proceedings of the august National Academy of Sciences: Pauling L, Corey RB. The pleated sheet, a new layer configuration of polypeptide chains. *Proc Natl Acad Sci USA*. 1951 May;37(5):251–56.

233 In 1951, the proceedings of the august National Academy of Sciences: Pauling L, Corey RB. The structure of feather rachis keratin. *Proc Natl Acad Sci USA*. 1951 May;37(5):256–61.

233 In 1951, the proceedings of the august National Academy of Sciences: Pauling L, Corey RB. The structure of hair, muscle, and related problems. *Proc Natl Acad Sci USA*. 1951 May;37(5):261–71.

233 In 1951, the proceedings of the august National Academy of Sciences: Pauling L, Corey RB. The structure of fibrous proteins of the collagen-gelatin group. *Proc Natl Acad Sci USA*. 1951 May;37(5):272–81.

233 In 1951, the proceedings of the august National Academy of Sciences: Pauling L, Corey RB. The polypeptide-chain configuration in hemoglobin and other globular proteins. *Proc Natl Acad Sci USA*. 1951 May;37(5):282–85.

237 It is regulating cell behavior: Langevin HM, Churchill DL, Wu J, Badger GJ, Yandow JA, et al. Evidence of connective tissue involvement in acupuncture. *FASEB J*. 2002 Jun;16(8):872–74.

237 It is regulating cell behavior: Ahn AC, Park M, Shaw JR, McManus CA, Kaptchuk TJ, Langevin HM. Electrical impedance of acupuncture meridians: the relevance of subcutaneous collagenous bands. *PLoS One*. 2010 Jul 30;5(7):e11907.

238 After all, as Becker pointed out in the book: Becker, Robert O., and Gary Selden. *The Body Electric*. CPA Books, Inc., 1985.

239 Dr. Davis is not the only expert to contend: Gandhi OP, Morgan LL, de Salles AA, Han YY, Herberman RB, Davis DL. Exposure limits: the underestimation of absorbed cell phone radiation, especially in children. *Electromagn Biol Med.* 2012 Mar;31(1):34–51.

239 Dr. Davis is not the only expert to contend: Davis DL, Kesari S, Soskolne CL, Miller AB, Stein Y. Swedish review strengthens grounds for concluding that radiation from cellular and cordless phones is a probable human carcinogen. *Pathophysiology.* 2013 Apr;20(2):123–29.

239 The World Health Organization has also issued a caution: Baan R, Grosse Y, Lauby-Secretan B, El Ghissassi F, Bouvard V, et al. Carcino-genicity of radiofrequency electromagnetic fields. *Lancet Oncol.* 2011 Jul;12(7):624–46.

240 The two men showed that the sickle-cell disease: Pauling L, Itano HA, et al. Sickle cell anemia, a molecular disease. *Science.* 1949 Apr 29;109(2835):443.

243 In humans, the evaluations note higher: Cai W, Ramdas M, Zhu L, Chen X, Striker GE, Vlassara H. Oral advanced glycation endproducts (AGEs) promote insulin resistance and diabetes by depleting the antioxidant defenses AGE receptor-1 and sirtuin 1. *Proc Natl Acad Sci USA.* 2012 Sep 25;109(39):15888–93.

243 In humans, the evaluations note higher: Münch G, Schinzel R, Loske C, Wong A, Durany N, et al. Alzheimer's disease—synergistic effects of glucose deficit, oxidative stress and advanced glycation endproducts. *J Neural Transm.* 1998;105(4–5):439–61.

244 As Prusiner demonstrated, the prions: Prusiner SB. Molecular biology of prion diseases. *Science.* 1991 Jun 14;252 (5012):1515–22.

244 Gajdusek traced the origin: Gajdusek DC, Zigas V. Degenerative disease of the central nervous system in New Guinea; the endemic occurrence of kuru in the native population. *N Engl J Med.* 1957 Nov 14; 257(20):974–78.

249 Higher levels of the estrogen hormone: Williams GP. The role of oestrogen in the pathogenesis of obesity, type 2 diabetes, breast cancer and prostate disease. *Eur J Cancer Prev.* 2010 Jul;19(4):256–71.

250 This suggested that the POPs: Lee DH, Lee IK, Jin SH, Steffes M, Jacobs DR, Jr. Association between serum concentrations of persistent organic pollutants and insulin resistance among nondiabetic adults: results from the National Health and Nutrition Examination Survey 1999–2002. *Diabetes Care.* 2007 Mar;30(3):622–28.

251 The two extended their studies to other countries: Park SK, Son HK, Lee SK, Kang JH, Chang YS, et al. Relationship between serum concentrations

of organochlorine pesticides and metabolic syndrome among non-diabetic adults. *J Prev Med. Public Health*. 2010 Jan;43(1):1–8.

251   The two extended their studies to other countries: Son HK, Kim SA, Kang JH, Chung YS, Park SK, et al. Strong associations between low-dose organochlorine pesticides and type 2 diabetes in Korea. *Environ Int*. 2010 Jul;36(5):410–14.

251   The connection between POPs and obesity: Kelishadi R, Poursafa P, Jamshidi F. Role of environmental chemicals in obesity: a systematic review of the current evidence. *J Environ Public Health*. 2013;2013:896789. Epub 2013 Jun 5.

252   In 2012, a landmark paper published in *JAMA:* Trasande L, Attina TM, Blustein J. Association between urinary bisphenol A concentration and obesity prevalence in children and adolescents. *JAMA*. 2012 Sep 19;308(11):1113–21.

252   In the same year, a study in China: Wang HX, Zhou Y, Tang CX, Wu JG, Chen Y, Jiang QW. Association between bisphenol A exposure and body mass index in Chinese school children: a cross-sectional study. *Environ Health*. 2012 Oct 19;11:79.

253   One of the most fascinating perspectives: Price, Weston. *Nutrition and Physical Degeneration*. New Canaan, CT: Keats Publishing, 2003.

254   Until recently it was thought: Giralt M, Villarroya F. White, brown, beige/brite: different adipose cells for different functions? *Endocrinology*. 2013 Jun 19. (Epub ahead of print.)

255   In other words, activating beige adipocytes: Spiegelman BM. Banting Lecture 2012: Regulation of adipogenesis: toward new therapeutics for metabolic disease. *Diabetes*. 2013 Jun;62(6):1774–82.

256   So you will not be surprised to learn: Rahman S, Lu Y, Czernik PJ, Rosen CJ, Enerback S, Lecka-Czernik B. Inducible brown adipose tissue, or beige fat, is anabolic for the skeleton. *Endocrinology*. 2013 Aug;154(8):2687–701.

257   The results showed two things: Holick MF, Lamb JJ, Lerman RH, Konda VR, Darland G, et al. Hop rho-iso-alpha acids, berberine, vitamin D3 and vitamin K1 favorably impact biomarkers of bone turnover in postmenopausal women in a 14-week trial. *J Bone Miner Metab*. 2010 May;28(3):342–50.

CHAPTER 11: A NEW APPROACH TO YOUR HEALTH

263   "Health," said the coordinating health authority: Preamble to the Constitution of the World Health Organization as adopted by the International Health Conference, New York, 19–22 June 1946; signed on 22 July 1946 by the representatives of the 61 states (Official Records of the World Health Organization, no. 2, p. 100) and entered into force on 7 April 1948.

269 The results, published in 2004: Knoops KT, de Groot LC, Kromhout D, Perrin AE, Moreiras-Varela O, et al. Mediterranean diet, lifestyle factors, and 10-year mortality in elderly European men and women: the HALE project. *JAMA*. 2004 Sep 22;292(12):1433–39.

271 The best advice I've heard on the subject: Eliot, Robert S. *Is It Worth Dying For? How to Make Stress Work for You—Not Against You*. New York: Bantam, 1985.

272 There is no technical solution to this: Hardin G. The tragedy of the commons. The population problem has no technical solution; it requires a fundamental extension in morality. *Science*. 1968 Dec 13;162(3859):1243–48.

CHAPTER 12: DEVELOPING YOUR BASELINE PROGRAM

276 Our researchers were aware: Tannenbaum BM, Tannenbaum GS, Anisman H. Impact of life-long macronutrient choice on neuroendocrine and cognitive functioning in aged mice: differential effects in stressor-reactive and stressor-resilient mouse strains. *Brain Res*. 2003 Sep 26;985(2):187–97.

280 We now know that lifestyle, diet, and environment: Needham BL, Adler N, Gregorich S, Rehkopf D, Lin J, et al. Socioeconomic status, health behavior, and leukocyte telomere length in the National Health and Nutrition Examination Survey, 1999–2002. *Soc Sci Med*. 2013 May;85:1–8.

280 We now know that lifestyle, diet, and environment: Paul L. Diet, nutrition and telomere length. *J Nutr Biochem*. 2011 Oct;22(10):895–901.

281 Yet another study, this one tracking 5,862 women: Sun Q, Shi L, Prescott J, Chiuve SE, Hu FB, et al. Healthy lifestyle and leukocyte telomere length in U.S. women. *PLoS One*. 2012;7(5):e38374.

281 Studies by Dean Ornish and Nobel laureate Elizabeth Blackburn: Ornish D, Lin J, Daubenmier J, Weidner G, Epel E, Kemp C, et al. Increased telomerase activity and comprehensive lifestyle changes: a pilot study. *Lancet Oncol*. 2008 Nov;9(11):1048–57.

281 The study also found that the greater the compliance: Ornish D, Lin J, Chan JM, Epel E, Kemp C, et al. Effect of comprehensive lifestyle changes on telomerase activity and telomere length in men with biopsy-proven low-risk prostate cancer: 5-year follow-up of a descriptive pilot study. *Lancet Oncol*. 2013 Oct;14(11):1112–20.

281 We also know that vitamins B3 (niacin): Kirkland JB. Niacin requirements for genomic stability. *Mutat Res*. 2012 May 1;733(1–2):14–20.

281 Michael Fenech, a senior scientist in nutrition: Fenech M. Folate (vitamin B9) and vitamin B12 and their function in the maintenance of nuclear and mitochondrial genome integrity. *Mutat Res*. 2012 May 1;733(1–2):21–33.

281 Michael Fenech, a senior scientist in nutrition: Bull C, Fenech M. Genome-health nutrigenomics and nutrigenetics: nutritional requirements or nutri-omes for chromosomal stability and telomere maintenance at the individual level. *Proc Nutr Soc.* 2008 May;67(2):146–56.

281 The telomeres were 5 percent longer: Xu Q, Parks CG, DeRoo LA, Caw-thorn RM, Sandler DP, Chen H. Multivitamin use and telomere length in women. *Am J Clin Nutr.* 2009 Jun;89(6):1857–63.

281 Longer telomeres were also noted in women: Cassidy A, De Vivo I, Liu Y, Han J, Prescott J, et al. Associations between diet, lifestyle factors, and telo-mere length in women. *Am J Clin Nutr.* 2010 May;91(5):1273–80.

282 Your goal is gradually to get to a point: Choi BC, Pak AW, Choi JC, Choi EC. Daily step goal of 10,000 steps: a literature review. *Clin Invest Med.* 2007;30(3):E146–151.

283 Studies on university students: Tully MA, Cupples ME. UNISTEP (uni-versity students exercise and physical activity) study: a pilot study of the effects of accumulating 10,000 steps on health and fitness among university students. *J Phys Act Health.* 2011 Jul;8(5):663–67.

283 achieving the target resulted in: Morgan AL, Tobar DA, Snyder L. Walk-ing toward a new me: the impact of prescribed walking 10,000 steps/day on physical and psychological well-being. *J Phys Act Health.* 2010 May;7(3):299–307.

283 achieving the target resulted in: Soroush A, Der Ananian C, Ainsworth BE, Belyea M, Poortvliet E, et al. Effects of a 6-month walking study on blood pressure and cardiorespiratory fitness in U.S. and Swedish adults: ASUKI step study. *Asian J Sports Med.* 2013 Jun;4(2):114–24.

283 achieving the target resulted in: Yates T, Haffner SM, Schulte PJ, Thomas L, Huffman KM, et al. Association between change in daily am-bulatory activity and cardiovascular events in people with impaired glucose tolerance (NAVIGATOR trial): a cohort analysis. *Lancet.* 2013 Dec 19. pii: S0140-6736(13)62061-9.

283 achieving the target resulted in: Cocate PG, de Oliveira A, Hermsdorff H, Alfenas RD, Amorim PR, et al. Benefits and relationship of steps walked per day to cardiometabolic risk factor in Brazilian middle-aged men. *J Sci Med Sport.* 2013 Jun 13. pii:S1440–2440(13)00104–7.

283 Here's even more proof: Knudsen SH, Hansen LS, Pedersen M, Dejgaard T, Hansen J, et al. Changes in insulin sensitivity precede changes in body composition during 14 days of step reduction combined with overfeeding in healthy young men. *J Appl Physiol.* 2012 Jul;113(1):7–15.

285 One study found that mindfulness-based cognitive therapy: White PD, Goldsmith KA, Johnson AL, Potts L, Walwyn R, et al. Comparison of

adaptive pacing therapy, cognitive behaviour therapy, graded exercise therapy, and specialist medical care for chronic fatigue syndrome (PACE): a randomised trial. *Lancet.* 2011 March 5;377(9768):823–36.

285 Another showed that mindfulness-based cognitive: Donta ST, Clauw DJ, Engel CC Jr, Guarino P, Peduzzi P, et al. Cognitive behavioral therapy and aerobic exercise for Gulf War veterans' illnesses: a randomized controlled trial. *JAMA.* 2003 Mar 19;289(11):1396–1404.

285 A randomized controlled trial of mindfulness-based: Collip D, Geschwind N, Peeters F, Myin-Germeys I, van Os J, Wichers M. Putting a hold on the downward spiral of paranoia in the social world: a randomized controlled trial of mindfulness-based cognitive therapy in individuals with a history of depression. *PLoS One.* 2013 Jun 27;8(6):e66747.

285 The therapy increased the expression of FKBP5: Levy-Gigi E, Szabó C, Kelemen O, Kéri S. Association among clinical response, hippocampal volume, and FKBP5 gene expression in individuals with posttraumatic stress disorder receiving cognitive behavioral therapy. *Biol Psychiatry.* 2013 Jul 12. (Epub ahead of print.)

285 They also demonstrate how mindfulness-based: Bothelius K, Kyhle K, Espie CA, Broman JE. Manual-guided cognitive-behavioural therapy for insomnia delivered by ordinary primary care personnel in general medical practice: a randomized controlled effectiveness trial. *J Sleep Res.* 2013 Jul 16. (Epub ahead of print.)

285 They also demonstrate how mindfulness-based: Schlögelhofer M, Willinger U, Wiesegger G, Eder H, Priesch M, et al. Clinical study results from a randomized controlled trial of cognitive behavioural guided self-help in patients with partially remitted depressive disorder. *Psychol Psychother.* 2013 May 17. (Epub ahead of print.)

286 Studies analyzing the composition of proteins: Herman RA, Price WD. Unintended compositional changes in genetically modified (GM) crops: 20 years of research. *J Agric Food Chem.* 2013 Feb 25. (Epub ahead of print.)

286 Studies analyzing the composition of proteins: Gong CY, Wang T. Proteomic evaluation of genetically modified crops: current status and challenges. *Front Plant Sci.* 2013;4:41.

287 Another question is whether GMO varieties: Ramesh SV. Non-coding RNAs in crop genetic modification: considerations and predictable environmental risk assessments (ERA). *Mol Biotechnol.* 2013 Feb 5. (Epub ahead of print.)

287 Another question is whether GMO varieties: Lupi R, Denery-Papini S, Rogniaux H, Lafiandra D, Rizzi C, et al. How much does transgenesis

affect wheat allergenicity? Assessment in two GM lines over-expressing endogenous genes. *J Proteomics*. 2013 Mar 27;80:281–91.

287   The duration of their exposure to GMO products: Arjó G, Capell T, Matias-Guiu X, Zhu C, Christou P, Piñol C. Mice fed on a diet enriched with genetically engineered multivitamin corn show no subacute toxic effects and no sub-chronic toxicity. *Plant Biotechnol J*. 2012 Dec;10(9):1026–34.

287   The duration of their exposure to GMO products: Zhu Y, He X, Luo Y, Zou S, Zhou X, et al. A 90-day feeding study of glyphosate-tolerant maize with the G2-aroA gene in Sprague-Dawley rats. *Food Chem Toxicol*. 2013 Jan;51:280–87.

287   A number of animal studies by prominent researchers: Tang X, Han F, Zhao K, Xu Y, Wu X. A 90-day dietary toxicity study of genetically modified rice T1C-1 expressing Cry1C protein in Sprague Dawley rats. *PLoS One*. 2012;7(12). (Epub 2012 Dec 27.)

287   A number of animal studies by prominent researchers: Yuan Y, Xu W, He X, Liu H, Cao S, et al. Effects of genetically modified T2A-1 rice on the GI health of rats after 90-day supplement. *Sci Rep*. 2013;3:1962.

287   And allergy testing of the GMO potato: Tu HM, Godfrey LW, Sun SS. Expression of the Brazil nut methionine-rich protein and mutants with increased methionine in transgenic potato. *Plant Mol Biol*. 1998 Jul;37(5):829–38.

287   And allergy testing of the GMO potato: Lehrer SB, Reese G. Recombinant proteins in newly developed foods: identification of allergenic activity. *Int Arch Allergy Immunol*. 1997 May-Jul;113(1–3):122–24.

287   And allergy testing of the GMO potato: Devos Y, Aguilera J, Diveki Z, Gomes A, Liu Y, et al. EFSA's scientific activities and achievements on the risk assessment of genetically modified organisms (GMOs) during its first decade of existence: looking back and ahead. *Transgenic Res*. 2013 Aug 21.

CHAPTER 13: PERSONALIZING YOUR HEALTH-CARE MANAGEMENT PROGRAM

305   The diet focused on lean protein: Hasper I, Ventskovskiy BM, Rettenberger R, Heger PW, Riley DS, Kaszkin-Bettag M. Long-term efficacy and safety of the special extract ERr 731 of *Rheum rhaponticum* in perimenopausal women with menopausal symptoms. *Menopause*. 2009 Jan–Feb;16(1):117–31.

305   The outcomes for the women in the study: Lukaczer D, Liska DJ, Lerman RH, Darland G, Schiltz B, et al. Effect of low glycemic index diet with soy protein and phytosterols on CVD risk factors in postmenopausal women. *Nutrition*. 2006 Feb;22(2):104–13.

306 The phytonutrient beta-sitosterol proved effective: Klippel KF, Hiltl DM, Schipp B. A multicentric, placebo-controlled, double-blind clinical trial of beta-sitosterol (phytosterol) for the treatment of benign prostatic hyperplasia. German BPH-Phyto Study group. *Br J Urol.* 1997 Sep;80(3):427–32.

308 But then along came Frances Moore Lappé: Lappé, Frances Moore. *Diet for a Small Planet.* New York: Ballantine Books, 1971.

309 I met Joe in 1983 shortly after he had published: Piscatella, Joseph. *Don't Eat Your Heart Out Cookbook.* New York: Workman, 1983.

311 One at the George Washington School of Medicine: Dipietro L, Gribok A, Stevens MS, Hamm LF, Rumpler W. Three 15-min bouts of moderate postmeal walking significantly improves 24-h glycemic control in older people at risk for impaired glucose tolerance. *Diabetes Care.* 2013 Jun 11. (Epub ahead of print.)

311 Even what Dr. Levine: McCrady-Spitzer SK, Levine JA. Nonexercise activity thermogenesis: a way forward to treat the worldwide obesity epidemic. *Surg Obes Relat Dis.* 2012 Sep–Oct;8(5):501–6.

312 Age-related macular degeneration (AMD) is the main cause: *National Eye Institute Statistics and Data.* http://www.nei.nih.gov/eyedata/pbd_tables.asp. Accessed 15 December 2013.

318 Moreover, studies have shown how and why: Yan H, Tang L, Chen T, Kral JG, Jiang L, et al. Defining and predicting complete remission of type 2 diabetes: a short-term efficacy study of open gastric bypass. *Obes Facts.* 2013;6(2):176–84.

318 Moreover, studies have shown how and why: Cohen RV, Pinheiro JC, Schiavon CA, Salles JE, Wajchenberg BL, Cummings DE. Effects of gastric bypass surgery in patients with type 2 diabetes and only mild obesity. *Diabetes Care.* 2012 Jul;35(7):1420–28.

318 Moreover, studies have shown how and why: Ghiassi S, Morton J, Bellatorre N, Eisenberg D. Short-term medication cost savings for treating hypertension and diabetes after gastric bypass. *Surg Obes Relat Dis.* 2012 May–Jun;8(3):269–74.

CHAPTER 14: YOUR HEALTH-CARE REVOLUTION

322 Again, not a moment too soon: The World Health Organization 2011 Summit: Bloom DE, Cafiero ET, Jané-Llopis E, Abrahams-Gessel S, Bloom LR, et al. *The Global Economic Burden of Noncommunicable Diseases.* Geneva: World Economic Forum, 2011.

322 In the United States as of 2012: Hurd MD, Martorell P, Delavande A, Mullen KJ, Langa KM. Monetary costs of dementia in the United States. *N Engl J Med.* 2013 Apr 4;368(14):1326–34.

322 In the United States as of 2012: Thies W, Bleiler L; Alzheimer's Association. *Alzheimers Dement.* 2013 Alzheimer's disease facts and figures. 2013 Mar;9(2):208–45.

322 At the famous Karolinska Institutet in Sweden: Lövdén M, Xu W, Wang HX. Lifestyle change and the prevention of cognitive decline and dementia: what is the evidence? *Curr Opin Psychiatry.* 2013 May;26(3):239–43.

323 A study at the Mayo Clinic concluded: Vemuri P, Lesnick TG, Przybelski SA, Knopman DS, Roberts RO, et al. Effect of lifestyle activities on Alzheimer disease biomarkers and cognition. *Ann Neurol.* 2012 Nov;72(5):730–38.

323 But numerous studies have indicated: Féart C, Samieri C, Allés B, Barberger-Gateau P. Potential benefits of adherence to the Mediterranean diet on cognitive health. *Proc Nutr Soc.* 2013 Feb;72(1):140–52.

323 But numerous studies have indicated: Vassallo N, Scerri C. Mediterranean diet and dementia of the Alzheimer type. *Curr Aging Soc.* 2012 Sep 27. (Epub ahead of print.)

323 But numerous studies have indicated: Allés B, Samieri C, Féart C, Jutland MA, Laurin D, Barberger-Gateau P. Dietary patterns: a novel approach to examine the link between nutrition and cognitive function in older individuals. *Nutr Res Rev.* 2012 Dec;25(2):207–22.

323 But numerous studies have indicated: Scarmeas N, Luchsinger JA, Stern Y, Gu Y, He J, et al. Mediterranean diet and magnetic resonance imaging–assessed cerebrovascular disease. *Ann Neurol.* 2011 Feb;69(2):257–68.

323 A 2013 study in the *New England Journal of Medicine:* Estruch R, Ros E, Salas-Salvadó J, Covas MI, Corella D, et al. Primary prevention of cardiovascular disease with a Mediterranean diet. *N Engl J Med.* 2013 Apr 4;368(14):1279–90.

323 Some of my own research: Minich DM, Bland JS. Dietary management of the metabolic syndrome beyond macronutrients. *Nutr Rev.* 2008 Aug;66(8):429–44.

Acknowledgments

As a man who considers himself extremely fortunate to be alive during this amazing time of transformation in health care, from the moment I wrote the first word of the first sentence of this book, I felt an overwhelming sense of indebtedness to the tens of thousands of health-care researchers and clinicians who are making the transformation happen. Their discoveries are shaping the future of global health and defining how medical care will be delivered to my children and grandchildren. Writing the book presented me with the humbling challenge to describe their work accurately and imposed on me a heavy sense of responsibility to do it well, for the work can profoundly reduce the incidence of unnecessary and premature disabilities and deaths associated with chronic diseases. So to the major innovators in this revolution, many of them noted in this book, and to the thousands of unnamed contributors who have dedicated their professional lives to this endeavor, I extend my first acknowledgement and my great gratitude.

In many ways, the process of writing the book was a personal and nostalgic "travelog," complete with sights, sounds, tastes, even smells, that transported me back through countless medical and scientific conferences, research briefings, formal discussions and casual conversations, meals shared with associates, presentations delivered and listened to, and heated debates with scientists and clinicians in the medical field about the future of health care. I consider myself blessed to have met and come to know so many people over the past thirty years and, logging more than 6 million miles of air travel, to have shared with them so many aha! moments about the revolution in health we are now living through. I claim very few original ideas, but rather I see myself as a "mosaic" of the thinking I've shared with these many associates, friends, colleagues, and family members over the years. I take responsibility for any errors in interpretation, but I honor them for stimulating the ideas in the book.

The first person to provide that stimulation was my mother, Marjorie Bland. Still a health advocate at eighty-eight years of age, as this book goes to press, she has been discussing health care with me for more than sixty-five years, asking hard questions and provoking hard thinking. My sister, Christie Clark, who has worked with us for the past thirty years, has taught me the power of the application of the lifestyle health-care model as she has applied it in her own family. Continuing to light the path of discovery for me is my wife, Susan, cofounder of the Institute for Functional Medicine and my essential sounding board and even more essential partner in life. My sons Kelly, Kyle, and Justin have contributed greatly to the evolution of my ideas and have always been an inspiration to me. Our daughters-in-law, Melissa Kiffin Bland, who worked for us for more than ten years in developing the medical food field, and Judith Bland are both exemplars of personal responsibility for health and are the mothers of health-conscious children who are carrying forward the concepts of personalized lifestyle health care in their own lives. Yet I think my most important teacher about health is my youngest son, Justin. His personal story of overcoming health challenges from birth to become an "old soul," as described in the book, has truly been a guide for me every day of his thirty-one years.

Reinforcing what I have learned from my family are special relationships with three amazing medical doctors: Graham Reedy, David Jones, and Scott Rigden. Dr. Reedy has been a friend, family doctor, medical innovator, visionary, and spiritual guide who taught me that a concept can be made real through dedicated, courageous commitment. Dr. Jones has been a comrade in arms in the creation of the functional medicine concept and in working with Susan and me in the establishment of the Institute for Functional Medicine in

1990 and serving as its president through 2013. Dr. Rigden and I first met in the late 1970s at the founding meeting of the American Holistic Medical Association, and we have been close friends and colleagues ever since. An expert in both chronic fatigue syndrome and obesity, Scott Rigden has also been a collaborator with me and my research group in many clinical research projects. I am grateful to all three of these friends for shaping my view of what constitutes good medicine and good medical practice. I also owe a deep debt of gratitude to Laurie Hofmann, MPH, chief executive officer of the Institute for Functional Medicine, for creating the organization that Susan, David, and I hoped for at its inception—one that contributes every day to the global revolution in health care.

Among the multitude of researchers, clinicians, and thought leaders from many different disciplines who have influenced my thinking—far too many to acknowledge individually—I extend particular thanks to those whose connection with me helped shape this book. First among them are two giants of science, Dr. Linus Pauling and Dr. Abram Hoffer, both of whom deeply imprinted my brain with "a better idea" for the future of medicine. Dr. Sidney Baker and Dr. Leo Galland, master clinicians, also became mentors to me and many others in the intellectual evolution of the medicine of our future. As told in these pages, Dr. Dean Ornish, whom I met in the early 1980s, set the standard for the importance of good clinical research in advancing a new approach to health care, while my friend Dr. Mehmet Oz has set the standard for courageous dedication in spreading the news about the power of the new medicine to address chronic illness. I am indebted to them all.

A chance meeting in 1976 with Dr. Joseph Pizzorno, founder and past president of Bastyr University, led to an essential intellectual collaboration in developing the model of health set forth in the book. It was through the efforts of Dr. Pizzorno and his naturopathic medicine colleagues that a scientifically sound approach to natural medicine was born.

Translating the science into effective systems for delivering care requires management skills and cross-disciplinary expertise. In 1994,

I met the special person with a natural talent for doing so, Dr. Mark Hyman, who has been as much a younger brother as a colleague ever since. Mark pioneered the evolution of functional medicine and is today acknowledged as such in his role as chairman of the board of directors of the Institute for Functional Medicine.

None of my work would have been possible had it not been for Dr. Darrell Medcalf, chairman of the chemistry department at the University of Puget Sound, who hired me in 1971 for my first academic position, and who gave me not only his friendship but, later, his business leadership when in 1990 he became the president of my first company, HealthComm International.

To the thousands of people who worked with me at Health-Comm International, to the thousands of health-care practitioners I have learned from around the world as a result of my founding the Institute for Functional Medicine, and to my colleagues at Metagenics and its research and development division, MetaProteomics, which I headed from 2000 to 2012, I extend my deepest thanks. My MetaProteomics research team, headed by Dr. Matthew Tripp, consisted of some of the most innovative, skilled, and productive researchers and clinicians I could ever have hoped to work with. To this group—including Deanna Minich, Robert Lerman, Jack Kornberg, Joseph Lamb, Daniel Lukaczer, Lincoln Bouillon, DeAnn Liska, Gary Darland, Veera Konda, Anu Desai, Margaret King, Barb Schiltz, Pamela Darland, Tracey Irving, Lewis Chang, Dennis Emma, Kim Koch, Jeff Hu, Lyra Heller, Brian Carroll, Jan Urban, Clinton Dahlberg, and Peter Nelson—my deepest thanks. I believe that the eighty peer-reviewed research publications and two hundred patent applications this group produced over a ten-year period helped define the field of nutritional medicine for all time.

Finally, I am glad to have the chance to acknowledge and thank the colleagues and collaborators who helped me bring this book from an idea to an expression of my view of the future of medicine. The thanks start with my colleague of more than fifteen years, Trish Eury, who has been the curator of my publications and of *Functional Medicine Update*, the audio newsletter that I have produced each month since 1982. As the director of content for the Personalized Lifestyle Medicine Institute, Trish has been my "second brain" in the writing and editing of this book. I also want to recognize the special contribution of my executive assistant, Kathy Sawyer, who for seventeen years has managed the complexity of my scheduling, professional connections, travel, and family life balance. Without her help, I never would have found time or space to write this book.

Nor would it ever have happened were it not for Robert Levine, my wonderful agent, who found a wonderful home for the book. I am grateful also to Susanna Margolis, who helped make my thoughts understandable, and to my amazingly talented and dedicated editor at HarperCollins, Karen Rinaldi, who was kind enough to support the book's message and tough enough to manage me and my ideas in the process of its development. Without all of these amazing people, the story I tell of the revolution in health care that we are now witnessing would not have seen the light of day. I am grateful.

JEFFREY BLAND
DECEMBER 2013

Index

Page numbers in *italics* refer to illustrations.

About the Author

Dr. Jeffrey S. Bland is known as the "father of functional medicine," a medical approach that focuses on the personalized prevention and treatment of chronic diseases. Over the past thirty-five years Dr. Bland has traveled more than six million miles, teaching more than a hundred thousand health-care practitioners in the United States, Canada, and more than forty other countries about Functional Medicine. He has been a university biochemistry professor, a research director at the Linus Pauling Institute of Science and Medicine, the cofounder of the Institute for Functional Medicine in 1991, and the founder/president of the Personalized Lifestyle Medicine Institute. He has authored more than one hundred scientific publications and ten books for health professionals and health consumers. He lives in Seattle, Washington, with his wife, Susan, and near his three sons and their families while pursuing his hobbies of boating, surfing, and scuba diving, as well as a lifelong passion for learning.